Supporting
Adolescents
with Language
Disorders

British Library Cataloguing in Publication Data

A catalogue record for this book is available from the British Library

Cover design: Jim Wilkie Cover image: Liliya Kulianionak/Shutterstock (used under license from Shutterstock.com)

Project management, typesetting and design: J&R Publishing Services Ltd, Guildford, Surrey, UK; www.jr-publishingservices.co.uk

Printed and bound by CPI Group (UK) Ltd, Croydon, CR0 4YY

Index: Terence Halliday hallidayterence@aol.com

Supporting Adolescents with Language Disorders

Sarah Spencer (Editor)

J&R Press Ltd

Contents

Part III School-level support for adolescents with language disorders

List of contributors

Karen Bryan, Professor, is Deputy Vice-Chancellor (Academic) at the University of Greenwich.

Judy Clegg is a Senior Lecturer in the Department of Human Communication Sciences at the University of Sheffield, UK. Judy is co-editor of the journal, *Child Language Teaching and Therapy,* a Fellow of the Royal College of Speech and Language Therapists and a Trustee of ICAN, the National Children's Communication Charity.

Susan Ebbels is Director of Research and Training at Moor House Research and Training Institute, Moor House School & College, Surrey, UK. She is also an honorary lecturer at University College London, UK.

Mary Hartshorne is Head of Evidence for I CAN, the national children's communication charity. A specialist speech and language therapist with many years experience of working in education, she leads I CAN's impact measurement and management.

During 2017/18 Mary led Bercow: Ten Years On – a national review of provision for children and young people with speech, language and communication needs (SLCN), the report of which was published in March 2018.

Lowry Hemphill is a Clinical Associate Professor in Literacy Education at Boston University, Wheelock College of Education & Human Development, USA.

Victoria Joffe is Professor, Enhancement of Child and Adolescent Language and Learning, Division of Language and Communication Science, School of Health Sciences, City, University of London, UK.

Hilary Lowe is an independent paediatric speech and language therapist and honorary research fellow at City, University of London. She was awarded a PhD in Language and Communication Science for her investigation into the effectiveness of classroom vocabulary intervention for adolescents with language disorder.

Rachel Mathrick is a Highly Specialist Speech and Language Therapist at St Catherine's School, Isle of Wight, UK.She is a contributor to LiLaC researcher-practitioner workshops UCL, and is a RCSLT Research Champion.

Courtenay Norbury is a Professor of Developmental Language and Communication Disorders at University College London and a Fellow of the Royal College of Speech Language Therapists. She is passionate about working with clinicians to improve understanding and use of research evidence through her Literacy, Language, and Communication (LiLaC) network (www.lilac-lab.org). Follow her on Twitter @lilaccourt

Martine Smith is an Associate Professor in Speech-Language Pathology in the Department of Clinical Speech and Language Studies in Trinity College Dublin, Ireland, with specific responsibility for teaching in developmental speech and language disorders and augmentative and alternative communication.

Catherine Snow is Patricia Albjerg Graham Professor of Education, at Harvard Graduate School of Education, Cambridge, USA.

Pamela Snow, Professor, is a speech pathologist and psychologist, and is Head of the La Trobe Rural Health School at La Trobe University in Australia.

Sarah Spencer is a speech and language therapist and lecturer in language development and disorders in the Department for Human Communication Sciences, University of Sheffield, UK.

Julia Starling, is a speech-language pathologist in Sydney, Australia. She has extensive clinical and research experience with populations of young people with language and literacy difficulties. She lectures at The University of Sydney and Macquarie University (Sydney).

Jenny Thomson is a Reader in Language and Literacy in the Department of Human Communication Sciences, University of Sheffield, UK.

Prologue

Ellie's Story

Hi, my name is Ellie.

I am 18 years old and I have speech and language difficulties.

At primary school, I just played and watched the other children and followed what was happening.

As I grew older and kids at school started to realise I had a problem, they would just carry on in their activities, I was finding it hard to communicate with them as the conversations was more older talk. When I tried to join in they had moved on to another subject.

At senior school I was in an integrated resource unit. I enjoyed my time in this unit with my peers and staff. It does segregate you from other pupils a little but I could communicate better with the staff than some of the pupils.

I've always tried my very hardest to communicate as I know this will help my difficulties.

Example, when I wanted some Battenberg cake I could only keep saying yellow pink and motion eat.

I always smiled through and been myself (Yorkshire Lass).

Whenever I went into the transition periods, this was always a problem when meeting new people that didn't know me and my problems.

My personality is always happy chappy.

I've felt very frustrated at times when people don't understand me. My family have always supported me and encouraged me in everything I've done. Also my mum as always said to me: them who love you understand you.

When I left school I went to college. I found this very difficult as there was no real structure to my time there. In my second year I was able to do an internship at a company. I really enjoyed my time there as I met some nice people who saw through my difficulties and encouraged me in a work environment, so much so that when my intern finished the people at the company asked if I would like to work there, so I am now on a 6 months part time contract.

Internship gave me lots of confidence, getting up and going to work gave me routine, these were missing when I was at college and on holiday, so my head began to become fuzzy and I started to make bad decisions.

One other thing that has happened that I thought would be a struggle is I now have a lovely boyfriend, who sees past my difficulties and is happy to take me anywhere and meet anyone.

Top tips for readers:
Encouragement and Believe

Part I

Understanding adolescents with language disorders

1 Adolescents with language disorders

Sarah Spencer

This introductory chapter will give an overview of *Supporting Adolescents with Language Disorders* and will enable readers to:

- Discuss the different terminology and criteria for children and adolescents with language disorders

- Present current knowledge about developmental trajectories of adolescents with language disorders

- Describe how intervention can target the needs of those with language disorders

- Discuss the rationale for supporting adolescents with language disorders by using teaching strategies in classrooms and by applying whole-school approaches.

This book invites the reader to consider how adolescents with language disorders can be better supported and how interventions can be designed to increase language abilities and maximize inclusion within education and beyond. Prevalence of language disorders is high, with international studies reaching a consensus that around 7% of all children will present with a disordered ability to understand or use language or both (Hannus, Kauppila, & Launonen, 2009; Norbury et al., 2016; Tomblin et al., 1997). For many people, language disorders persist beyond childhood into adolescence and adulthood (Beitchman et al., 2001; Stothard et al., 1998). Government statistics from the UK show that 10.5% of adolescents have a recorded primary special educational need related to speech, language and communication during the first year of secondary school (reducing to 7.8% in the final year of school) (Department for Education, 2017). Despite the fact that language disorders are relatively common (e.g., seven times more common than autistic spectrum disorders (Baird et al., 2006)), public awareness is low, research funding is limited (Bishop, 2010), and there are persisting concerns regarding access to quality interventions and educational support (Nippold, 2010).

These issues apply to children of all ages, but are particularly salient in relation to older children and adolescents, as research and clinical practice tends to focus on early childhood (Cirrin & Gillam, 2008; Dockrell et al., 2006). We know that too many adolescents have unsupported, undiagnosed language disorders (e.g., Cohen et al., 2013; Hughes et al., 2017) and we know that those who have recognized difficulties often struggle to access speech and language therapy and specialist educational services (Bercow, 2008; Dockrell et al., 2006).

This book aims to bring together what we know about adolescents with language disorders in order to argue for increased access to quality assessment, intervention services, and to robust educational support. Chapters in Part 1 summarize what we know about this population and present the challenges faced by young people with language disorders during this unique life stage. Chapters in Part II provide examples of interventions which have a sound theoretical rationale and evidence base. Chapters in Part III discuss ways that schools can support adolescents with language disorders through collaboration with speech and language therapists. This introductory chapter gives an overview of these themes and contextualizes the ideas and arguments developed in later chapters.

What is a language disorder?

Children with language disorders are defined as those who have difficulties acquiring language, leading to functional impairments in everyday life in terms of social interaction and education (Bishop, 2017). Adolescents with language disorders, like younger children, are a heterogeneous group and present with a wide range of difficulties across different aspects of language. These difficulties can occur across the following domains of language (Bishop et al., 2017):

- Phonology, impacting on the speech sound system

- Syntax, impacting on the use and understanding of grammatical structures and sentences

- Semantics and word finding, impacting knowledge and use of vocabulary and accessing known words respectively

- Pragmatics and social use of language, impacting on language skills in interactions across different contexts and social situations

- Discourse, impacting on extended use and comprehension of linguistic discourses such as narratives, debates, and explanations

- Verbal learning and memory, for example impacting on the ability to retain and recall sounds or words over a short period of time or learning information about new words and their meaning

- Reading and writing: there are close associations between oral and written language and many adolescents with language disorders will have difficulties in areas such as phonological skills, language comprehension and vocabulary knowledge which will impact on reading and writing ability.

Various systems of sub-grouping children with language difficulties have been put forward, but finding a robust approach to classification over time is difficult (Conti-Ramsden & Botting, 1999). Language disorders that occur without a known cause (e.g., despite typical hearing, intelligence, and physical development) may have been given a diagnosis of specific language impairment (SLI). SLI has been the subject of much debate. Certainly the criteria used for its diagnosis are notoriously varied (Bishop et al., 2016). There are a variety of contesting theories about the underlying cause of SLI, for example that there is a core difficulty with language acquisition (and in particular grammar) or that there is a general difficulty with information processing or with working memory (Marinis, 2011). Terminology used is also inconsistent across research studies, and clinical and educational practice (Bishop et al., 2017). However, there is consensus that (a) language disorders are heterogeneous, and (b) prognosis is generally poor, with difficulties often persisting throughout childhood, during adolescence and into adulthood (Bishop, 2017).

There have been calls to revise both the criteria used in diagnosing SLI and the label itself (Bishop et al., 2016, 2017). A review of literature found that over 130 terms were used to describe children who had difficulties with receptive and expressive language (Bishop, 2014). Following an international and cross-disciplinary consultation exercise, developmental language disorder (DLD) has become the agreed term, replacing SLI and functioning in its stead as a diagnostic label that can be used consistently across research and clinical practice (Bishop et al., 2017; see also the discussion in Snow and Bryan, this volume).

The argument for replacing SLI with DLD has been driven in part by a challenge to the prior inclusion of nonverbal skills in the diagnosis of developmental language disorders. Traditionally, for a diagnosis of SLI to be made, there needed to be a discrepancy between verbal and nonverbal skills, with stronger nonverbal reasoning (hence the 'specificity' of specific language impairment). However, this criterion proved difficult to apply, with unresolved issues around the assessment tools used to assess the constructs of language versus nonverbal skills, and the thresholds applied (e.g., how low language ability scores had to be, and the minimum nonverbal score required to rule out an alternative diagnosis of general learning difficulties). The magnitude of a discrepancy between verbal and nonverbal skills that was required for a diagnosis of SLI was also unclear. Furthermore, in cases where nonverbal skills were low in relation to expected norms, but where verbal skills were lower still, it was unclear whether a diagnosis of SLI was still appropriate.

A further complication is that several longitudinal studies of children with language disorders have reported that performance on nonverbal assessments can decline in later childhood and adolescence (Botting, 2005; Conti-Ramsden, St Clair, Pickles, & Durikin, 2012; Tomblin, Freese, & Records, 1992) or fluctuate over time (Clegg, Hollis, Mawhood, & Rutter, 2005; Krassowski & Plante, 1997). It is not clear why this is the case for some children; one possibility is that language ability mediates many forms of learning and that over time a disorder of language will impact on supposedly nonverbal reasoning tasks (Conti-Ramsden et al., 2012). It may also be that tests used to measure cognition rely increasingly on verbal mediation (Tomblin, Zhang, Buckwalter, & O'Brien, 1999). It therefore seems sensible that a verbal–nonverbal IQ discrepancy should not be used to determine diagnosis or eligibility for intervention services.

Language disorders can also form part of the profile of difficulties with other associated developmental disorders such as autism spectrum disorder (ASD), intellectual disability, genetic conditions such as Down syndrome, cerebral palsy, brain injury, neurodegenerative conditions and hearing loss. Accompanying the argument that SLI be replaced with DLD, it is suggested that children and young people with such co-occurring conditions are not diagnosed with DLD but 'language disorder associated with x' where, x is the differentiating condition (Bishop et al., 2017: 4).

A further term used, particularly in UK schools, when describing adolescents with language disorders is Speech, Language and Communication Needs (SLCN). This umbrella term is used in relation to children and young people who struggle to communicate, whether this is due to "social or environmental causes, neuro-developmental difficulties or sensory impairment" (Bercow, 2008: 3). The term includes those with complex needs and those with what has historically been referred to as SLI. It is a term applied without diagnostic or exclusion criteria and is therefore thought to facilitate shared understanding and communication between staff across different levels of service provision (McKean et al., 2017). It is recommended by the CATALISE project as a super-ordinate category, encompassing all difficulties with communication (e.g., DLD, fluency, voice, speech sound disorders, mild language difficulties which do not require specialist support, and language disorders associated with biomedical conditions). Furthermore, it is argued that this term is useful for engaging with policymakers, though it is less suitable for use when working with families or within research. It has the advantage of encompassing a larger population of children with communication difficulties, with clear resource implications for policymakers and those commissioning services (Bishop et al., 2017).

Throughout this volume, chapters vary in terms of the terminology used. This reflects continuing variation across the broader community of researchers and practitioners. Some authors in the current collection apply terminology in line with the consensus achieved by Bishop et al. (2017) and as such refer to developmental language disorder and/or language disorder (see chapters by Spencer and Clegg; Bryan and Snow; Ebbels and Spencer). Others use the umbrella term SLCN, which is particularly common in education settings in the UK (see chapters by Clegg; Hartshorne; Mathrick and Norbury). The chapter by Starling uses the descriptive term 'language-based learning difficulty' in reference to education-based interventions in Australia, and Joffe and Lowe refer to 'language impairment' in their chapter on multi-level vocabulary interventions. As a group of authors, we felt that the variation in terminology used also reflects differences in the young people we describe in terms of the global setting, the level of severity of the disorders diagnosed, and the level of intervention required (e.g., some interventions may be universal for all adolescents or targeted at adolescents who need support to continue to develop speech, language and communication skills despite the absence of a clinically relevant disorder). In all chapters, reference is made to research and policy which uses terms other than those adopted by the authors.

Part I: Understanding adolescent language disorders

Part 1 of this book summarizes our understanding of adolescents with language disorders. In Chapter 2, I describe the biological, psychological and social transitions of adolescence, drawing from interdisciplinary research In Chapter 3, Spencer and Clegg consider what young people can tell us themselves about living with a language disorder, summarizing research which has listened to adolescents' own perspectives. The chapter argues for the importance of going beyond listening towards working *with* adolescents to facilitate change in terms of understanding adolescent language disorders, person-centred planning for intervention and support, and strategic planning of services and policies.

In Chapter 4, Snow and Bryan present our understanding of language disorders within youth justice contexts, examining the complex biosocial factors that result in the increased likelihood of language disorders in this population. The chapter discusses the complexity of these young people's lives, contextualizing language disorders with higher rates of socioeconomic disadvantage, previous educational failure and disengagement, and complex and chaotic personal lives. Approaches to providing support for young offenders with language disorders are discussed.

In Chapter 5, Clegg unpicks the complex associations between language disorders and mental health and wellbeing. The chapter details why adolescence is a risk period for mental health problems such as psychoses, conduct disorders, anxiety, depression and eating disorders, as well as for behaviour such as substance misuse and criminal behaviour. These issues are discussed in relation to young people with speech, language and communication needs, using two case studies to illustrate the challenges and complexities of providing effective support.

In what follows I contextualize these three chapters, offering a broad overview of our understanding of adolescents with language disorders.

Diagnosed versus unsupported adolescent language disorders

Research has concentrated on two populations of adolescents with language disorders: (1) those with a diagnosis in early childhood who have persisting difficulties throughout childhood and into adolescence and beyond; and (2) those who reach adolescence without a formal diagnosis but are later identified as having difficulties with language. Longitudinal studies of children known to speech and language therapy services have shown that language disorders can result in persisting difficulties (Beitchman et al., 1996; Clark et al., 2007).

Research has also found that many adolescents with language disorders do not have a previous diagnosis or access to specialist support or interventions. Much of this work has examined prevalence of language disorders in specific populations of adolescents, such as those who are: at risk of exclusion from school for behavioural difficulties (Clegg et al., 2009); in contact with the youth justice system (Hopkins et al., 2017; Hughes et al., 2017); accessing mental health services (Cohen et al., 2013; Cohen, Barwick et al., 1998; Cohen, Menna et al., 1998); considered at risk of educational underachievement (Spencer et al., 2017), and attending school in areas of general socioeconomic disadvantage (Spencer, Clegg, & Stackhouse, 2012).

Findings from these studies with different groups considered to be vulnerable confirm that adolescents may well have language disorders which are not diagnosed or supported. For example, one study reports that 45% of adolescents who were attending mental health services had 'higher order language impairments' which had not been identified. Similarly, over 25% of adolescents in a young offender institution in England met criteria for having a language disorder, and only 25% of these had previously accessed speech and language services (Hughes et al., 2017).

The reasons why language disorders remain undetected and unsupported are poorly understood (Hollo, Wehby, & Oliver, 2010). It may be that some children with language disorders are able to manage in earlier childhood, but have increasingly significant functional difficulties during adolescence when the linguistic demands of school and social life increase (Nippold, 2004). It may also be that some of the adolescents with unsupported language disorders within research studies meet criteria for language disorder using standardized assessment scores but may not have the 'scholastic deficits', 'abnormalities in interpersonal relationships' or emotional or behavioural disturbances that typify clinical case status, according to the ICD-10 (WHO, 1992: 233). It also seems likely that the lack of awareness of adolescent language difficulties and reduced access to speech and language services and specialist educational input contribute to high incidence of unsupported language disorders during adolescence across vulnerable populations (Joffe, 2015).

Trajectories of children diagnosed with language disorders through adolescence

Longitudinal studies have typically followed up adolescents with a childhood diagnosis of specific language impairment (e.g., Botting & Conti-Ramsden,

1999) or those who were identified as having a language disorder by a teacher during childhood (e.g., Dockrell & Lindsay, 2001). For example, the Manchester Language Study (MLS) investigated 50% of all 7-year-olds with a diagnosis of specific language impairment who attended specialist language units in the UK (Conti-Ramsden & Botting, 1999). Language units are specialist classrooms within mainstream schools that are designed to provide support, education and interventions for children with developmental language disorders. Participants took part in the study when they were aged 7 (n=242), 8 (n=232), 11 (n=200), 14 (n=113), 16 (n=139), 17 (n=85) and 24 (n=84). This study has afforded rich insights into reported outcomes for these young people, ranging from the development of friendships to academic attainment, learning to drive, and use of social media. The study has also examined developmental trajectories of expressive and receptive language skills and nonverbal assessment scores over time. Expressive and receptive abilities are reported to remain stable over time as does level of severity. In other words, children who had poorer language assessment scores when they were 7 years maintained this relative position into adulthood and vice versa (Conti-Ramsden, St Clair, Pickles, & Durkin, 2012). One-third of participants no longer met traditional criteria for SLI in later childhood and adolescence due to low nonverbal assessment scores, despite having nonverbal scores within the typical range when aged 7 years (Conti-Ramsden et al., 2012).

Covering a similar period of time in their own longitudinal study, Dockrell and Lindsay (2001) recruited 69 monolingual 8-year-old children with primary difficulties in speech and language, as identified by the teachers, educational psychologists, and speech and language therapists who worked with them. These children attended mainstream and special schools in two areas in England (one rural and one urban). Participants were followed up when they were around 10 years old (10;2-11;4), upon starting secondary school at around 12 years old (11;3-12;6) and then again when they were around 13 (13;4-14;10). Academic outcomes and language assessment scores for 62 participants were also analyzed when they were aged around 16 years (15;2-16;4), which was when they reached the end of compulsory education. At this time, pupils were still performing significantly below the norm on measures of language and literacy, and performed lower than expected in terms of educational attainment (Dockrell, Lindsay & Palikara, 2011).

These findings are in line with another follow-up study which found that early childhood language difficulties were associated with language outcomes in adolescence. Stothard et al. (1998) followed up children who had been assessed when aged 4 and 5;6 years. At 15-16 years of age, the study assessed 26 participants who were thought to have resolved their language difficulties by age 5;6; 30 participants who had persisting language difficulties at 5;6; and 15 participants who had a general delay. These groups were compared to a control group of 49 adolescents with no history of language difficulties. Results suggested that in adolescence the group with 'resolved' language difficulties did not differ from controls on measures of vocabulary or language comprehension but did differ on tests of literacy and phonological processing. The group with persisting language difficulties at 5;6 years performed significantly below controls on all language and literacy measures, as did the group with the general delay. Effectively, these results suggested that, in these latter two groups, vocabulary growth fell further behind their peers over time. Therefore, there is robust evidence that language disorders in early childhood do persist into adolescence, and can have consequences for literacy skills even when the language impairment appears to have resolved.

Language disorder as a risk factor for emotional and social development

Persisting language disorders are known to have significant and negative consequences for emotional and social development in adolescence. In terms of mental health, there have been reported associations with attention deficit disorder (Beitchman et al., 1996); anxiety disorder (Conti-Ramsden & Botting, 2008) and aggressive behaviour (Brownlie, Bao, & Beitchman, 2004). The Manchester Language Study found that participants had increased risk of emotional difficulties compared to adolescents without a history of SLI, although direct causality was not established in results (Botting & Conti-Ramsden, 2000). At 19 years of age, a history of early language difficulties may be associated with a 2.7-fold increase in social anxiety disorder (Voci et al., 2006). A longitudinal study of 68 children aged 8 to 12 years identified high levels of behavioural, emotional and social difficulties in those with language difficulties (Lindsay, Dockrell, & Strand, 2007). Studies also suggest that adolescents with a history of language difficulty have a greater risk of poorer quality friendships than those without (Durkin & Botting, 2007). Moving to mid-adulthood, a history of language difficulties was associated with greater risk of depression, anxiety and personality disorders (Clegg et al., 2005).

Difficulties with peer relationships are also reported for a higher proportion of young people with language disorders (Mok et al., 2014; St Clair et al.,

2011). The profiles of a sub-cohort of the Manchester Language Study (177 participants tracked between ages 7 years and 16 years) were analyzed, looking at questions related to peer relations and prosocial behaviour on teacher questionnaire measures and the associations with assessments of nonverbal, language and literacy (Mok et al., 2014). A sizable proportion displayed no difficulties with peer relations (22.2%). A further 12.3% had difficulties only in childhood that were resolved by the time they started secondary school. However, two-thirds of the sample had persisting difficulties with peer relations, including 26.3% who had difficulties that began during adolescence. Scores on measures of expressive and receptive language were not related to the likelihood of difficulties with peer relations, nor were nonverbal abilities or literacy measures. However, teacher ratings of pragmatic difficulties were significant, with children rated as having pragmatic difficulties being 2.5 times more likely to have persistent difficulties with peers. This study is based on teacher rating only, and peer report and parent perspectives may offer different or additional insight. The teachers rated the young people on items related to being bullied, bullying other children, being well liked by children and having at least one good friend. The study highlights the importance of supporting friendships for young people with language disorders, even if children appear to have no issues before the onset of adolescence.

Research has shown that childhood language disorders persist into and beyond adolescence, even in the context of high levels of specialist support. Detailed investigations of psychosocial trajectories have consistently shown increased risk of poor outcomes, such as in relation to mental health, wellbeing, friendships, and educational outcomes. It is important to note that this is about increased risk only: it is by no means inevitable that adolescents with language disorders will have poor outcomes of this sort. Further research is needed to unpick risk and resilience and to understand how to support adolescents to maximize positive outcomes.

Part II: Interventions for adolescent language disorders

Part II of this book is made up of five chapters, each detailing approaches to specialist interventions for adolescents with language disorders.

In Chapter 6, Ebbels and Spencer describe available grammar interventions, including details of Shape Coding by Susan Ebbels®. The chapter then goes on to evaluate the evidence base for providing intervention, in relation to specific syntax targets.

In Chapter 7, Joffe provides a detailed rationale for placing storytelling at the centre of interventions for adolescents with language disorders. The evidence base for narrative approaches to intervention is presented and critiqued. The chapter offers many ideas for using storytelling for language assessment and for targeting and enhancing skills in reasoning, nonverbal communication, structural elements of language, conversation skills, and inferential language.

In Chapter 8, Lowe and Joffe present the case for the critical importance of vocabulary interventions for adolescents. Robust intervention strategies and programmes are presented in detail and related to this age group. The chapter also discusses options for delivering support and intervention at universal, targeted and specialist levels, and presents the process for considering which level of intervention may be most appropriate.

Chapter 9 then details two innovative intervention programmes, designed, delivered and evaluated in a busy school. Mathrick and Norbury present the rationale for providing specialist interventions for social communication skills, in order to support the period of transition when young people leave school. This is followed by a programme to develop interview skills, and a programme that uses song lyrics to scaffold understanding of non-literal and figurative language. The process of evaluating the impact of these new programmes is also described, providing useful insights and techniques for readers who wish to evaluate complex and new interventions within their workplace.

In Chapter 10, Smith discusses the factors to be taken into consideration when working with adolescents with language disorders to incorporate augmentative and alternative communication (AAC) into their lives. The chapter outlines four principles for designing interventions with teenage AAC users: vocabulary; building social networks; links to the curriculum; and supporting independence, autonomy and choice.

These five chapters provide a detailed insight into evidence-based practice for developing the skills of adolescents with language disorders. To help frame these chapters, I now offer a short discussion of the rationale for providing specialist interventions during this life stage, when resources and time are often in short supply. This discussion also considers how evidence-based interventions can target adolescent language disorders.

The rationale for intervention for adolescents with language disorders

It is important to provide interventions for adolescents with language disorders because:

1. Language disorders do not always resolve by adolescence. Despite the potential for early intervention and support in childhood to advance language abilities, many adolescents still have language disorders.

2. Adolescent language disorders are very unlikely to resolve without intervention.

3. For some, language disorders will have pervasive and significant consequences for literacy, academic attainment, engagement with education, employment status and quality of employment, self-esteem and behaviour. It is therefore important to provide intervention for adolescents with language disorders in order to prevent long-term negative outcomes (see also Ehren & Whitemire, 2009).

4. The distinct challenges of the secondary or high-school educational phase also give a compelling reason to provide support and intervention for adolescents.

5. Research has shown that intervention can indeed be effective in increasing adolescents' language abilities.

Despite these arguments in favour of intervention which are well rehearsed in the literature, many adolescents with language disorders do not have access to a comprehensive, appropriate, evidence-based programme of assessment, support, and intervention. It would seem that further concerted effort is needed to develop and assert a clear case for evidence-based practice in relation to adolescents with language disorders. This will be required to convince stakeholders (e.g., service managers, school headteachers, commissioners and policymakers) to fund services for this population.

Evidence-based interventions for adolescents with language disorders

Evidence-based practice (EBP) is defined as the "conscientious, explicit, and judicious use of current best evidence in making decisions about the care of individual patients" (Sackett et al., 1996: 71). EBP is traditionally associated with medicine, but has increasing importance in education and social policy (causing concern amongst some commentators in disciplines that are not informed by a medical model (Gillies, Edwards, & Horsley, 2017)). A commonly-applied EBP framework brings together clinical expertise, best available research evidence, and patient rights and predicaments in order to inform clinical decision-making (Sackett et al., 1996). This basic model has been debated and adapted, for example to include greater emphasis on patient choice and autonomy (Haynes, Devereaux, & Guyatt, 2002).

Figure 1.1 is an adapted model describing how EBP might be implemented for adolescents with language disorders. Decisions must be primarily based on the profile of language disorder; that is to say, the adolescents' strengths and difficulties and access to activities and participation, for example socially and in relation to education. This needs to be considered in relation to the adolescents' circumstances, for example their age, location, ability to access local services, educational engagement, mental health, and so on. The options for assessment, support and intervention then need to be considered in relation to the best research evidence available, considering information about intervention programmes and strategies of support in terms of efficacy (if the intervention works in ideal circumstances), effectiveness (if the intervention is likely to be successful in the current context), and efficiency (whether the intervention warrants the investment of time and funding available). The adolescents' own perspectives and priorities are also very important, and the views of family might also be considered here (see Spencer and Clegg, this volume). Positioned at the centre of these considerations is the professional expertise of the team involved in supporting the young person, who bring together relevant information and use it to recommend and plan next actions. In the original medical model from which this EBP process is adapted, Haynes et al. (2002) term this professional input 'clinical expertise'. However, in relation to language disorders, this is likely to involve a collaborative team of school staff and speech and language therapists, along with any other involved professionals (such as professionals in mental health or youth justice, psychologists, and occupational therapists). Such models of EBP are put forward as a means of integrating research evidence into making decisions about service delivery. Research studies are only one component of this EBP decision-making process. Although EBP is often discussed in relation to control trials of intervention programmes, wider research can also inform EBP decision making. For example, the established evidence that childhood language disorders persist into adolescence with significant impact on a range of psychosocial outcomes can be used to build a rationale for delivering specialist interventions and educational support throughout adolescence.

Implementing evidence-based practice means combining theory, research evidence and clinical knowledge. Ebbels (2017) adapts the 'virtuous circle' described by Snowling and Hulme (2011), where theory is used to design interventions, which are then evaluated in robust intervention studies, which then inform the development of theory. Ebbels proposes that clinical expertise is central to this process, and to the development of practical, deliverable interventions (Ebbels, 2017). Results of evaluations then feed back into clinical practice and the application of theory to support adolescents with language disorders.

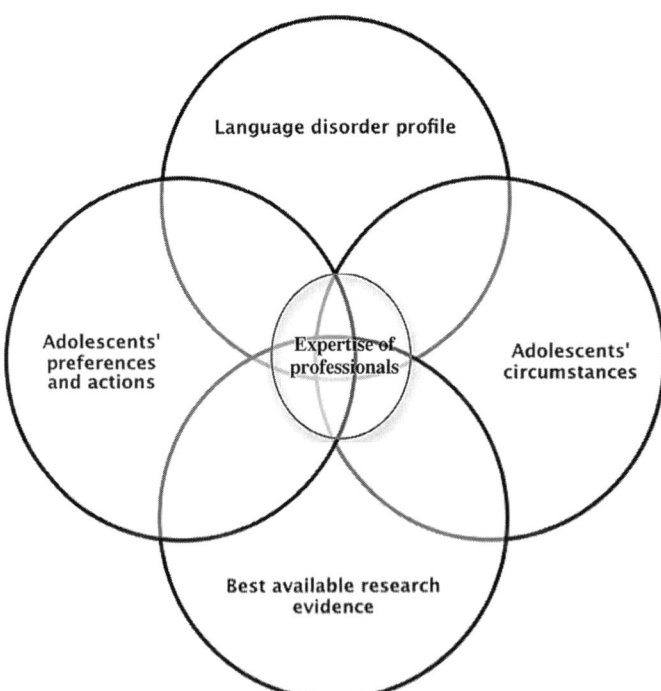

Figure 1.1 An adapted model for evidence-based decisions regarding adolescent language disorders (based on Haynes et al., 2002: 1350).

Intervention approaches

Adolescents with language disorders need access to theoretically grounded intervention programmes and support strategies that match their profiles of strengths and difficulties and fit well with their circumstances and preferences. A range of resources is available offering advice or manual-based instruction for providing interventions for adolescents with language disorders. Some examples include Paul and Norbury (2012), Joffe (2011a, 2011b), and Nippold and Scott (2010).

Paul and Norbury (2012) offer advice and detailed examples of how to assess language and communication skills right from infancy through to adolescence. Theirs is an excellent resource for professionals, and includes lists of standardized assessments, informal observation schedules, and many practical ideas for supporting children's and adolescents' written and oral language.

Joffe (2011a, 2011b) provides plans for intervention sessions to target narrative skills, understanding figurative language and idioms, and vocabulary, which are accompanied by a range of engaging resources. The two manuals by Joffe can be used by speech and language therapists, as well as other professionals working in schools, ideally in partnership with a language specialist.

Nippold's extensive research with adolescents can also be used to select specific targets to work on and to design intervention sessions. For example, her work on expository discourse can be used to examine how adolescents use language to explain complex ideas, and to then support them to increase their skills in this area (Nippold & Scott, 2010; Nippold, Mansfield, Billow, & Tomblin, 2008). Nippold has also used fables to assess critical thinking and syntactic skills, by asking adolescents to reflect on the moral messages of these fables and on characters' thoughts and behaviours. This approach could be used to work on listening skills, systematic reflection, and expressive language (Nippold et al., 2015).

Professionals also need access to high-quality studies that examine the impact of programmes and strategies so that they can be confident that resources are being best used. There are long-standing concerns about the paucity of intervention studies for children and young people with language disorders (Ebbels, 2014; Law, Garrett, & Nye, 2003). However, there is now an established and growing body of research to guide evidence-based interventions for adolescents with language disorders. Studies have shown the impact of intervention for older children and adolescents in relation to: vocabulary and word learning (Lowe, Henry, Muller, & Joffe, 2017; Spencer, Clegg, Lowe, &

Stackhouse, 2017; Wright, Pring, & Ebbels, 2017); word finding (Ebbels et al., 2012); and production and understanding of specific syntactic targets (see Ebbels and Spencer, this volume). There is also some limited evidence that reading interventions can be effective for this age group (Paul & Clarke, 2016) and that oral language interventions (including strategy use, vocabulary, figurative language, and spoken narrative) can improve reading for younger children (Clarke, Snowling, Truelove, & Hulme, 2010).

Speech and language therapy in general (rather than in relation to one specific target) can be effective when delivered to adolescents with language disorders within a special school (Ebbels et al., 2017). Over one school term, a study monitored the progress of 72 pupils aged between 9 and 17 years. Therapists worked with pupils individually on 120 targets, including vocabulary, comprehension of 'before' and 'where' questions, idioms, inference skills, verbs within narratives, and a variety of grammatical targets addressed using the Shape Coding by Susan Ebbels' method. Progress was demonstrated on bespoke outcome measures, with greater progress on targeted rather than control items. The study concludes that direct, specialist speech and language therapy can be effective for older children and adolescents in relation to all areas of language.

Nonetheless, more evidence of what works in supporting adolescents' language skills is required. There are still relatively few robust trials designed to examine the efficacy, effectiveness, and efficiency of interventions for adolescents in relation to all aspects of language disorders. Further research is also needed to unpick and understand the elements of successful interventions. For example, future studies could: investigate the long-term impact of intervention, examine the important features of interventions, examine the effect of treatment density and duration, and investigate the impact of oral language interventions on reading and other outcomes. Research is also needed into how best to support adolescents in relation to functional targets, whether this is in relation to socialization (e.g., asking and answering questions, telling anecdotes), education (e.g., interpreting plays, making persuasive speeches, understanding assessment instructions), or future employment (e.g., performing in job interviews, dealing with customers and colleagues) (Nippold, 2010; see also Mathrick and Norbury, this volume).

The trajectory of current research is promising, with a clear ongoing and international commitment to expanding what we know about assessment and interventions for adolescent language disorders (Nippold, 2010). The chapters in this volume detail how to design robust interventions to support adolescents to target and improve the use and understanding of grammatical constructs, narratives, vocabulary, social communication skills, and the implementation of AAC.

Part III: School-level support for adolescents with language disorders

Part 3 of this book is made up of three chapters which discuss evidence-based approaches to providing school-level support for adolescents with language disorders.

In Chapter 11, Starling argues for the importance of collaborative practice between speech and language therapists and teaching staff. She draws from an evaluated collaborative programme that targets teachers' oral and written instructional language. This chapter introduces strategies and ideas for increasing adolescents' engagement and learning in the classroom.

In Chapter 12, Hartshorne describes *Secondary Talk*, a three-tier approach to supporting adolescents' language skills at the whole-school level. The evidence for whole-school programmes to support language is summarized. The chapter then focuses on the process of evaluating whole-school programmes, identifying the challenges of demonstrating that programmes' impact upon both oral language skills and broader educational attainment. Ideas for overcoming these challenges are put forward, using a theory of change approach.

In Chapter 13, Thomson, Hemphill and Snow discuss evidence for schools supporting written language difficulties. They present the evidence-based Strategic Reading Intervention (STARI) programme and give details of how the programme works.

The final section of this chapter now considers why whole-school interventions are required and how these fit within broader service delivery models.

The impact of language disorders in secondary schools

Whole-school support for language disorders is needed to reduce the impact on educational engagement and achievement. There is good research evidence to suggest that there are associations between adolescents' language skills and their academic outcomes across the curriculum (Spencer et al., 2017).

Research indicates that language disorders in particular impact on academic attainment (Conti-Ramsden, Durkin, Simkin, & Knox, 2009; Dockrell et al., 2007; Durkin, Simkin, Knox, & Conti-Ramsden, 2009; Knox, 2002; Snowling et al., 2001). For example, nearly one-quarter of a cohort of 120 adolescents aged 16 and 17 years with a history of language disorders were not entered for any examinations (Conti-Ramsden et al., 2009). Forty-four percent of the group with a history of SLI attained at least one GCSE A* to C or equivalent. This represents a considerable achievement, although it is half the percentage of those without language disorders. Educational outcomes measured in young adulthood have also suggested lower attainment for those with a history of language difficulties (Clegg et al., 2005; Johnson, Beitchman, & Brownlie, 2009).

Although the mechanisms by which language ability impacts upon educational attainment are not fully understood, they are likely to involve vocabulary skills because of: (a) the complex and abstract vocabulary used in the curriculum (Nagy & Townsend, 2012), and(b) the impact of vocabulary learning on reading comprehension and writing (e.g., Catts et al., 2014; Chall, Jacobs, & Baldwin, 1990; Snow, Porche, Tabors, & Harris, 2007; see Thomson, Hemphill and Snow, this volume). Oral language comprehension and expression is also key to learning by teacher talk and pupil discussion (Dockrell, Lindsay, & Palikara, 2011), particularly during adolescence when understanding and contributing to debate and discussion features increasingly as a mode of learning (Paul & Norbury, 2012).

The challenges of secondary/high school

Adolescents with language disorders need whole-school support in order to overcome the unique challenges presented by secondary or high schools. Referring to UK schooling, Joffe (2015) gives a convincing overview of the additional language demands of the classroom during adolescence:

> "Entry into secondary school brings with it new and more complex challenges that pupils are required to navigate, including larger class sizes, multiple teaching styles, an increasingly complex education curriculum, abstract reasoning and idiomatic understanding, heavy reliance on literacy as the medium of learning, and a greater need for independent working and self-reflection" (Joffe, 2015: 80).

The challenges of the language environment of secondary schools are outlined by Starling, Munro, Togher and Arciuli (2012). The increased complexity of timetabling in schools can make it difficult to schedule adolescents to leave lessons for group or individualized support. Adolescents will typically have a far greater number of teachers than younger children, making collaborative practice and joint working more difficult to deliver. High-stakes exams may result in reluctance to miss lesson content for specialist support, although targeted skills can impact positively on curriculum learning.

A strong foundation of universal support is important in secondary schools, involving ongoing discussions about making classroom learning accessible, making any specialist interventions relevant for the curriculum, responding to arising difficulties in school such as bullying, ability to complete coursework, and preparation for exams, and integrated service delivery opportunities. This is important for children with language disorders of all ages, and particularly during adolescence, given the particular challenges of secondary school. Strong collaborations between speech and language therapists and teachers are therefore required to situate specialist interventions within a context of communication-supporting classrooms.

Levels of intervention within secondary school

Models of service delivery for children and adolescence with language disorders typically involve a tiered approach consisting of: (1) universal provision for all children; (2) targeted provision for children with specific difficulties or vulnerabilities; and (3) specialist services for those requiring direct and intense intervention (Law, Reilly, & Snow, 2013). The specialist tier can also be divided into direct, individualized intervention delivered by a specialist, and intervention managed by a specialist but delivered indirectly by others (Ebbels et al., 2017). While all three tiers of intervention might require similar levels of speech and language therapist input, the proportion of SLT time per child will increase from universal to specialist tiers, as outlined by Gascoigne (2006, 2011).

Similarly, in the USA and beyond, a Response to Intervention (RTI) service delivery model is frequently used to support school-aged children with special educational needs in schools (Bjorn et al., 2016; Fuchs & Fuchs, 2006) and has been put forward as a model for use in youth justice contexts (Snow et al., 2015). This framework also uses a tiered approach (also referred to as levels):

> **Tier 1** (general support) is for all students and involves screening to identify children at risk of educational under-achievement. This tier also

includes differential instruction and delivering evidence-based strategies and programmes by classroom teachers, with some group-based interventions. At-risk children are monitored to see if they respond to universal provision, and if a child does not make progress they move into Tier 2.

Tier 2 (intensified support) is therefore for children who have received universal interventions but have not made expected progress. It usually involves more specialist and more intensive intervention, though these may be delivered at whole-class or in small groups. If a child does not make progress, they move on to Tier 3.

Tier 3 (special support) involves more continued and intensive intervention, often tailored for individuals and based on research (Fuchs, Fuchs, & Compton, 2012).

These three tiers form a multilevel approach to ensuring that all children have access to high-quality instruction and interventions, while identifying and providing increasingly intense and specialist support for struggling learners (Ehren & Whitmire, 2009). Although a tiered model may imply a linear journey through different tiers, there should be overlap. For example, students receiving specialist interventions at Tier 3 would still receive high-quality instruction in the classroom (Tier 1).

Ehren and Whitmere (2009) argue for the importance of speech and language therapist/pathologist input into RTI for secondary schools, proposing that speech and language therapists/pathologists need to: (a) orient their work towards the curriculum and towards literacy; (b) increase their visibility within busy schools; (c) go beyond a traditional pull-out model to work within classrooms, and work indirectly, provide consultation, and be present in classrooms; and (d) move from a caseload to a workload approach, scheduling tasks both with and on behalf of students. Ehren and Whitmere (2009) stress that speech and language therapists/pathologists should work collaboratively with other professionals, should focus on literacy as well as language, and should broaden the concept of services to include adolescents without a diagnosis of language disorders. Although put forward in relation to RTI, these suggestions are relevant for all professionals wanting to deliver educationally relevant and high-impact services in schools.

The relationship between different levels of service delivery is not unproblematic: there is inconsistency of terminology used in tiered or RTI approaches across SLT services and within education, a lack of clarity about specific professional roles within service delivery options, and too few robust research studies demonstrating the efficiency of resources allocated across different levels (Ebbels et al., 2017). Despite these issues, collaborative practice between speech and language therapists and teachers is needed to facilitate inclusion for adolescents with language disorders. Emerging evidence has shown that high-quality training, with follow-up support and collaborative practice, can have an impact on secondary school students' language and literacy skills (Snow, Lawrence, & White, 2009; Starling et al., 2012). The last three chapters of this book detail how speech and language specialists can work with teachers to increase educational access for all, drawing from three evidence-based programmes.

Conclusion

Language disorders are common, persistent, and have significant impacts on broader psychosocial outcomes. Many of the issues raised in Part I of this chapter will be familiar from Ellie's story which is told in the Preface. Ellie describes issues such as the enduring nature of difficulties, the impact on friendships and relationships, the need for support around times of transition, resilience as well as risk, the importance of and the role of specialist resource units.

Studies have designed, delivered and evaluated the impact of interventions for different dimensions of language functioning during adolescence. It is well known that theoretically-driven support strategies and interventions are needed for adolescents with language disorders. And there is emerging evidence that they can indeed be effective. People working with adolescents have access to evidence-based interventions for a range of language targets, and there is recognition that oral language work can impact on reading and writing skills. Collaboration between professionals is essential to delivering high-quality support, both in terms of specialist, individualized interventions and classroom-based and whole-school approaches to maximizing inclusion. This book presents theoretically-driven ways to support adolescents with language disorders, both in relation to specialist interventions and whole-school strategies and programmes.

Reflective questions

1. How would you describe Developmental Language Disorder to a parent who had not heard of the diagnosis?

2. How would you convince a head teacher to commission specialist provision for adolescents with developmental language disorder within their mainstream school?

3. How do you apply evidence-based practice to your current work? What changes could you make to ensure evidence-based practice is at the centre of your practice?

References

Beitchman, J.H., Wilson, B., Brownlie, E.B., Walters, H., & Lancee, W. (1996). Long-term consistency in speech/language profiles: I. Developmental and academic outcomes. *Journal of the American Academy of Child & Adolescent Psychiatry, 35*(6), 804-814.

Bishop, D.V.M. (2014). Ten questions about terminology for children with unexplained language problems. *International Journal of Language & Communication Disorders, 49*(4), 381-415.

Björn, P.M., Aro, M.T., Koponen, T.K., Fuchs, L.S., & Fuchs, D.H. (2016). The many faces of special education within RTI frameworks in the United States and Finland. *Learning Disability Quarterly, 39*(1), 58-66.

Botting, N. & Conti-Ramsden, G. (2008). The role of language, social cognition, and social skill in the functional social outcomes of young adolescents with and without a history of SLI. *British Journal of Developmental Psychology, 26*(2), 281-300.

Botting, N., Toseeb, U., Pickles, A., Durkin, K., & Conti-Ramsden, G. (2016). Depression and anxiety change from adolescence to adulthood in individuals with and without language impairment. *PloS one, 11*(7), e0156678.

Brownlie, E.B., Bao, L., & Beitchman, J. (2016). Childhood language disorder and social anxiety in early adulthood. *Journal of Abnormal Child Psychology, 44*, 1061–1070.

Catts, H.W., Fey, M.E., Weismer, S., & Bridges, S.M. (2014). The relationship between language and reading abilities. In J.B.Tomblin & M.A. Nippold (Eds), *Understanding Individual Differences in Language Development across the School Years* (pp.144-165). New York: Psychology Press/Taylor & Francis.

Cirrin, F.M. & Gillam, R.B. (2008). Language intervention practices for school-age children with spoken language disorders: A systematic review. *Language, Speech, and Hearing Services in Schools, 39*(1), S110-S137.

Clark, A., O'Hare, A., Watson, J., Cohen, W., Cowie, H., Elton, R., ... & Seckl, J. (2007). Severe receptive language disorder in childhood - familial aspects and long-term outcomes: Results from a Scottish study. *Archives of Disease in Childhood, 92*(7), 614-619.

Cohen, N.J., Davine, M., Horodezky, N., Lipsett, L., & Isaacson, L. (1993). Unsuspected language impairment in psychiatrically disturbed children: Prevalence and language and behavioral characteristics. *Journal of the American Academy of Child & Adolescent Psychiatry, 32*(3), 595-603.

Cohen, N.J., Menna, R., Vallance, D.D., Barwick, M.A., Im, N., & Horodezky, N.B. (1998). Language, social cognitive processing, and behavioral characteristics of psychiatrically disturbed children with previously identified and unsuspected language impairments. *The Journal of Child Psychology and Psychiatry and Allied Disciplines, 39*(6), 853-864.

Cohen, N.J., Farnia, F., & Im-Bolter, N. (2013). Higher order language competence and adolescent mental health. *Journal of Child Psychology and Psychiatry, 54*(7), 733-744.

Conti-Ramsden, G. & Botting, N. (2008). Emotional health in adolescents with and without a history of specific language impairment (SLI). *Journal of Child Psychology and Psychiatry, 49*(5), 516-525.

Conti-Ramsden, G., Durkin, K., Simkin, Z., & Knox, E. (2009). Specific language impairment and school outcomes. I: Identifying and explaining variability at the end of compulsory education. *International Journal of Language & Communication Disorders, 44*(1), 15-35.

Conti-Ramsden, G., Durkin, K., Mok, P.L., Toseeb, U., & Botting, N. (2016). Health, employment and relationships: Correlates of personal wellbeing in young adults with and without a history of childhood language impairment. *Social Science & Medicine, 160*, 20-28.

Department for Education. (2017). Statistics: Special Educational Needs. London: Department for Education, accessed online at: https://www.gov.uk/government/collections/statistics-special-educational-needs-sen

Dockrell, J.E., Lindsay, G., Letchford, B., & Mackie, C. (2006). Educational provision for children with specific speech and language difficulties: Perspectives of speech and language therapy service managers. *International Journal of Language & Communication Disorders, 41*(4), 423-440.

Dockrell, J.E., Lindsay, G., & Palikara, O. (2011). Explaining the academic achievement at school leaving for pupils with a history of language impairment: Previous academic achievement and literacy skills. *Child Language Teaching and Therapy, 27*(2), 223-237.

Durkin, K. & Conti-Ramsden, G. (2007). Language, social behavior, and the quality of friendships in adolescents with and without a history of specific language impairment. *Child Development, 78*(5), 1441-1457.

Durkin, K. & Conti-Ramsden, G. (2010). Young people with specific language impairment: A review of social and emotional functioning in adolescence. *Child Language Teaching and Therapy, 26*(2), 105-121.

Durkin, K., Simkin, Z., Knox, E., & Conti-Ramsden, G. (2009). Specific language impairment and school outcomes. II: Educational context, student satisfaction, and post-compulsory progress. *International Journal of Language & Communication Disorders, 44*(1), 36-55.

Durkin, K., Toseeb, U., Botting, N., Pickles, A., & Conti-Ramsden, G. (2017). Social confidence in early adulthood among young people with and without a history of language impairment. *Journal of Speech, Language, and Hearing Research, 60*(6), 1635-1647.

Ebbels, S H. (2017). Intervention research: Appraising study designs, interpreting findings and creating research in clinical practice. *International Journal of Speech-Language Pathology, 19*(3), 218-231.

Ebbels, S.H., McCartney, E., Slonims, V., Dockrell, J.E., & Norbury, C. (2017). Evidence based pathways to intervention for children with language disorders. PeerJ Preprints 5:e2951v1 https://doi.org/10.7287/peerj.preprints.2951v1

Ehren, B.J. & Whitmire, K. (2009). Speech-language pathologists as primary contributors to response to intervention at the secondary level. *Seminars in Speech and Language, 30*(2), 90-104.

Fuchs, D. & Fuchs, L.S. (2006). Introduction to response to intervention: What, why, and how valid is it? *Reading Research Quarterly, 41*(1), 93-99.

Fuchs, D., Fuchs, L.S., & Compton, D.L. (2012). Smart RTI: A next-generation approach to multilevel prevention. *Exceptional Children, 78*(3), 263-279.

Gascoigne, M. (2006). Supporting children with speech, language and communication needs within integrated children's services. *RCSLT Position Paper.* London: Royal College of Speech and Language Therapists. http://www. rcslt. org/docs/free-pub/ Supporting_children-website. pdf

Gascoigne, M. (2008). Change for children with language and communication needs: Creating sustainable integrated services. *Child Language Teaching and Therapy, 24*(2), 133-154.

Gascoigne, M. (2011). The Balanced System. Accessed online at: https://www.mgaconsulting. org.uk/the%20balanced%20system%20outline%20v3%202011.pdf

Hannus, S., Kauppila, T., & Launonen, K. (2009). Increasing prevalence of specific language impairment (SLI) in primary healthcare of a Finnish town, 1989–99. *International Journal of Language & Communication Disorders, 44*(1), 79–97.

Haynes, R.B., Devereaux, P.J., & Guyatt, G.H. (2002). Physicians' and patients' choices in evidence based practice: Evidence does not make decisions, people do. *BMJ: British Medical Journal, 324*(7350), 1350.

Hollo, A., Wehby, J.H., & Oliver, R.M. (2014). Unidentified language deficits in children with emotional and behavioral disorders: A meta-analysis. *Exceptional Children, 80*(2), 169-186.

Hughes, N., Chitsabesan, P., Bryan, K., Borschmann, R., Swain, N., Lennox, C., & Shaw, J. (2017). Language impairment and comorbid vulnerabilities among young people in custody. *Journal of Child Psychology and Psychiatry, 58*(10), 1106-1113.

Im-Bolter, N., Cohen, N.J., & Farnia, F. (2013). I thought we were good: Social cognition, figurative language, and adolescent psychopathology. *Journal of Child Psychology and Psychiatry, 54*(7), 724-732.

Joffe, V. (2011a). *Narrative Intervention Programme.* Milton Keynes: Speechmark.

Joffe, V.L. (2011b). *Vocabulary Enrichment Intervention Programme.* Milton Keynes: Speechmark.

Justice, L.M. (2006). Evidence-based practice, response to intervention, and the prevention of reading difficulties. *Language, Speech, and Hearing Services in Schools, 37*(4), 284-297.

Knox, E. (2002). Educational attainments of children with specific language impairment at year 6. *Child Language Teaching and Therapy, 18*(2), 103-124.

Law, J., Garrett, Z., & Nye, C. (2003). Speech and language therapy interventions for children with primary speech and language delay or disorder. *The Cochrane Database of Systematic Reviews, 3.* Accessed online at: http://onlinelibrary.wiley.com/doi/10.1002/14651858. CD004110/pdf/

Law, J., Reilly, S., & Snow, P.C. (2013). Child speech, language and communication needs re-examined in a public health context: A new direction for the speech and language therapy profession. *International Journal of Language & Communication Disorders, 48*(5), 486–496.

Lowe, H., Henry, L., Müller, L.M., & Joffe, V.L. (2017). Vocabulary intervention for adolescents with language disorder: A systematic review. *International Journal of Language & Communication Disorders.* doi: 10.1111/1460-6984.12355

Mok, P.L., Pickles, A., Durkin, K., & Conti-Ramsden, G. (2014). Longitudinal trajectories of peer relations in children with specific language impairment. *Journal of Child Psychology and Psychiatry, 55*(5), 516–527.

Nippold, M.A. (2014a). *Language Sampling with Adolescents: Implications for Intervention (2nd ed.).* San Diego, CA: Plural.

Nippold, M.A. (2014)b. Language intervention at the middle school: Complex talk reflects complex thought. *Language, Speech, and Hearing Services in Schools, 45*(2) 153–156.

Nippold, M.A. (2016). *Later Language Development: School-age Children, Adolescents, and Young Adults (4th ed.).* Austin, TX: Pro-Ed.

Nippold, M.A. & Scott, C.M. (Eds) (2010). *Expository Discourse in Children, Adolescents, and Adults: Development and Disorders.* New York, NY: Psychology Press/Taylor & Francis.

Nippold, M.A., Frantz-Kaspar, M.W., Cramond, P.M., Kirk, C., Hayward-Mayhew, C., & MacKinnon, M. (2015). Critical thinking about fables: Examining language production and comprehension in adolescents. *Journal of Speech, Language, and Hearing Research, 58*(2), 325–335.

Nippold, M.A., Mansfield, T.C., Billow, J.L., & Tomblin, J.B. (2008). Expository discourse in adolescents with language impairments: Examining syntactic development. *American Journal of Speech-Language Pathology, 17,* 356–366.

Norbury, C.F., Gooch, D., Wray, C., Baird, G., Charman, T., Simonoff, E., ... & Pickles, A. (2016). The impact of nonverbal ability on prevalence and clinical presentation of language disorder: Evidence from a population study. *Journal of Child Psychology and Psychiatry, 57*(11), 1247–1257.

O'Donnell, P.S. & Miller, D.N. (2011). Identifying students with specific learning disabilities: School psychologists' acceptability of the discrepancy model versus response to intervention. *Journal of Disability Policy Studies, 22*(2), 83–94.

Pickles, A., Durkin, K., Mok, P.L., Toseeb, U., & Conti-Ramsden, G. (2016). Conduct problems co-occur with hyperactivity in children with language impairment: A longitudinal study from childhood to adolescence. *Autism & Developmental Language Impairments, 1,* 2396941516645251.

Sackett, D.L., Rosenberg, W.M., Gray, J.M., Haynes, R.B., & Richardson, W.S. (1996). Evidence based medicine: What it is and what it isn't. *BMJ: British Medical Journal, 312,* 71–72.

Snow, C.E., Lawrence, J.F., & White, C. (2009). Generating knowledge of academic language among urban middle school students. *Journal of Research on Educational Effectiveness*, *2*(4), 325-344.

Snowling, M.J., Adams, J.W., Bishop, D.V.M., & Stothard, S. (2001). Educational attainments of school leavers with a preschool history of speech-language impairments. *International Journal of Language & Communication Disorders*, *36*(2), 173-183.

Starling, J., Munro, N., Togher, L., & Arciuli, J. (2012) Training secondary school teachers in instructional language modification techniques to support adolescents with language impairment: A randomised control trial. *Language, Speech and Hearing Services in Schools*, *43*, 474-495.

Stothard, S.E., Snowling, M.J., Bishop, D.V., Chipchase, B.B., & Kaplan, C.A. (1998). Language-impaired preschoolers: A follow-up into adolescence. *Journal of Speech, Language, and Hearing Research*, *41*(2), 407-418.

Tomblin, J.B., Records, N.L., Buckwalter, P., Zhang, X., Smith, E., & O'Brien, M. (1997). Prevalence of specific language impairment in kindergarten children. *Journal of Speech, Language, and Hearing Research*, *40*(6), 1245-1260.

Wright, L., Pring, T., & Ebbels, S. (2017). Effectiveness of vocabulary intervention for older children with (developmental) language disorder. *International Journal of Language & Communication Disorders*. doi: 10.1111/1460-6984.12361

World Health Organization (WHO). (1992). *The ICD-10 Classification of Mental and Behavioural Disorders: Clinical Descriptions and Diagnostic Guidelines* (Vol. 1). Geneva: World Health Organization.

WHO (2012) Expanding access to contraceptive services for adolescents. Geneva: WHO. Accessed online at: http://apps.who.int/iris/bitstream/10665/75160/1/WHO_RHR_HRP_12.21_eng.pdf?ua=1

WHO (2015). Adolescent development. Geneva: WHO. Accessed online at: http://www.who.int/maternal_child_adolescent/topics/adolescence/development/en/

2 Multidisciplinary perspectives on adolescence

Sarah Spencer

This chapter will enable readers to:

- Describe the complex and multilayered development that occurs during adolescence, in terms of:

  - Puberty

  - Neuro-maturation and cognitive changes

  - Social transitions

  - Identity formation

  - Language development

  - Use of linguistic features to signal social meaning.

- Apply a multidisciplinary account of adolescence to a case example of an adolescent with language disorders.

Introduction

The adolescent life stage marks the official transition from childhood to adulthood and results from a combination of biological, psychological, and social transitions (Kirkham & Moore, 2013; Steinberg, 2010). It is characterized as the most turbulent phase in life, one where teens are physically, physiologically, socially, intellectually and linguistically in a constant state of flux (Tagliamonte, 2016). It is also conceptualized as a time of risk, due to the perception that biological maturity can precede psychosocial maturity (WHO, 2012).

A biopsychosocial or bioecological framework (Bronfenbrenner & Morris, 2006; Dodge & Pettit, 2003) is often applied to adolescence to examine the dynamic interplay between factors influencing young people, including the interpersonal and the environmental, and to examine the integration of psychological and contextual effects on adolescent outcomes (see also Clegg, this volume). For example, factors such school climate (size, location, quality of education provided) may interact with factors such as the adolescents' orientation to their future outcomes to influence problem behaviours (Chen & Vazsonyi, 2013). It is beyond the scope of this book to go into detail about the developments and demands of the adolescent life stage and, indeed, very good texts are dedicated to doing just that (e.g., Arnett, 2014; Steinberg, 2010). However, this chapter does include a brief overview of adolescent development from a multidisciplinary perspective to enable the reader to apply research regarding cognitive, social, and linguistic changes to those with language disorders.

What do we mean by *adolescence*?

Adolescence is a life stage that stretches from somewhere between the ages of 11 and 21 or 22, or between 13 and 19 if adolescence is deemed synonymous with teenage years. The exact definition of adolescence has "long posed a conundrum" (Sawyer et al., 2018: 1) since, as indicated above, it is a life stage influenced by biological changes and social transitions, both of which are influenced by societal factors. For example, the age of onset of puberty is now lower globally as a result of improved health and nutrition. Many role transitions which are markers of adulthood are occurring later than a generation ago, such as completing education, marriage, living outside the parental home, and parenthood. If adolescence is accepted as a distinct stage falling between childhood and adulthood, there is an argument that the definition of this stage will shift as biological and life stage norms themselves adjust. Accordingly, Sawyer et al. (2018) propose that adolescence is now to be defined as lasting between 10 and 24 years in terms of legal markers, social policy and access to services.

The fluidity of the boundaries that define adolescence has implications for those working with adolescents with language disorders. Young people should be viewed within their own context, that is to say, within the life transitions and challenges that they are experiencing at any given time. There are also implications for service delivery. Statutory care for care leavers and young people with special educational needs now extends to 24 years in the UK but many young people with language disorders will not qualify for access to services. Speech and language therapy services typically only offer assessment and intervention until the end of compulsory schooling, despite considerable evidence that language disorders continue to impact on outcomes up to the age of 24 years and beyond (e.g., Conti-Ramsden et al., 2017).

Puberty

Puberty is a central part of adolescence. Young people's bodies transform due to hormonal changes linked to the development of primary and secondary sex characteristics; the former referring to the production of eggs and sperm and the development of the sex organs, and the latter to other changes to the body not related to reproduction. Levels of sex hormones (androgens and estrogens) rise and physical growth increases in terms of height, muscle and fat mass, and organ growth. The order of events during puberty is predictable, though when puberty starts and how long it lasts varies. There are also cultural influences on puberty, with the onset of puberty occurring earlier when nutrition and medical care are good. It is important that adolescents have timely information about the biological changes they are experiencing, as well as the psychological and social implications of puberty for them and their peers (Arnett, 2014). For adolescents with language disorders, it is important that this information is accessible and adapted to their language abilities and difficulties.

Neuro-maturation

We now know that the adolescent brain continues to develop, resulting in substantial neurodevelopmental changes alongside increased reasoning skills. There appear to be three main areas of brain development:

1. Overproduction of the connections – synapses – between neurons in the brain. This occurs in many parts of the outer grey matter at around the onset of puberty (about 11 or 12 years). In the years that follow, synaptic pruning takes place, which reduces the connections and reduces grey matter by around 10% (Sowell et al., 1999a, 1999b). This synaptic pruning allows brain pathways to become more specialist and efficient.

2. White matter volume increases into adulthood. This is thought to be caused by increases in axonal caliber (e.g., how thick or thin axons are) and increased myelination (e.g., more myelin, a fatty white substance which surrounds the axon of some nerve cells, resulting in increased speed of nerve impulse) (Fuhrmann, Knoll, & Blakemore, 2015).

3. Growth in the cerebellum continues well into the 20s. This is part of the lower brain, beneath the cortex. As well as being involved in basic functions like movement, the cerebellum is also important for higher functioning cognitive tasks such as decision making, mathematical reasoning, and some social skills (Tiemeier et al., 2010).

Neuro-maturation is particularly pronounced in the frontal and temporal brain regions (Tamnes et al., 2010). For example, the limbic system develops: a region associated with pleasure seeking, reward processing, emotional responses and sleep regulation. The prefrontal and parietal cortices also change, these being associated with higher cognitive skills and executive functioning (including skills such as relational reasoning, decision making, organization, and future orientation) (Fuhrmann et al., 2015; WHO, 2015). The frontal regions also become better connected with other brain regions, with resulting improvement to response inhibition (Steinberg, 2004).

Research is starting to piece together associations between the trajectories of 'typical' adolescent behaviour such as responses to risk and associated neuro-cognitive maturation. For example, there is overlapping adolescent development in terms of social cognition (including skills such as joint attention, face recognition, inferencing, attributing mental states to others), structural brain development in regions associated with 'the social brain network', and in the nature and impact of social relationships (e.g., responding to peer judgement or social decision-making) (Kilford, Garrett, & Blakemore, 2016).

Recent attempts to examine neuropsychological testing and neuroimaging data alongside one another have led to insights into the associations between changes to the adolescent brain and related cognitive skills. For example, a study of 185 12–14-year-olds found that thinner cortices (due to increased myelination and pruning of unnecessary synaptic connections) in the right and left inferior parietal lobe and the right superior parietal lobe, were related to verbal learning and memory (Squeglia et al., 2013). Development in social cognition has also been attributed to developments to the structure and activity in the medial prefrontal cortex (Dumontheil, Apperly, & Blakemore, 2010). However, future longitudinal study into developmental trajectories of both neuro-maturation and neuro-cognition is needed to investigate causal relationships between brain development and skills in adolescence.

Neurodevelopment in adolescence has important consequences for providing support and protection for adolescents. Research has shown that adolescence is a period of neural plasticity (where the brain changes according to internal or external influences), and for that reason is thought to be a particularly sensitive period. The brain may be more vulnerable to the impact of stress, with long-term consequences for mental health (Fuhrmann et al., 2015). Drug use and alcohol intake may also have a heightened impact on cognitive development at this stage (Squeglia, Jacobus, & Tapert, 2009a; Squeglia et al., 2009b). In a more positive light, adolescence may be a particularly promising period for training in abilities such as working memory, which would build on development in frontal areas of the brain (Løhaugen et al., 2011).

Cognitive changes

Ongoing cognitive development occurs throughout adolescence, alongside neuro-maturation. Selective attention develops, memory improves, and processing speed becomes faster. Executive functioning advances, meaning that adolescents are more able to manage and control their own cognitive processes (Blakemore & Choudhury, 2006). Critical thinking skills develop, particularly where foundational knowledge is in place and educational contexts provide opportunities and support for developing analytical skills. Adolescents become more able to analyze and make judgements about information, and to analyze their own understanding of the information that they scrutinize.

Early adolescence marks the beginning of Piaget's formal operational stage, which lasts until somewhere between 15 and 20 years. Formal operational thought is associated with the ability to think about abstract concepts and display logical thought, deductive reasoning, and systematic planning (Piaget, 1977). The facility for what is called 'scientific thought' develops, and adolescents become increasingly adept at applying scientific reasoning (or hypothetical-deductive reasoning) to test possible solutions to problems and defend the resulting solutions. Adolescents also become more able to reflect on their own thoughts as metacognitive skills develop, enabling them to reason and monitor their thinking processes.

Researchers have also examined 'post-formal thought' in late adolescence and early adulthood. This type of reasoning involves a greater awareness of the complexity of real-life situations and factors which influence responses. Dialectical thought emerges, involving a growing awareness that opposing opinions or alternatives can each have their own range of advantages and disadvantages. Adolescents and young adults become increasingly adept at addressing problems without all of the information they would have in an ideal world (see Arnett, 2014, for a summary).

Social cognition develops during adolescence, involving increasingly sophisticated ways of thinking about other people, their social relationships, and others' perspectives. Theory of mind is the ability to attribute mental states to others (such as beliefs, feelings, or intentions). While much development occurs in early childhood, adolescents continue to develop their theory of mind abilities into late adolescence. For example, adolescents are increasingly able to consider a speakers' perspective (e.g., what objects they can see from their position) when using that speaker's instructions to guide their own behaviour (Dumontheil et al., 2010).

Adolescents also become more able to consider interpretive diversity (the idea that there is variation and ambiguity in others' thoughts). For example, when considering questions and scenarios such as "Could two people watch the same thing happen and both see and hear everything, but remember it very differently?", older adolescents are more likely to give answers which attributed interpretive diversity, including descriptions of active mental processing (e.g., an answer such as "Yes, if one person sees things positively and the other negatively") (Weimer et al., 2017). As social metacognition develops, adolescents may have difficulties distinguishing between their thinking about their own thoughts from their thinking about the thoughts of others. Adolescents may conclude that others think of them with similar intensity as they think about their self, leading to 'adolescent egocentrism' (Arnett, 2014).

Cognitive development has been examined in relation to cultural context and variation (Arnett, 2012). Indeed, cognition can be considered inseparable from culture, as people use their cognitive skills in their daily activities. The unique social transitions made during adolescence form one level of cultural context, as do personal relationships and social institutions.

Social transitions

> "While the 'raging hormones' of puberty may well be a source of difficulty, the social construction of this life stage is sufficiently elaborate to make the effects of biology seem trivial." (Eckert, 2000: 10).

Adolescence is a time of social change, within education, families, and friendships. The life stage typically involves the transition from primary (or junior) school to secondary (or high) school and then the transition from compulsory education to whatever lies ahead, including further education, employment or training (or, indeed, a lack of these options).

Secondary schooling typically brings greater independence, autonomy and opportunities to tailor learning to pupils' own interests and strengths. The secondary school environment is a demanding space with a shift towards taking increased responsibility for learning and conduct, multiple teachers and teaching styles, and increased educational demands and pressures. Adolescence often features decision making about which areas of education to specialize in and then preparation for high-stakes examinations and assignments (the demands of secondary school are also discussed in Part III of Chapter 1).

Adolescence is characterized as a period of disequilibrium in the family unit. There are a range of changes which may lead to conflict within families: puberty; changing perceptions regarding parents' abilities; renegotiation of expectations and boundaries; increased social attachments outside the family; parents' own transition to middle age – to name but a few. However, research has indicated that in fact the 'storm and stress' within families is often minor. Families frequently maintain agreement on core values and remain a source of love, advice and support for adolescents (Arnett, 2014).

Typically, autonomy increases, young people develop wider contacts, and there is a move towards being more independent from parents, with increased solidarity among friends (Tagliamonte, 2016). Friendships and peer relationships become more important. This can be positive, with intensified friendship groups, clear group identity, and increased sense of belonging. However, it may not be plain sailing as "the peer social order…is fraught with conflict, competition, and emotional volatility" (Eckert, 2000: 4). Adolescents navigate a peer-controlled arena of identities where they compete for popularity with friends and potential romantic partners, and prepare themselves for college and employment (Eckert, 2000). Globally, adolescents are increasingly sexually active (WHO, 2012), with sexual behaviour being influenced by physiological development (e.g., hormone profiles and gender differences) alongside psychosocial factors (Pringle et al., 2017).

Adolescence is often characterized as a time of risk in terms of behaviours such as excessive alcohol intake, lack of contraceptive use, violence, and drug abuse. International evidence shows that the inclination towards risky behaviour and real-world risk taking peaks during late adolescence, despite cultural variation in norms and opportunities for risk taking (Duell et al., 2017). Research has explored the complex factors which underpin increased risky behaviours, including neural mechanisms (Blankenstein et al., 2018), cognitive factors (Harden et al., 2017), and social processes (Hoorn, Crone, & Leijenhorst, 2017).

Identity development

Adolescents take on the task of identity development, constructing self and world views in relation to social and cultural contexts (Trommsdorff, 2012). In Erik Erikson's classic work on developmental stages, the central task of adolescence is to create a coherent identity and avoid identity confusion (Erikson, 1950, 1968). Adolescents develop goals, values and beliefs to shape their decisions and to position themselves in relation to social groups. Of course, identity issues are not unique to adolescence, occurring across the lifespan as people fit within their worlds in different ways. However, adolescence has long been considered an important time for identity development, and one which often includes exploration and participation in a range of identities without commitment (Marcia, 1966). Thus, adolescents may try out different educational pathways, employment options, peer groups, styles, etc. Successful adolescent identity formation is important as it impacts on a variety of outcomes such as wellbeing, academic engagement, and interpersonal relationships (Klimstra & van Doeselaar, 2017).

The field of identity studies now involves alternative neo-Eriksonian theories of how identities form and are maintained and revised. For example, Luyckx et al. (2006, 2011) put forward a four-dimensional model of identity formation during adolescence including: (a) commitment making; (b) identification with commitment; (c) exploration in depth; and (d) exploration in breadth. According to this model, exploration is defined as questioning and experimenting with different identity alternatives. Exploration in depth examines one identity from a range of options, whereas exploration in breadth involves experimentation with a range of different identities. Commitment is when choices are made in identity relevant areas. Identification with commitment relates to personal expressiveness and is concerned with how well an adolescent feels secure with an identity and how well it fits with their values and standards. Commitment-exploration cycles repeat, leading to dynamic shifts in identity formation across adolescence and, indeed, the lifespan.

A narrative identity is the internal story that we develop, reflecting on the past and imagined future, constructing a coherent sense of purpose and meaning (Singer, 2004). Adolescents' use of personal stories to create a coherent identity has been researched, with adolescents becoming more able to use stories to process experiences and make sense of their feelings and reactions (McAdams & McLean, 2013). This is linked to cognitive development, as adolescents become more able to represent their identity in abstract ways and to cope with inconsistencies and tensions in everyday life. Also, adolescence is often a time of broadening social networks. Therefore, adolescence can involve more opportunities for presenting and explaining yourself in conversations with diverse audiences. Conversations are therefore key opportunities for explaining who you are and sharing memories through stories. Attentive listeners can shape the importance of a shared story for identity formation, leading to a developed idea of who the person is and how they came to be (McAdams & McLean, 2013; see also Joffe, this volume).

The concept of identity is not a straightforward one and use of 'identity' varies across and within academic disciplines (Moore & Podesva, 2009). Identities can be constructed in relation to demographic categories, local and specific cultural positions, or interactionally specific stances and roles (Bucholtz & Hall, 2005). Individuals develop a range of identities, which may vary across contexts. For example, in relation to education, adolescents develop their identity through their selection of study areas, commitment to subjects, and applications for further and higher education. Educational identity does not evolve in isolation. Factors such as friendships are important, with nurturing, balanced friendships forming a safe environment for making educational choices (van Doeselaar et al., 2016). People may present different aspects of their self to friends, family, colleagues, and so on. Talk is a central way of engaging with identity work, not only through stories and conversations as outlined above, but also through the use of linguistic features (across all levels from phonetic to discourse), because speakers "will be appropriating and constructing social meanings in ways which identify them to relative micro-, meso-, and macro- identity frames" (Moore & Podesva, 2009: 449).

Language development

Language continues to develop during adolescence. This is often overlooked, given that many 5-year-old children can produce and understand long and complex utterances. However, language skills do continue to develop throughout late childhood, adolescence and into adulthood (Nippold, Frantz-Kaspar, & Vigeland, 2017). This development is less obvious in terms of speed, saliency and substance when compared to the linguistic gains of infancy and early childhood (Nippold, 2016). However, adolescent language development is equally important, given the impact on education, employment, relationships, and wellbeing.

It is important to understand typical language development of older children so that appropriate and challenging assessments and interventions can be planned and delivered. However, this chapter will give only a very brief overview of adolescent language development, given that (a) Marilyn Nippold has written a comprehensive and detailed textbook on the subject based on her extensive research in this area (Nippold, 2016), and (b) many adolescents with language disorders will not yet have reached the stage of developing the linguistic skills expected during adolescence but will be building foundational language skills which typically emerge in earlier childhood.

Adolescent language development is evident in range of areas (see Nippold, 2016) such as:

- Word knowledge (see also Lowe and Joffe, this volume), including new words (e.g., interpretation, icon, juxtapose) and developing knowledge of polysemous words (e.g., those with physical and psychological meaning, such as cold or hard, or related to mathematical, spatial and musical concepts such as volume). It is estimated that a 10-year-old has knowledge of at least 20,000 words, increasing to 30,000 by 15 years and 50,000 by 25 years (Nippold, 2016).

- Derivational morphology (e.g., understanding and using the suffix -ly to move between adjective and adverb, such as personal to personally).

- Metacognitive verb production, for example words such as *believe* versus *know* (Nippold, Vigeland, & Frantz-Kaspar, 2017a).

- Word definitions, which increasingly mention subordinate category classification and more subtle aspects of meaning between ages 12 and 23 years (Nippold et al., 1999). At 15 years, definitions of abstract nouns typically involve key features, while by 25 years the Aristotelian form of definitions is applied (e.g., 'Democracy is a system of government in which the whole population has a role, typically through elected representatives').

- Figurative expressions (Levarato & Cacciari, 2002; Nippold & Taylor, 2002). Adolescents can understand, reflect upon, and explain the meaning of increasingly abstract metaphors and idioms.

- Ambiguity and sarcasm, with increasing understanding, even without contextual cues and intonation.

- Syntax (see also Ebbels and Spencer, this volume), in terms of cohesion within and across sentences as well as syntactic complexity and utterance length (Nippold et al., 2017a). The length of each clause (including all modifiers, known as the c-unit) increases from 7+ at 10 years, to 8+ at 15 years, and 9+ at 25 years during conversation (it is around two words longer during expository discourse) (Nippold, 2016).

- Conversation, narrative, and expository discourses (see also Joffe, this volume). Strategies to engage listeners increase in efficiency, for example through humour, drama, and elaborate stories (e.g., with more episodes, more detail, embedded events, and explicit emotional states). Adolescents are increasingly able to collaborate with peers to produce joint narratives.

- Reading and writing: Proficiency in critically analyzing meaning increases – including understanding authors' conflicting opinions, identifying fact from opinion, understanding technical material and reflecting on themes and implied meaning. Writing becomes longer and contains more complex ideas. Persuasive writing develops, as does expository writing. Proficiency in using literate vocabulary in formal speaking and writing increases.

There are also significant interactions between linguistic areas. For example, lexical and syntactic components of language develop in association with one another, a phenomenon referred to as the 'lexicon-syntax interface' (Nippold et al., 2017b). Adult-like competence regarding figurative language is based on metalinguistic and metasemantic awareness, closely linked to the ability to reflect on language as a complex cognitive and interpersonal phenomenon (Levorato & Cacciari, 2002). Morphological analysis relies on an extensive vocabulary to draw from, the ability to draw from syntactic cues about a word's meaning, alongside integrated knowledge of the interrelations between lexical convention, semantic content, and formal structure (Larsen & Nippold, 2007).

The processes driving language change during adolescence (Nippold, 2016). For example, they are more individualistic, driven by teenagers' academic choices and specialisms, as well as personal interests and in-depth engagement in literacies. Language relies on metalinguistic competence, and the ability to reflect on new meanings, to scrutinize linguistic contexts, and to update interpretations and understandings. Abstract thought is important, as teenagers access concepts with less concrete meanings (e.g., resilience, relevance, stimulating, pedagogy). Social perspective-taking also develops in this age group, with implications for language development, particularly in relation to pragmatic skills and the ability to adapt their communication to others' thoughts, feelings and views (Nippold, 2016).

Given the range and complexity of the changes summarized above, it is essential that people working with adolescents with language disorders understand typical language development in this population to ensure that assessment and interventions are adequately designed to target the linguistic skills that adolescents need. Language deficits may not be obvious during casual conversation, but language skills may nevertheless be impaired during explanations or other challenging speaking and writing tasks (Nippold et al., 2008). Detailed knowledge of adolescent language development is the foundation for analyzing language samples as part of assessment and target setting (Nippold, 2014; Nippold et al., 2017).

Language and identity – insights from sociolinguistics

Sociolinguistic research has looked at how adolescent language is used to form and express aspects of identity that are related to social groups and networks (for detailed accounts of adolescence and sociolinguistic research, see Kirkham & Moore, 2013; Tagliamonte, 2016). Language plays a key role in creating and maintaining adolescent peer groups, and is used to accomplish status, cohesion, trust, and entitlement to knowledge (Bucholtz, 1999; Eckert, 2003). Adolescents jointly create distinctiveness, via the comparison of distinct social groups within the same 'social landscape'. Groups differentiate themselves from each other, as well as in opposition to adults and children (Kirkham & Moore, 2013). Vernacular language features tend to be associated with an anti-institutional stance, local orientation, and local innovation in contrast to the educational and institutional affiliation of Standard English, which tends to be conservative. However, the choice between vernacular and Standard English is not a binary one: they are not two alternatives but are resources for the construction of more complex styles, rich in social meaning (Eckert, 2003). Such styles draw from voice quality, prosody, phonology, morphology, syntax, discourse, lexicon, and speech acts. Within groups, individual identities are nested and complemented with an inner hierarchy, often signalled linguistically (Eckert, 2003).

Emma Moore's work is considered here in detail to examine how adolescents use language to signal social meaning (Moore, 2004, 2010, 2012). Moore's ethnography examined use of non-standard 'were' ('I were so drunk'), tag questions ('it was mainly Natalie, wasn't it?'), right dislocation ('it was new, that skirt') and negative concord ('I didn't say nothing') in a longitudinal study of girls aged 13 and 14 years at the start of the study (school year 9), and 14 and 15 years at the end of the study (year 10). The study identified four communities of practice: 'Populars', 'Geeks', 'Eden Village' and 'Townies'. A community of practice can be briefly defined as a people who are grouped according to their joint engagement in social practice rather than to their membership of decontextualized social structures (such as social class or ethnic group) (Moore, 2004: 381). Townies were characterized by attending local parks and streets to socialize, wearing certain branded clothing, and by risk behaviours such as engaging in sexual activity and heavy alcohol and illegal drug consumption, while Populars socialized in cinemas and shopping centres, drank less alcohol and avoided illegal drugs, had more engagement with school, and were less committed to wearing certain brands of clothing. Eden Village girls were named after the exclusive area where they lived, and they were more engaged with school, socializing by shopping and having sleepovers. The Geek girls engaged in extra-curricular activities such as orchestra and sport and were most conformist to school values.

Whilst both Popular and Townie girls used non-standard linguistic forms, results indicate that the Townie girls used more non-standard forms, in line with their more extreme social behaviours and their orientation to the local community. Nonetheless, both groups used the same linguistic resources in subtly different ways, making it simplistic to talk of Popular versus Townie variants. Moore's analysis demonstrates how these two distinct social groups both manipulate linguistic features to create separate styles. For example, Popular girls used non-standard 'were' in tag questions ('it were that new t-shirt, weren't it?') far less than Townie girls year 9. However, by year 10, the Popular girls had dramatically increased their use of tag questions and, specifically, their use of 'were' tag questions. In contrast, the Townie girls had dramatically decreased their use of 'were' tag questions. This demonstrates reciprocal negotiation between social groups: as Populars "encroach on what might have been described as Townie linguistic territory…the Townies respond to this by retreating from non-standard 'were' in this context" (Moore, 2004: 392). Moore attributes the Populars' increased stylization of tag questions to the fact that they are not stigmatized in institutional discourse, unlike the more visible morphosyntactic features such as negative concord.

Further analysis of the discourse structure, grammatical form and topic of tag questions across all of the social groups studied showed that, although different social groups all used tag questions, stylistic composition varied along with the frequency of use (Moore & Podesva, 2009). The Eden Village girls used grammatically standard tag questions, with agreement from the interlocutor often overlapping with the tag question itself (e.g., 'I know you've spoken to Danny, haven't you?'). This hyper-collaborative style could be interpreted as 'female' in line with the 'girly girl' identity of the group. The Popular girls – who employed far more tag questions than the other groups – used non-standard tag questions to talk about people outside their own social group. The tag questions allowed the Populars to evaluate others and be critical (e.g., 'they changed for the worse, some of them, didn't they?'). The Townies mostly used tag questions when talking about their own group members, often in relation to boys and 'rebellious' behaviours such as flirting online. The questions were used to invite others to take part in the story (e.g., 'cos you left me, didn't you?'). They included vernacular features such as nonstandard 'were', deleted word final /t/ and dropping word initial /h/. Moore's study presents evidence of how adolescents manipulate linguistic variants in relation to local context in order to create unique social meanings. These meanings can be in relation to stance (e.g., the cool critical stances of the Populars), persona (e.g., rebel, geek), and social type (e.g., experienced, polite) negotiated in relation to socially meaningful units like styles and social categories (females, social class groups).

Adolescent language is central to the emergence of social distinctions within peer groups. Nonetheless, as yet, very little – if any – research has studied how adolescents with speech and language disorders participate in such dynamic use of linguistic variation to index different levels of social meaning. Research into how adolescents without language disorders use linguistic features to signal social meaning has implications for supporting those adolescents with disorders: most obviously, non-standard features of language must be viewed within a local social context. Standard English forms (e.g., in terms of phonology or syntax) will not always be appropriate targets for intervention. Furthermore, sociolinguistic research into adolescence provides an important reminder that adolescents with language disorders need to apply their linguistic skills to do complex identity work in every interaction.

Conclusion

This chapter has offered brief insights into adolescence through a multidisciplinary lens. It is important that adults working with adolescents understand that this is a time of rapid development across all aspects of life

(WHO, 2015). Although this chapter has presented biological, psychological and social developments separately, the advancements of adolescents blur these distinctions: age differences in behaviours that have strong roots in biology are ultimately shaped by the contexts in which young people grow up (Duell et al., 2017: 18).

Adolescence is a time of contradiction. It is a time of both new-found freedom and constraint. Typically, good health and fitness is experienced alongside increased risk of the onset of mental illness, injury and substance use disorders. It is characterized as a period of rebellion, innovation, and hedonism, but it also often includes preparation for high-stakes examinations and goal-planning for the future. Of course, not all adolescents fit the above descriptions: like any other social grouping, adolescence "is a simplification, which erases diversity of experience" (Kirkham & Moore, 2013: 286). However, this simplification is useful for understanding changes in how adolescents think and act in order to mediate the relative vulnerability that adolescence can bring.

There is a chronic lack of services for many adolescents with language disorders (Joffe & Nippold, 2012; Nippold et al 2017; Paul & Norbury, 2012). Yet the unique nature and importance of adolescence demands systematic, specific, intensive interventions and support. Oral language is a central part of the navigation through adolescence. Talk is the primary means of learning in classrooms (Silver & Lwin, 2013); is used to initiate and maintain friendships (Marton, Abramoff, & Rosenzweig, 2005); is a means of negotiation when dealing with new roles, responsibilities, and boundaries within families; and, finally, talk is used to create linguistic identities within groups, form alliances and establish distance, and negotiate stance (Eckert, 2003). It is therefore essential that adolescents with language disorders have access to adequate and sensitive support and intervention during this important life stage. The dynamic nature of adolescence and the potential for rapid and extensive development – cognitively, linguistically, socially – form an important rationale for providing effective language interventions for this age group.

Reflective questions

1. Adolescents need to understand the processes taking place during this life stage. How would you explain them to an adolescent with a language disorder?

2. By what mechanisms does adolescent development impact on adolescent health and wellbeing?

3. Reflect on the following case study of Joe and apply your reading by considering the following questions.

Joe

Joe is 20 years old and he attends a specialist college for young adults with complex needs where he has been enrolled for two years. Joe has diagnoses related to learning difficulties and mental illness. He had a difficult time in his mainstream secondary school but has been very happy in college. He attends college some 90 miles away from his home town and lives with a host family during the week. His funding to attend college is being cut and he has one more term left before he will stop attending and return to live full time at his family home. Joe is very distressed about leaving behind the good friends he has made at college. Staff at college are prioritizing work on skills related to independent living, including accessing public transport and household budgeting. Joe is unsure about what he wants to do next, or what his options are in terms of employment or further education.

- Joe is not a teenager. What are the factors which lead to his current life stage still being considered 'adolescent'?

- This is an important time of transition for Joe. What challenges does he face?

- Joe's tutor at college is working with him to plan his immediate future and to put some positive steps in place. How can research on identity formation be applied in this situation?

References

Arnett, J.J. (2011). Bridging cultural and developmental psychology: New syntheses in theory, research, and policy. In L.A. Jensen (Ed.), *Emerging Adulthood(s): The Cultural Psychology of a New Life Stage* (pp.255–275). New York: Oxford University Press.

Arnett, J. J. (2014). *Adolescence and Emerging Adulthood*. Boston, MA: Pearson.

Blakemore, S.J. & Choudhury, S. (2006). Development of the adolescent brain: Implications for executive function and social cognition. *Journal of Child Psychology and Psychiatry*, *47*(3-4), 296-312.

Blankenstein, N.E., Schreuders, E., Peper, J.S., Crone, E.A., & van Duijvenvoorde, A.C.K. (2018). Individual differences in risk-taking tendencies modulate the neural processing of risky and ambiguous decision-making in adolescence. *NeuroImage*, *172*, 663-673.

Brechwald, W.A. & Prinstein, M.J. (2011). Beyond homophily: A decade of advances in understanding peer influence processes. *Journal of Research on Adolescence*, *21*(1), 166-179.

Bronfenbrenner, U. & Morris, P.A. (2006). The bioecological model of human development. In R.M. Lerner (Ed.), *Handbook of Child Psychology, 6th edition – Volume 1: Theoretical Models of Human Fevelopment* (pp.793-828). Hoboken, NJ: John Wiley & Sons.

Bucholtz, M. (1999). "Why be normal?": Language and identity practices in a community of nerd girls. *Language in Society*, *28*(2), 203-223.

Chen, P. & Vazsonyi, A.T. (2013). Future orientation, school contexts, and problem behaviors: A multilevel study. *Journal of Youth and Adolescence*, *42*(1), 67-81.

Conti-Ramsden, G., Durkin, K., Toseeb, U., Botting, N., & Pickles, A. (2017). Education and employment outcomes of young adults with a history of developmental language disorder. *International Journal of Language & Communication Disorders* (in press).

Dodge, K.A. & Pettit, G S. (2003). A biopsychosocial model of the development of chronic conduct problems in adolescence. *Developmental Psychology*, *39*(2), 349.

Duell, N., Steinberg, L., Icenogle, G., Chein, J., Chaudhary, N., … Chang, L. (2017). Age patterns in risk taking across the world. *Journal of Youth and Adolescence*, 1-21. Accessed online at: https://link-springer-com.sheffield.idm.oclc.org/article/10.1007/s10964-017-0752-y

Dumontheil, I., Apperly, I.A., & Blakemore, S.J. (2010). Online usage of theory of mind continues to develop in late adolescence. *Developmental Science*, *13*(2), 331-338.

Eckert, P. (2000). *Language Variation as Social Practice: The Linguistic Construction of Identity in Belten High*. London: Wiley-Blackwell.

Eckert, P. (2003). Language and adolescent peer groups. *Journal of Language and Social Psychology*, *22*(1), 112-118.

Fuhrmann, D., Knoll, L.J., & Blakemore, S.-J. (2015). Adolescence as a sensitive period of brain development. *Trends in Cognitive Sciences*, *10*, 558–566.

Harden, K.P., Kretsch, N., Mann, F.D., Herzhoff, K., Tackett, J.L., Steinberg, L., & Tucker-Drob, E.M. (2017). Beyond dual systems: A genetically-informed, latent factor model of behavioral and self-report measures related to adolescent risk-taking. *Developmental Cognitive Neuroscience*, *25*, 221-234.

Haynes, R.B., Devereaux, P.J., & Guyatt, G.H. (2002). Physicians' and patients' choices in evidence based practice: Evidence does not make decisions, people do. *BMJ: British Medical Journal, 324*(7350), 1350.

Hoorn, J., Crone, E.A., & Leijenhorst, L. (2017). Hanging out with the right crowd: Peer influence on risk-taking behavior in adolescence. *Journal of Research on Adolescence, 27*(1), 189-200.

Joffe, V.L. & Nippold, M.A. (2012). Progress in understanding adolescent language disorders. *Language, Speech, and Hearing Services in Schools, 43*(4), 438-444.

Keating, D.P., Lerner, R.M., & Steinberg, L. (2004). Cognitive and brain development. *Handbook of Adolescent Psychology, 2*, 45-84.

Kilford, E.J., Garrett, E., & Blakemore, S.J. (2016). The development of social cognition in adolescence: An integrated perspective. *Neuroscience & Biobehavioral Reviews, 70*, 106-120.

Kirkham, Sam & Moore, Emma (2013). Adolescence. In J.K. Chambers & N. Schilling-Estes (Eds), *The Handbook of Language Variation and Change, 2nd ed.* (pp.277-296). Malden, MA: Wiley-Blackwell.

Klimstra, T.A. & van Doeselaar, L. (2017). Identity formation in adolescence and young adulthood. In J. Specht (Ed.), *Personality Development Across the Lifespan* (pp.293-308) London: Academic Press.

Larsen, J.A. & Nippold, M.A. (2007). Morphological analysis in school-age children: Dynamic assessment of a word learning strategy. *Language, Speech, and Hearing Services in Schools, 38*(3), 201-212.

Levorato, M.C. & Cacciari, C. (2002). The creation of new figurative expressions: Psycholinguistic evidence in Italian children, adolescents and adults. *Journal of Child Language, 29*(1), 127-150.

Løhaugen, G.C., Antonsen, I., Håberg, A., Gramstad, A., Vik, T., Brubakk, A.M., & Skranes, J. (2011). Computerized working memory training improves function in adolescents born at extremely low birth weight. *The Journal of Pediatrics, 158*(4), 555-561.

Luyckx, K., Goossens, L., Soenens, B., & Beyers, W. (2006). Unpacking commitment and exploration: Preliminary validation of an integrative model of late adolescent identity formation. *Journal of Adolescence, 29*, 361-378.

Luyckx, K., Schwartz, S.J., Goossens, L., Beyers, W., & Missotten, L. (2011). Processes of personal identity formation and evaluation. In S.J. Schwartz, K. Luyckx, & V.L. Vignoes (Eds), *Handbook of Identity Theory and Research* (pp.77-98). New York, NY: Springer.

Marcia, J.E. (1966). Development and validation of ego-identity status. *Journal of Personality and Social Psychology, 3*(5), 551.

Marton, K., Abramoff, B., & Rosenzweig, S. (2005). Social cognition and language in children with specific language impairment (SLI). *Journal of Communication Disorders, 38*(2), 143-162.

McAdams, D.P. & McLean, K.C. (2013). Narrative identity. *Current Directions in Psychological Science, 22*(3), 233-238.

Moore, E. (2004). Sociolinguistic style: A multidimensional resource for shared identity creation. *Canadian Journal of Linguistics/Revue canadienne de linguistique, 49*(3-4), 375-396.

Moore, E. (2010). The interaction between social category and social practice: Explaining *was/were* variation. *Language Variation and Change, 22*, 347-371.

Moore, E. (2012). The social life of style. *Language and Literature, 21*(1), 66-83.

Moore, E. & Podesva, R. (2009). Style, indexicality, and the social meaning of tag questions. *Language in Society, 38*(4), 447-485.

Nippold, M.A. (2014a). *Language Sampling with Adolescents: Implications for Intervention, 2nd ed.* San Diego, CA: Plural.

Nippold, M.A. (2014b). Language intervention at the middle school: Complex talk reflects complex thought. *Language, Speech, and Hearing Services in Schools, 45*(2) 153-156.

Nippold, M.A. (2016). *Later Language Development: School-age Children, Adolescents, and Young Adults, 4th ed.* Austin, TX: Pro-Ed.

Nippold, M.A. & Berman, R.A. (2004). Research on later language development: International perspectives. *Language Development Across Childhood and Adolescence, 3*, 1-8.

Nippold, M.A. & Scott, C.M. (Eds) (2010). *Expository Discourse in Children, Adolescents, and Adults: Development and Disorders.* New York, NY: Psychology Press/Taylor & Francis.

Nippold, M.A., Frantz-Kaspar, M.W., & Vigeland, L.M. (2017). Spoken language production in young adults: Examining syntactic complexity. *Journal of Speech, Language, and Hearing Research, 60*(5), 1339-1347.

Nippold, M.A., Frantz-Kaspar, M.W., Cramond, P.M., Kirk, C., Hayward-Mayhew, C., & MacKinnon, M. (2015). Critical thinking about fables: Examining language production and comprehension in adolescents. *Journal of Speech, Language, and Hearing Research, 58*(2), 325-335.

Nippold, M.A., Mansfield, T.C., Billow, J.L., & Tomblin, J.B. (2008). Expository discourse in adolescents with language impairments: Examining syntactic development. *American Journal of Speech-Language Pathology, 17*, 356-366.

Nippold, M.A., Vigeland, L.M., & Frantz-Kaspar, M.W. (2017a). Metacognitive verb production in adolescents: The link to complex syntax. *Clinical Linguistics & Phonetics, 10*, 761-776.

Nippold, M.A., Vigeland, L.M., Frantz-Kaspar, M.W., & Ward-Lonergan, J.M. (2017b). Language sampling with adolescents: Building a normative database with fables. *American Journal of Speech-Language Pathology, 26*(3), 908-920.

Parker, J., Mitchell, A., Kalpakidou, A., Walshe, M., Jung, H.Y., … Allin, M. (2008). Cerebellar growth and behavioural and neuropsychological outcome in preterm adolescents. *Brain, 131*(5), 1344-1351.

Piaget, J. (1977). *Epistemology and Psychology of Functions* (Vol. 23). Springer Science & Business Media.

Pringle, J., Mills, K., McAteer, J., Jepson, R., Hogg, E., Anand, N., & Blakemore, S.J. (2016). A systematic review of adolescent physiological development and its relationship with health-related behaviour: A protocol. *Systematic Reviews, 5*(1), 3.

Pringle, J., Mills, K.L., McAteer, J., Jepson, R., Hogg, E., Anand, N., & Blakemore, S.J. (2017). The physiology of adolescent sexual behaviour: A systematic review. *Cogent Social Sciences, 3*(1), 1368858.

Reyna, V.F. & Farley, F. (2006). Risk and rationality in adolescent decision making: Implications for theory, practice, and public policy. *Psychological Science in the Public Interest, 7*(1), 1-44.

Sawyer, S.M., Afifi, R.A., Bearinger, L.H., Blakemore, S.J., Dick, B., Ezeh, A.C., & Patton, G.C. (2012). Adolescence: A foundation for future health. *The Lancet, 379*(9826), 1630-1640.

Sawyer, S.M., Azzopardi, P.S., Wickremarathne, D., & Patton, G.C. (2018). The age of adolescence. *The Lancet: Child and Adolescent Health.* Early view accessed online at: http://www.thelancet.com/pdfs/journals/lanchi/PIIS2352-4642(18)30022-1.pdf

Silver, R.E. & Lwin, S.M. (2013). *Language in Education: Social Implications.* London: Bloomsbury.

Singer, J.A. (2004). Narrative identity and meaning making across the adult lifespan: An introduction. *Journal of Personality, 72*(3), 437-460.

Snowling, M.J., Adams, J.W., Bishop, D.V.M., & S.E. Stothard (2001). Educational attainments of school leavers with a preschool history of speech-language impairments. *International Journal of Language & Communication Disorders, 36*(2), 173-183.

Sowell, E.R., Thompson, P.M., Holmes, C.J., Batth, R., Jernigan, T.L., & Toga, A.W. (1999a). Localizing age-related changes in brain structure between childhood and adolescence using statistical parametric mapping. *Neuroimage, 9*(6), 587-597.

Sowell, E.R., Thompson, P.M., Holmes, C.J., Jernigan, T.L., & Toga, A.W. (1999b). In vivo evidence for post-adolescent brain maturation in frontal and striatal regions. *Nature Neuroscience, 2*(10), 859.

Squeglia, L.M., Jacobus, J., & Tapert, S.F. (2009a). The influence of substance use on adolescent brain development. *Clinical EEG and Neuroscience, 40*(1), 31-38.

Squeglia, L.M., Spadoni, A.D., Infante, M.A., Myers, M.G., & Tapert, S.F. (2009b). Initiating moderate to heavy alcohol use predicts changes in neuropsychological functioning for adolescent girls and boys. *Psychology of Addictive Behaviors, 23*(4), 715.

Squeglia, L.M., Jacobus, J., Sorg, S.F., Jernigan, T.L., & Tapert, S.F. (2013). Early adolescent cortical thinning is related to better neuropsychological performance. *Journal of the International Neuropsychological Society, 19*(9), 962-970.

Steinberg, L. (2010). *Adolescence, 9th ed.* New York, NY: McGraw-Hill Higher Education.

Steinberg, L. (2004). Risk taking in adolescence: what changes, and why? *Annals of the New York Academy of Sciences, 1021*(1), 51-58.

Tagliamonte, S.A. (2016). *Teen Talk: The Language of Adolescents.* Cambridge: Cambridge University Press.

Tamnes, C.K., Østby, Y., Fjell, A.M., Westlye, L.T., Due-Tønnessen, P., & Walhovd, K.B. (2010). Brain maturation in adolescence and young adulthood: Regional age-related changes in cortical thickness and white matter volume and microstructure. *Cerebral Cortex, 20*(3), 534-548.

Tiemeier, H., Lenroot, R.K., Greenstein, D.K., Tran, L., Pierson, R., & Giedd, J.N. (2010). Cerebellum development during childhood and adolescence: A longitudinal morphometric MRI study. *Neuroimage, 49*(1), 63-70.

Trommsdorff, G. (2012). Cultural perspectives on values and religion in adolescent development: A conceptual overview and synthesis. In G. Trommsdorff (Ed.), *Values, Religion and Culture in Adolescent Development* (pp.3-45). New York: Cambridge University Press.

van Doeselaar, L., Meeus, W., Koot, H.M., & Branje, S. (2016). The role of best friends in educational identity formation in adolescence. *Journal of Adolescence, 47*, 28-37.

Walther, A. (2006). Regimes of youth transitions: Choice, flexibility and security in young people's experiences across different European contexts. *Young, 14*(2), 119-139.

Weimer, A.A., Dowds, S.J.P., Fabricius, W.V., Schwanenflugel, P.J., & Suh, G.W. (2017). Development of constructivist theory of mind from middle childhood to early adulthood and its relation to social cognition and behavior. *Journal of Experimental Child Psychology, 154*, 28-45.

WHO (2012). Expanding access to contraceptive services for adolescents. Geneva: WHO. Accessed online at: http://apps.who.int/iris/bitstream/10665/75160/1/WHO_RHR_HRP_12.21_eng.pdf?ua=1

WHO (2014). Adolescents' health-related behaviors. Accessed online (03.03.2018): http://apps.who.int/adolescent/second-decade/section4

WHO (2015). Adolescent development. Geneva: WHO. Accessed online at: http://www.who.int/maternal_child_adolescent/topics/adolescence/development/en/

3 Young people's own perspectives and experiences of living with a language disorder

Sarah Spencer and Judy Clegg

Learning outcomes

At the end of this chapter, readers will be able to:

- Summarize the importance of listening to young people about their experiences of living with a language disorder

- Describe practical techniques and strategies for researching young people's perspectives

- Discuss insights gained from previous research which has listened to adolescents with language disorders.

Introduction

It is important to listen to young people with language disorders in order to understand the impact of their abilities and difficulties, and to gain insight into their daily lived experiences. However, we need to go *beyond listening*, to embed young people's perspectives within person-centred target setting and in service planning, delivery and evaluation. The chapter reviews research that has previously sought the perspectives of young people with language disorders. Challenges to accessing the voices of young people with language disorders are considered and addressed, with an outline of practical strategies and methods for inclusive listening and facilitating active participation in research, educational provision and clinical intervention.

Reference to children and young people's views and perspectives increasingly feature in research, policy, service evaluation, and legislation. The 1989 United Nations Convention of the Rights of the Child (UNICEF, 1989) was an important turning point for listening seriously to children and young people. The Article 12 document sets out children's right to be listened to, the right to form his or her own views, and to express these views freely in all matters affecting their lives (p.4). The Convention has increased efforts to incorporate children's rights and empowerment in communication and advocacy activities within both academia and services for children (Porter, Townsend, & Hampshire, 2012).

The drive to ensure children and young people are heard and fully involved in decision making in matters affecting their lives has also been driven by re-conceptualizations of childhood (Christensen & James, 2008). Four ways of seeing children and childhood are put forward: child as object, child as subject, child as social agent, and child as participant and co-researchers (Christensen & Prout, 2002). Traditionally, research has presented children in a passive role within predictable trajectories of biological or psychological development. Childhood was studied from an adult perspective. Within the discipline of childhood studies, there has been increasing recognition that children are social agents who have important and unique insights into their own lived and daily experiences (Christensen & James, 2008):

Children are seen to act, take part in, change and become changed by the social and cultural world they live in (Christensen & Prout, 2002: 481). Research has thus moved from being *about* children to being designed *with* children as active participants (Wickenden, 2011), with some studies going further to facilitate research *by* children (Alderson, 2000). The move towards listening to children and young people fits well with a social constructivist view of childhood. This puts the emphasis on children as being active participants in their own knowledge and having an active role in constructing their own understanding and in the meaning-making process (James & James, 2004).

This dual shift in both legislation and childhood research has resulted in an increase in listening to children and young people in order to both respect their rights and to benefit from their experiences to drive policy and practice change. Listening to the views, experiences and perspectives of adolescents with language disorders is important in order to: (a) develop theoretical understandings and insights into childhood and disability in relation to language disorders; (b) design appropriate and person-centred clinical and educational interventions; and (c) influence service planning, delivery, and evaluation.

Insights into young people's experiences of living with language disorders

It is important to understand how young people experience daily life with language disorders, because the prevalence is so high (McLeod, 2011). Within the context of mainstream research and policy-making claims to be listening to the views of children and young people, it would be unfair to exclude the large proportion of children and young people with some form of language disorder. Merrick (2011) argues that there is an ethical imperative not to exclude children with language disorders from research due to the perceived levels of competence required for participation. In addition, a further driver is that we know that the impact of language disorders is pervasive, with effects on relationships, education, mental health and wellbeing (Clegg et al., 2005). Increasing our understanding of young people's lived experiences of language disorders is essential in order to provide social, clinical, and educational responses that reduce negative impacts and promote social justice (McLeod, 2011).

A growing body of research has examined the experiences of children with a range of speech, language and communication needs (see Roulstone & McLeod, 2011 for an overview). For example, Owen, Hayett and Roulstone (2004) interviewed 12 children aged between 6 and 11 years about their speech and language therapy sessions in school. The children reported concerns about the impact of their speech difficulties on friendships, interactions, and educational outcomes. Children as young as 2 years, who have communication disabilities, have been supported to reflect on their experiences of early intervention (Carroll & Sixsmith, 2016).

Very little research has specifically investigated the experiences and perspectives of adolescents with language disorders. Some research has investigated the perspectives of adolescents who use alternative and augmentative communication systems by using an ethnographic approach, with detailed observation and narrative conversations using visual techniques such as photography (Wickenden, 2011). This research looked at issues of the young people's identities, with young people reporting that they were ordinary teenagers first and foremost but that people typically focused on their disabled identities. They did not see their disabled status as the most important part of them. Their selfhood was viewed in relation to gender, family, and teenage interests such as supporting Chelsea or 'being a laugh'. People close to them viewed them in relation to qualities such as being fun, feisty, beautiful... or lazy, stubborn or cheeky. In contrast, the 'personhood' – how they were viewed by others who were not close to them – emphasized not who they are but what they could or *could not* do. The research highlighted the young people's priorities: their 'normal' adolescence, unsupervised friendships with people their own age, and identities beyond their disability (see also Smith, this volume).

We also have some insight into the views of adolescents with language disorders around the time of transition into post-16 education, training and work from school. A study interviewed 54 adolescents with a diagnosis of specific language impairment about their abilities and educational provision, within a broader longitudinal project (Palikara, Lindsay, & Dockrell, 2008). The study aimed to access the views of young people with language disorders as they entered. A structured interview with standard prompts was used to access views, with some semi-structured elements to allow young people to explore issues that were most relevant to them. Results indicated that the children were able to describe their special educational needs and their feelings towards their difficulties. While some participants were accepting of their skills (e.g., "I tried not to focus so much on my special needs but to do my best in order to overcome these difficulties", p.62), around a quarter reported negative feelings such as shame, worry or frustration. Most young people (46/54) were positive about their educational experiences and the support that they received, though the need for consistent and high-quality support was emphasized and critiqued by some participants. The support of family and friends and social networks was emphasized in overcoming the challenges faced by the young people, in relation to both school and post-16 options.

Listening to adolescents to understand lived experiences: Graham

Graham is 17 years old and has diagnosed speech, language and communication needs. He currently attends a specialist college, having previously been included within a mainstream school. In the interview extracts below, Graham describes how he has experienced bullying in school, how he had limited friendships until late in his teens, and how this impacted on his wellbeing.

Bullying

First school, erm what it is, is cos it was a mainstream school, and obviously I've got Aspergers syndrome, I didn't fit in, I wasn't accepted in the same way as other students were and erm I were just, the word, bullied.

Everyday coming to school I know that I've got it in the front of my head that something's gonna happen to me today, am I gonna get hit, and I gonna get verbally abused, it's gonna be either or and erm, it were just hell, in one word, hell. And erm, then I moved to [another school] which was the equivalent of heaven at the time.

Social confidence

Err things for me that I find difficult, err, probably well at first, probably going out socially, you know, being in public. That's the word, public. Before I was my old school – house – school – house that's it. But I used to find going out really hard, you know if we were in a public place I used to be conscious watching people left-right, left - right.

Friendships

At [my old] school I had no friends, hand on heart I can say that, no friends at all.

And since I've come here [specialist college] I've got more friends now. I can't even count how many I've got er,so I mean the friends have been probably one of the biggest confidence boosters, besides the staff, erm just knowing that you've got people there for you that can back you up if you've got any problems or anything, you know.

It's just brilliant but it's probably my first experiences of true friendship.

For more information about Graham, see Teen Talk (Clegg & Spencer, 2017). Teen Talk is a free online learning resource for professionals working with teenagers and young adults with language disorders.

Placing young people's views at the centre of intervention

It is important that young people with language disorders can influence the interventions and educational support that they receive. Their perspectives, views and priorities should be central to specialist services at each stage: assessment, identifying targets and goals, joint decision making, taking action, completing interventions and evaluating progress and next steps. A handful of studies have listened to the views of children and their families about goals for speech and language therapy interventions (Hambly, Coad, Lindsay, & Roulstone, 2011; Lyons, O'Malley, O'Connor, & Monaghan, 2010; Pratt, Botting, & Conti-Ramsden, 2006; Roulstone et al., 2012b). However, very little empirical research has investigated how we can incorporate the views of children and their families into the implementation of speech and language therapy interventions.

The need to involve young people and their families in decisions is now a feature of educational policy. For example, consulting young people and their families is a key part of the Special Educational Needs reforms that came into place in 2014 in England, as a result of the Children and Families Act of March 2014. The guidelines for SEN provision emphasize the importance of children's views regarding the assessment of their education, health and care plans: "The assessment includes talking to you and your child and finding out from you what support you think your child needs, and what aspirations you and your child have for his or her future" (Department for Education, 2014: 23). The SEN guidelines also outline the need to listen to the perspectives of children and young people in service delivery and decisions about provision:

When making decisions about SEN or disabilities, your local authority must:

- Have regard to the views, wishes and feelings of children, their parents and young people

- Make sure that children, their parents and young people participate as fully as possible in decisions that affect them

- Provide support to children, their parents and young people so that children and young people do well educationally and can prepare properly for adulthood.

Parents should have a real say in decisions that affect their children, should have access to impartial information, advice and support and know how to challenge decisions they disagree with. Local authorities must also involve children, their parents and young people in developing local provision and services for children with special educational needs and disabilities. (Department for Education, 2014: 11).

Person-centred planning is one approach to putting the needs of young people at the centre of planning targets for intervention and support. The National Autistic Society (www.autism.org.uk) detail the following five features of person-centred planning:

1. The person is at the centre of the planning process.

2. Family and friends are partners in planning.

3. The plan shows what is important to a person now and for the future, and what support they need.

4. The plan helps the person to be part of a community of their choosing and helps the community to welcome them.

5. The plan puts into action what a person wants for their life and keeps on listening: the plan remains 'live'.

A person-centred approach is designed to be specific to each individual. It takes into account individual circumstances, perspectives and aims, and allows for meaningful and relevant targets to be created; importantly, it also allows for these targets to be developed with time, in order to ensure continued progress and relevance. Listening to the views and perspectives of young people with language disorders (and their families) will be central to person-centred approaches.

Listening to adolescents as part of a language assessment process

Any intervention with adolescents needs to take into account adolescents' own views of their language skills and their own ideas about goals and targets. Adolescents' own views can be used as part of the assessment process to gain unique insights into perceived impairments, barriers to participation, and priorities for intervention and support. Spencer, Clegg and Stackhouse (2010) use two case studies to give a worked example of how interviews with adolescents can be used to identify and discuss levels of communicative competence in different contexts. An interview schedule is provided, asking young people to reflect on their own talking, their own understanding, the words that they know and use, and how their talking is understood by others. Paul and Norbury (2012) also report that a student-centred approach to assessment with adolescents is essential in order to:

- Establish a cooperative partnership between the adult and the adolescent that they are working with

- Gain additional insight into the adolescents' abilities

- Plan intervention in a team, with shared responsibilities and accountability

- Increase motivation for both assessment and intervention

- Gain insight into the adolescents' perceptions of their difficulties in context.

A self-assessment is recommended as part of the goal-setting process and an example is provided (Paul & Norbury, 2012: 541). The young person is asked to rate their abilities on a five-point scale (from 'I'm Good' to 'Argh! Help! Help!') in relation to 22 learning skills related to both oral and written language. Examples of learning skills include: 'finding main ideas in textbooks', 'asking questions when I don't understand', and 'vocabulary'. The textbook also recommends that adolescents be asked about the writing demands of their curriculum (Paul & Norbury, 2012: 564) so that language disorders can be assessed in relation to adolescents' own views about the functional skills that they require in the classroom.

Listening to adolescents to inform clinical practice: Lucy

Lucy is a 15-year-old girl who attends mainstream school. She does not have any access to speech and language therapy or specialist educational support in school. Language assessment scores show that she has significant speech, language and communication needs. In her interview, Lucy reflects on areas of difficulties and talks about the strategies that she uses to cope in class (see Spencer, Clegg, & Stackhouse, 2010: 154).

Sarah: So when you are listening to people can you understand what people are saying?

Lucy: Yeah but sometimes if it comes through a teacher, I'll always ask them to repeat it. Or if I don't get it, I'll ask them to come and ask tell me on my own – tell me what to do, say if it's work I'll ask them to show me, instead of listening to them.

Sarah: What makes [teachers] hard to understand?

Lucy: Because they're grown-ups. They blabber on and on and on just to think that we're gonna learn all these words when we don't know what they mean… (Sarah: what kind of words then?) Like persistent – [a teacher] said that before and I don't even know what it means.

….

[I don't understand] when teacher shout at you. They're like 'it's not appropriate, you do understand that what you're doing is blah de blah de blah'. Carry on, it's going in one ear and back out. I don't get a word they're saying. They just get it over with and then whatever you're doing, just do it.

This sort of consultation could be used to plan how to best facilitate inclusion within school. The extract reveals information about the strategies that Lucy currently uses to support her own understanding (asking teachers to repeat information and come and explain individually) that could be acknowledged and built upon. It could be used to identify targets for intervention (perhaps vocabulary work starting with 'persistent'!) and to inform collaborations with teachers so that they are aware of Lucy's needs and how to best support her. It could be used (with Lucy's permission) as a starting point for discussions with teachers about using accessible language to engage Lucy in learning.

For more information about Lucy, see Spencer, Clegg and Stackhouse, 2010.

Service planning, delivery, and evaluation

Research has suggested that children with speech, language and communication needs are able to reflect upon intervention sessions and that insights gained from consulting children could be used to improve approaches to intervention (Owen, Haylett, & Roulstone, 2004; McCormick et al., 2010; Simkin et al., 2009). There are multiple practical benefits of listening to adolescents with language disorders in relation to service-level provision, including:

- The ability to gain valuable insights into service provision (Clegg, Ansorge, Stackhouse, & Donlan, 2012; Palikara et al., 2008)

- Enhancing accountability in order to identify areas for improvement and ensure resources are allocated effectively (Hartas & Lindsay, 2011)

- The potential to improve the quality of service provision and school life for other students (Tangen, 2009)

- Increasing a sense of ownership with a school or provision by involving young people in decision making (Hartas & Lindsay, 2011)

- Facilitating cooperative ventures between adults and young people. In a school context, this may lead to higher enjoyment of school via more consistent and better teacher–student relationships and more equitable respect (Gorard & See, 2011).

One of the Better Communication Research Programme's key recommendations is that services and schools should systematically collect evidence of children's and young people's outcomes that include the perspectives of children, young people and their parents (Roulstone & Lindsay, 2012).

Interestingly, studies within youth justice systems have advocated the use of interviews in understanding and profiling adolescents' language skills and difficulties as part of an assessment and for service delivery planning (Bryan, 2004). For example, Sanger et al. (2003) used interviews to investigate language difficulties in 13 female adolescents who had committed crime, triangulating findings with assessment data and school records. Themes that emerged from interviews included: communication with friends, parents and authority; participant views about themselves; and learning in school. Participants described difficulties with understanding jokes, teachers' oral instructions and vocabulary. Literacy was also described by some participants as an area of difficulty. The authors describe the implications for professionals working with this population, contrasting participants' own concerns regarding vocabulary and comprehension with the focus on pragmatic and social use of language found in many intervention programmes designed for incarcerated adolescents.

Sanger et al. (2003: 480) conclude that interview "findings provide important clues for advancing research and planning better programs".

Hopkins, Clegg, and Stackhouse (2016) interviewed 31 young offenders on court orders about their literacy and communication skills to understand how they perceive these abilities and their experiences of 'communication' in the youth justice system. Communication and literacy were considered important skills and being good communicators with good literacy skills was important to their engagement with youth justice services. However, the young people did not perceive themselves as literate or competent communicators and expressed a desire to improve this. The young people reported a long history of communication difficulties starting in school with teachers and people in positions of authority. Listening and attending was difficult and this was not supported by teachers and schools, resulting in frustration, failure, disengagement and anger. Confrontation and conflict persist through their lives with communication and avoidance of communication central to this. These young people find using communication to resolve disagreements and conflict difficult with subsequent negative communication used such as shouting, swearing and being unable to use communication to seek support, disclose and confide in others. School was a very challenging environment for these young people as children whereas the youth offending services was perceived more positively with case workers highlighted as being able to listen and explain themselves well by using less complex language.

There is now more recognition of the speech, language and communication needs of young offenders and how youth justice services need to be more communication-friendly. In the Hopkins et al. (2016) study, the findings supported the commissioning of the equivalent of a full-time speech and language therapist who works into the youth offending service. This support enables staff to be trained in the identification of SLCN and to provide a communication-friendly environment where staff are able to communicate more effectively with the young people. This was summarized succinctly by the service manager (personal communication, October 2017).

> "This is a young person who is very challenging and we had struggled to meet his needs. Despite how he presented, I finally understood that I needed to talk to him in a different way. Once I did this, our interactions became more productive as I now realise he could understand what we were saying and asking him to do as well as listening

to him. I met him downstairs in the building once and he was really angry but I managed to support him this time by thinking about how I was communicating with him and changing this. He then became more responsive to me and it's improved, not completely but it's better."

Listening to adolescents to gain insights into specialist provision

In England, Education Authorities aim to educate children and young people with language disorders in mainstream provision with or without support rather than in specialist education provision. The number of children and young people boarding in residential special schools has reduced considerably from 7600 in 2010 to 4878 in 2017 yet the number of children with Education and Health Care Plans (EHCP) or Statements of Special Educational Need (SEN) has increased.

Despite changes to specialist educational provision, there are still some primary and secondary schools that specialize in education for children with language disorders at primary, secondary and post-16 years, usually offered by charitable organizations through non-maintained status. The perspectives of these children and young people about their experiences of specialist provision are relatively unexplored. A very recent government review of all residential special schools in England surveyed parents, school staff and local authorities but surveying or gaining the perspectives of the children or young people in the schools was not evident (Lenehan & Geraghty, 2017). It is a challenge to gain these perspectives, especially so for children and young people with communication impairments. However, recent studies have overcome this by adhering to accessible information guidelines and amending research protocols to enable participation.

Twenty-six young adults between the ages of 18 and 36 years who had attended a specialist residential school for children and young people with communication impairments (Clegg et al., 2012) were interviewed about their experiences. Fifteen parents of the adults were also interviewed separately. The interview methodology was adapted to enable full participation through the use of accessible information guidelines in the writing of information letters and consent forms about their participation. Visual support through the use of symbols and other aided communication systems was also used during the interviews as well as scheduling and timing of the interviews to enable breaks and pauses and an interviewer trained in knowing how to communicate effectively with adults with language disorders.

The ex-pupils highlighted both the advantages and disadvantages of specialist educational provision. Advantages included smaller class sizes, increased support to manage the educational demands, less bullying than experienced in previous schools and specialist support including speech and language therapy. The school enabled a shared community of children and young people with similar needs, thus facilitating friendships and reducing bullying. The main disadvantage was perceived as being away from the family home and community, particularly for the adults who had stayed in the residential provision due to the distance of the school from their family home. The transition from specialist educational provision was particularly challenging and heightened by the lack of support for adults with language disorders in terms of education, health and social services. Friendships made through the school disappeared as a result of the distance, and integration back into the family home was challenging for the individual and their family, resulting in feelings of loneliness and exclusion. The adults changed how they viewed their language disorder and resulting communication impairment during their time in the school compared to when they left. The adults did not always identify themselves as having language disorders or communication impairments but instead described the functional impact of their experiences in relation to their employment and everyday life. Difficulties with reading documents in the workplace and learning new words specific to their work were described, as well as experiences of victimization from people in the workplace about their communication.

The interviews with the parents of the ex-pupils highlighted shared and differing perspectives. The adults agreed with their parents about the positive and negative aspects of special educational provision. Differing perspectives were identified around the transition back to the family home and area with parents finding this more challenging than the adults due to parental concerns about the future. Parents were more aware of the lack of support for their grown-up children and perceived the impact of their communication impairments on employment, independence and wellbeing as more severe. The study enabled the school to develop their strategies around pupil wellbeing and transition to prepare pupils and their families for the transition away from the school. The voice of the ex-pupils and their parents confirms the valuable role specialist educational provision has in the lives of children, adolescents and adults with language disorders.

Listening to adolescents to gain insights into specialist provision: An example

James attended the specialist residential school at the age of 8 years after several years in a mainstream primary school, He described this time as 'very difficult' as he had no friends and 'no one helped him'. James talked about not wanting to go to school and then refusing to go to school:

> "I just didn't want to go and I wouldn't. Mum was really upset and everyone was really cross."

James then attended the specialist residential school and boarded during the week.

> "I missed my family and I would be really upset on Sundays when I knew I had to go back to school. I cried in the taxi on the way back."

The school was positive and James enjoyed being at school, wanting to learn and being part of a community of school pupils.

> "I got on with the teachers…they helped me and wanted to be with me. I had friends for the first time and we used to do stuff like and be with each other."

James entered the post-16 years provision at the school, attending a local college as well during this time. James left school with National Vocational Qualifications and went on to Catering College and now works as an assistant chef while living in the family home.

Listening to adolescents to evaluate interventions: The impact of a word learning group

We designed, delivered and evaluated a vocabulary intervention programme for teenagers with low vocabulary skills (Spencer et al., 2017). Alongside using detailed and specific outcome measures, we also asked the young people to give us feedback on the programme. On the whole, they rated the intervention positively, with 93% reporting that they enjoyed the sessions (64% said they enjoyed the session a lot) on a Lickert scale. However, much richer information and insights were gained when we asked the young people to talk to us and tell us about the programme. By listening to what they said, we gained insights into their learning. We learned:

- The young people could report clearly what they gained from the intervention in relation to our targets. For example, a young person said, "I learned loads – many new words like interpret, or sustain, and others. I heard of them but never really understood what it meant. I found it useful." Others reported about increased understanding of words (not just learning new words): "I know exactly what discrimination means now."

- But they also reminded us that the outcomes of the intervention went beyond what we captured with our outcome measure. We targeted one word per session but learning went beyond this. As one young person said: "We learned loads of different words every week, like generate and influence. We definitely learned more than one word in a lesson."

- The functionality of the new words taught (at the heart of our design but not really reflected on the outcome measure we used) was also highlighted. For example, one young person said: "We used the words we learned. For example, we wrote a letter to the head teacher about non-uniform day using the words that we'd been learning." Others said that they used the words to get better in English. While this was positive, it also reminded us that we needed to continue to highlight the application of the taught words across the curriculum.

- Some young people said that their learning went beyond vocabulary. For example, one young person said she learned not to bully or swear in class. Another reported that they became more confident in talking to other people.

- When we asked the young people how to improve the intervention programme, we were reminded about the importance of working with young people to plan the delivery of sessions. Very little feedback was given regarding the content of sessions (our priority as researchers) but we were reminded of the importance of negotiating the timing and logistics of the sessions in partnership with participants (e.g., avoiding missing cooking sessions in the technology curriculum and ensuring that friendship groups were respected when timetabling small group work).

For more information about the word learning groups, see Spencer et al. (2017) and visit the project's website at: https://adolescentvocabulary. wordpress.com/

Challenges of listening to the views of adolescents with language disorders

It is important to acknowledge the challenges of involving children and young people in decision making and facilitating participation in matters affecting their own lives. Practical barriers may include: a lack of staff or researcher resources; insufficient time to implement true collaboration and participation; insufficient time to develop children and young people's skills; a lack of skills in listening and working partnerships; and difficulties with ensuring true informed consent (Franklin & Sloper, 2009). Once children are viewed as social agents, new ethical dilemmas and responsibilities are created (Christensen & Prout, 2002), increasing the need for ongoing dialogue with children throughout the research process (Christensen & Prout, 2002). It can be challenging to overcome power inequalities in adult–child interactions and to step away from 'schooled' ways of being, related to deference, compliance and meeting adult expectations (Curtin 2001; Hurley & Underwood, 2002). It is important to avoid the temptation to invite the views of young people but then ignore or subvert voices according to adult-led agendas (Lewis & Porter, 2004). Asking young people for their views is not in itself necessarily 'empowering' or transformative. Therefore, as well as planning for listening, there must be a clear pathway of outcomes following young people's participation in research into their perspectives, feelings and experiences.

These challenges can feel amplified when working with young people with language disorders, due to the nature of their difficulties. There are issues around gaining consent and assent for participation and ensuring true and informed decision making where young people may have impairments in language comprehension (Merrick, 2011). Young people may have limited understandings of what involvement means, especially where this information is not provided in accessible formats (Franklin & Sloper, 2009). Then, due care must be given to both methods of elicitation and means of interpreting young people's responses (Dockrell & Lindsay, 2011). The cognitive and linguistic demands of interviews and participatory research methods may be at odds with the profiles of language strengths and difficulties associated with language disorder. Dockrell and Lindsay (2011) summarize some relevant challenges, such as:

- When responding to questions, children will typically provide an answer to an adult even when they are not able to understand the question.

- Open questions are more demanding for young people with language disorders. However, they are more likely to result in an accurate answer than closed questions. When interviewing young people with language disorders, the interviewer may not know whether a non-response or undeveloped answer is due to language barriers (e.g., not being able to understand the question or explain the answer) or due to the respondent not knowing the answer or having an opinion. Further scaffolding or rephrasing of the question may lead the young person to fabricate a response.

- Memory difficulties may impact on recalling specific events, situations, or feelings in relation to scenarios or periods of time.

- Autobiographical accounts can be influenced by the way that they are questioned about the events.

- There may not be shared understandings of key words or concepts used in the interview (or other method).

- Data collection may have pragmatic demands that are challenging for young people with language disorders. Familiarity with the researcher can impact on participants' responses.

Table 3.1 Examples of strategies for enabling adolescents with language disorders to share their experiences.

Strategy	Rationale	Considerations
Use accessible information, with pre-planning of use of strategies in correspondence with the young person, family and professionals.	For example, a visual prompt sheet might be used to support interview topics, giving greater time for asking questions and processing interviewer questions, repeating and rephrasing questions, giving rest breaks during data collection. Such techniques can be planned and used as a technique to increase accessibility of language in interviews (Carroll & Dockrell, 2009).	Resources need to be well designed, matched to the young person's level of need and visually appealing to the age group. Pre-planning use of strategies will require 'data collection' about level of language abilities and difficulties before true data collection begins. This may be demanding in terms of time and resources. More importantly, it may result in an over-emphasis on the young person's impairment as described by others before the data collection (rather than centralising the young person's own perceptions and experiences).
Involve a familiar adult, such as a parent, in data collection.	This can overcome difficulties of an unfamiliar researcher working directly with a young person and may be able to offer practical support in developing effective communication (Goldbart & Marshall, 2011; Merrick, 2011).	It is important not to centralise adult accounts and to disentangle the views of the adult from those of the young person (Merrick, 2011).
Collaborate with young people with language disorders from throughout the research process.	Young people can help design the project with professional researchers in order to increase accessibility. Examples of roles could include: contributing to aims, designing or co-designing any interview schedules or arts-based measures, advising on the procedure (e.g., length of sessions, location), and participating in making adaptations for different profiles of strengths and difficulties.	It is important to address the underlying assumptions of participatory research with children and young people with language disorders. For example, disbursement of power between researcher and researcher-participants needs to be acknowledged and negotiated (Miskelly & Roulstone, 2011)..
Use of 'interrupted interviews', augmenting semi-structured interviews with activities such as collages, card sorting, and walking. interviews (Shepherd, 2015).	This is argued to be a good way of facilitating the participation of young people with social communication needs such as Autistic Spectrum Disorder by taking the direct focus away from the social interaction and towards the tasks (Shepherd, 2015).	Scaffolding the interviews with collages and cards does involve pre-determined choices. This risks being prescriptive and limiting options for expression.

- Young people's meta-cognition and comprehension monitoring will have implications for interviews. Young people will have varying levels of insight into their understanding of a situation and will have varying ability to reflect on research materials and interview questions.

Enabling adolescents with language disorders to share their experiences and perspectives

Listening to the voices of children and young people with language disorders may be challenging, but it is certainly possible, given a commitment to developing appropriate methodologies, developing mutual understanding, establishing relationships, and building rapport. Considerable investment of time, resources and expertise may be required, but young people with language disorders – and indeed those with profound and complex disabilities – can participate, be heard, and have influence (Wickenden, 2011).

An overview of some strategies to support young people with language disorders to have their voices heard is given in Table 3.1.

Next steps: From listening to young people to enabling their participation in decision making

This chapter has argued for the importance of listening to young people with language disorders across different levels: individual, service, and strategic. Much has been written about methods and theoretical approaches for working with children and young people to increase knowledge and expertise in their experiences. There has also been some discussion of facilitating participation of children with disabilities in making decisions about their own lives. Gradually, research is emerging which considers the views of children and young people with language disorders.

However, this research is in its infancy. Very little empirical research – if any – has investigated the process of facilitating children or adolescents with language disorders to participate fully in joint decision making in relation to their own specialist interventions. There are very few examples of young people with language disorders taking a central role in service planning, or the development of strategy or policy development. Rarely have young people with language disorders been involved in setting research agendas, generating study aims, determining methods and outcomes. As McLeod reflects: "The future of our research with children and young people with speech, language and communication needs will facilitate the sharing of power and responsibility, ideally in ways that will be conducive to them having a voice in their own lives" (McLeod, 2001: 35). Developing research to support the lives of these children will only have an impact if their voices are heard.

References

Alderson, P. (2000). 12 children as researchers: The effects of participation rights on research methodology. In P. Christensen & A. James (Eds), *Research with Children: Perspectives and Practices*. London: Falmer Press.

Bryan, K. (2004). Preliminary study of the prevalence of speech and language difficulties in young offenders. *International Journal of Language & Communication Disorders*, 39(3), 391-400.

Carroll, C. & Dockrell, J. (2011). Listening to post-16 transition experiences of young people with Specific Language Impairment. In S. Roulstone & S. McLeod (Eds), *Listening to Children and Young People with Speech, Language and Communication Needs*. Guildford: J&R Press.

Carroll, C. & Sixsmith, J. (2016). Exploring the facilitation of young children with disabilities in research about their early intervention service. *Child Language Teaching and Therapy*, 32(3), 313-325.

Christensen, P. & James, A. (Eds.). (2008). *Research with Children: Perspectives and Practices*. London: Routledge.

Christensen, P. & Prout, A. (2002). Working with ethical symmetry in social research with children. *Childhood*, 9(4), 477-497.

Clegg, J. & Spencer, S. (2017). Teen Talk. Accessed online at: https://teen-talk.group.shef.ac.uk/

Clegg, J., Ansorge, L., Stackhouse, J., & Donlan, C. (2012). Developmental communication impairments in adults: Outcomes and life experiences of adults and their parents. *Language, Speech and Hearing Services in Schools*, 43, 521-535.

Clegg, J., Hollis, C., Mawhood, L., & Rutter, M. (2005). Developmental language disorders – A follow-up in later adult life. Cognitive, language and psychosocial outcomes. *Journal of Child Psychology and Psychiatry*, 46(2), 128-149.

Curtin, C. (2001). Eliciting children's voices in qualitative research. *American Journal of Occupational Therapy*, 55(3), 295-302.

Department for Education (2014). Special Educational Needs and Disability: A Guide for Parents and Carers. London: Department for Education. Accessed online at: https://www.gov.uk/government/uploads/system/uploads/attachment_data/file/417435/Special_educational_needs_and_disabilites_guide_for_parents_and_carers.pdf

Dockrell, J.E. & Lindsay, G. (2011). Cognitive and linguistic factors in the interview process. In S. Roulstone & S. McLeod (Eds), *Listening to Children and Young People with Speech, Language and Communication Needs*. Guildford: J&R Press.

Franklin, A. & Sloper, P. (2009). Supporting the participation of disabled children and young people in decision-making. *Children & Society, 23*, 3–15.

Goldbart, J. & Marshall, J. (2011). Listening to proxies for children with speech, language and communication needs. In S. Roulstone & S. McLeod (Eds), *Listening to Children and Young People with Speech, Language and Communication Needs*. Guildford: J&R Press.

Gorard, S. & See, B.H. (2011) How can we enhance enjoyment of secondary school? The student view. *British Educational Research Journal, 37*(4), 671-690.

Hambly, H., Coad, J., Lindsay, G., & Roulstone, S. (2011). Listening to children and young people's desired outcomes. In S. Roulstone & S. McLeod (Eds), *Listening to Children and Young People with Speech, Language and Communication Needs*. Guildford: J&R Press.

Hartas, D. & Lindsay, G. (2011). Young people's involvement in service evaluation and decision making. *Emotional and Behavioural Difficulties, 16*(2), 129-143.

Hopkins, T., Clegg, J., & Stackhouse, J. (2016). Young offenders' perspectives on their literacy and communication skills. *International Journal of Language & Communication Disorders, 51*(1), 95-109.

Hurley, J.C. & Underwood, M.K. (2002). Children's understanding of their research rights before and after debriefing: Informed assent, confidentiality, and stopping participation. *Child Development, 73*(1), 132-143.

James, A. & James, A. (2004). *Constructing Childhood: Theory, Policy and Social Practice*. London: Macmillan.

Lenehan, C. & Geraghty, M. (2017). *Good Intentions, Good Enough? A Review of the Experiences and Outcomes of Children and Young People in Residential Special Schools and Colleges*. London: Department for Education.

Lewis, A. & Porter, J. (2004). Interviewing children and young people with learning disabilities: Guidelines for researchers and multi-professional practice. *British Journal of Learning Disabilities, 32*(4), 191-197.

Lyons, R., O'Malley, M.P., O'Connor, P., & Monaghan, U. (2010). 'It's just so lovely to hear him talking': Exploring the early-intervention expectations and experiences of parents. *Child Language Teaching and Therapy, 26*(1), 61-76.

McCormack, J., McLeod, S., McAllister, L., & Harrison, L.J. (2010). My speech problem, your listening problem, and my frustration: The experience of living with childhood speech impairment. *Language, Speech, and Hearing Services in Schools, 41*(4), 379-392.

McLeod, S. (2011). Listening to children and young people with speech, language and communication needs: Who, why and how? In S. Roulstone & S. McLeod (Eds), *Listening to Children and Young People with Speech, Language and Communication Needs*. Guildford: J&R Press.

Merrick, R. (2011). Ethics, consent and assent when listening to children with speech, language and communication needs. In S. Roulstone & S. McLeod (Eds), *Listening to Children and Young People with Speech, Language and Communication Needs*. Guildford: J&R Press.

Miskelly, C. & Roulstone, S. (2011). Issues and assumptions of participatory research with children and young people with speech, language and communication needs. In S. Roulstone & S. McLeod (Eds), *Listening to Children and Young People with Speech, Language and Communication Needs*. Guildford: J&R Press.

Owen, R., Hayett, L., & Roulstone, S. (2004). Children's views of speech and language therapy in school: Consulting children with communication difficulties. *Child Language Teaching and Therapy, 20*(1), 55-73.

Palikara, O., Lindsay, G., & Dockrell, J.E. (2009). Voices of young people with a history of specific language impairment (SLI) in the first year of post-16 education. *International Journal of Language & Communication Disorders, 44*(1), 56-78.

Paul, R. & Norbury, C. (2012). *Language Disorders from Infancy Through Adolescence (E-Book): Listening, Speaking, Reading, Writing, and Communicating*. New York: Elsevier Health Sciences.

Porter, G., Townsend, J., & Hampshire, K. (2012) Children and young people as producers of knowledge, *Children's Geographies, 10*(2), 131-134.

Pratt, C., Botting, N., & Conti-Ramsden, G. (2006). The characteristics and concerns of mothers of adolescents with a history of SLI. *Child Language Teaching and Therapy, 22*(2), 177-196.

Roulstone, S., Coad, J., Ayre, A., Hambly, H., & Lindsay, G. (2012). *The Preferred Outcomes of Children with Speech, Language and Communication Needs and Their Parents*. London: Department for Education.

Roulstone, S. & McLeod, S. (Eds). (2011). *Listening to Children and Young People with Speech, Language and Communication Needs*. Guildford: J&R Press.

Sanger, D., Moore-Brown, B.J., Montgomery, J., Rezac, C., & Keller, H. (2003). Female incarcerated adolescents with language problems talk about their own communication behaviors and learning. *Journal of Communication Disorders, 36*(6), 465-486.

Shepherd, J. (2015). 'Interrupted Interviews': Listening to young people with autism in transition to college. *Exchanges: The Warwick Research Journal, 2*(2), 249-262.

Spencer, S., Clegg, J., & Stackhouse, J. (2010). 'I don't come out with big words like other people': Interviewing adolescents as part of communication profiling. *Child Language Teaching and Therapy, 26*(2), 144-162.

Spencer, S., Clegg, J., Lowe, H., & Stackhouse, J. (2017). Increasing adolescents' depth of understanding of cross-curriculum words: An intervention study. *International Journal of Language & Communication Disorders, 52*(5), 652-668.

Tangen, R. (2009). Conceptualising quality of school life from pupils' perspectives: A four-dimensional model. *International Journal of Inclusive Education, 13*(8), 829-844.

UNICEF. (1989.) *Convention on the Rights of the Child.* New York: UNICEF.

Wickenden, M. (2011). Talking to teenagers: Using anthropological methods to explore identity and the lifeworlds of young people who use AAC. *Communication Disorders Quarterly, 32,* 151-163.

4 Supporting adolescents with language impairments in the youth justice system

Pamela C. Snow and Karen Bryan

Learning outcomes

This chapter will enable readers to:

- Describe the complex biopsychosocial factors that contribute to the combined outcome of suboptimal expressive and receptive language skills (often not formally diagnosed in childhood), early academic disengagement, and involvement with the youth justice system in adolescence.

- Discuss the interface between child protection and youth justice, and the over-representation (but often under-diagnosis) of neurodevelopmental disabilities, and the typically chaotic and economically struggling families in which young offenders are reared.

- Appreciate the role of school suspensions and exclusions in the histories of adolescents in the youth justice system.

- Understand the implications of impoverished language skills in youth offenders, with particular emphasis on ways that vulnerable children and adolescents can be supported, (a) in the early years of school (socially and academically); (b) in their interface with criminal justice personnel (e.g., police and court officials); (c) in participation in restorative justice conferencing; and (d) in engaging with literacy and other verbally mediated interventions designed to reduce re-offending.

- Critically engage with inconsistencies in reported prevalence rates of language impairment in youth offenders, together with methodological and definitional tensions that account for these, with a focus on (a) the interface between low socio-economic status (SES) and youth offending, and (b) classification/diagnostic cut-off differences in the determination of what constitutes language disorder in an already vulnerable population.

Introduction

Adolescents in the youth justice system are among the most vulnerable and most challenging of any community. Recent international research highlights the role of impaired language functioning in this population, and this is the focus of the current chapter. Before examining prevalence rates of language disorder in youth offenders, however, we must consider some important definitional issues. These contribute to methodological discrepancies between studies and are important to resolve if aetiological pathways are to be better understood, and intervention targets are to be operationalized, for both clinical and research purposes.

What is 'language disorder'?

This is a significant question for the whole field of child and adolescent language development and disorders, and has been the subject of recent international debate. A special forum in the *International Journal of Language and Communication Disorders* (Volume 49, no. 4, 2014) entitled 'The SLI Debate' canvassed the complexities and tensions for researchers and clinicians regarding appropriate terminology to classify and describe young people whose language skills are not within what is considered 'normal range' for their age, based on standardized measures. It became apparent in the course of this debate that the term 'Specific Language Impairment' (SLI) has significant limitations, particularly regarding constraints imposed by the meaning of the modifier 'specific'. Whilst efforts have been made since the 1980s by researchers to reserve this term for children whose language difficulties are not accounted for by low IQ or other known neurodevelopmental disorders, it has had less traction with clinicians who must deal with the everyday reality of common co-morbidities with developmental language disorders, e.g., attentional difficulties and social-emotional-behavioural disturbances. Interested readers are referred to Bishop (2014) and Reilly et al. (2014) and associated commentaries for further detail on the debate concerning the appropriateness or otherwise of the term SLI going forward. Readers should also consult two important open-access papers that report on the response to this debate by an international consortium: Bishop, Snowling, Thompson, Greenhalgh et al. (2016) addressing identification of children with language difficulties, and Bishop, Snowling, Thompson, Greenhalgh et al. (2017) on terminological challenges and inconsistencies, and their resolution. In line with the consensus achieved by Bishop et al. (2017), we will refer in this chapter to developmental language disorder and/or language disorder. We note, however, that much of the literature we review uses terms other than these.

This debate is relevant to consideration of language skills in young offenders, because these young people typically come from low-SES backgrounds, which (as outlined below) is often sufficient in itself to create language profiles that fall below so-called 'normal' performance on standardized measures. Certain neurodevelopmental disorders are also over-represented in young offender samples, and these are independent risk factors for compromised language skills.

Low socio-economic status: Where impoverished language skills and youth offending coalesce

Hart and Risley (1995) conducted influential work in the United States on language development and socio-economic status, when they recruited 42 families with infants aged 10 months, across three SES strata (professional parents, working-class parents and parents on welfare benefits) and recorded monthly samples of child-directed language from when the children were aged 10 months to 36 months. They concluded that children of professional parents hear (i.e., have directed to them) a little over 2000 words per hour, and children of parents on welfare benefits hear only slightly more than 600 words per hour, with children of working-class parents falling in between, hearing a little over 1000 words an hour. Further, Hart and Risley reported important qualitative differences in language input across the SES strata, with children of professional parents hearing significantly more encouraging and expansive utterances than their peers from lower-SES backgrounds. Famously, Hart and Risley equated the discrepancy between the lowest and highest SES families to a 30-million word gap by the time children are aged 4.

Hart and Risley's work has been has been criticized on sociolinguistic grounds for taking a deficit view of difference (e.g., Michaels, 2013) and also on methodological grounds (e.g., Dudley-Marling & Lucas, 2009) regarding its relatively small and biased sample. On the latter, a key point is the fact that only six low-SES families were studied, and in all cases these were Black. Further, the possibility that the presence of observers may have had differential effects on families from different social strata was not controlled. It cannot be assumed from the Hart and Risley findings that all low-SES families provide linguistically impoverished environments, any more than we can assume that all high-SES families provide linguistically enriching environments. As Willingham (2012) points out, other influences on children's early development include physical health and nutrition, access to primary healthcare, exposure to psychological stress, and the amount of time that parents spend with them – all factors that reflect human and social capital as well as economic wellbeing. Further, Bishop (2014) has observed that low SES and parental education level may be consequences of, rather than contributors to, language impairment, and may have a common underlying genetic basis. Notwithstanding these caveats, reduced performance on standardized measures of expressive and receptive language skills in low-SES samples has been observed by a number of subsequent workers employing a range of methodologies (e.g., Hoff, 2003; Locke, Ginsborg, & Peers, 2002; Roy & Chiat, 2013; Spencer, Clegg, & Stackhouse, 2012; Weisleder & Fernald, 2013). These studies affirm the importance of SES when examining the language and academic skills of adolescents in the youth justice system, as such young people overwhelmingly come from lower-SES and more disadvantaged communities (Australian Institute of Health and Welfare, 2015; Ministry of Justice, 2014), thus raising questions as to whether what is being observed by language researchers in this population is simply a manifestation of their low-SES and reduced exposure to more elaborate (perhaps 'middle class') linguistic forms (vocabulary, syntactic structures, idioms).

However, there is evidence from two Australian studies which employed comparison groups from low-SES backgrounds (Snow & Powell, 2004, 2008) that SES, in itself, is not the explanatory mechanism for poor language skills in young offenders. In fact, in their 2008 study, Snow and Powell reported that their low-SES control group was on average *a year younger* than the young offenders, yet they out-performed the offender group on all language and social skill measures. Clearly then, being a young offender is associated with threats to language competence that extend beyond explanations afforded by low-SES alone. Factors that may need to be considered include early trauma exposure and parent-child relationships that are characterized by various forms of maltreatment (neglect and/or abuse). This is important in light of the fact that the same conditions that support early language development also support the development of early secure attachment to primary caregivers and the beginnings of empathy (Cohen, 2001; Snow, 2009). This is borne out by the over-representation of adolescents in the youth justice system who have histories of involvement with child protection agencies (Stewart, Dennison, & Waterson, 2002) and also the higher rates of language impairment that have been reported for young offenders who have experienced out-of-home care placements compared to youth offending peers who have not (Snow & Powell, 2011).

In addition to low-SES as an aggregate risk for both youth offending and sub-optimal language development, it is important to consider the contribution made to both by adverse childhood experiences (ACEs). ACEs include all forms of maltreatment (abuse and/or neglect): physical, sexual, emotional, social, and/or educational, and have been extensively studied regarding their impact on childhood mental and physical health, as well as their implications for health and wellbeing across the lifespan (e.g., Schilling, Aseltine, & Gore, 2007).

The fact that the overwhelming majority of adolescents in the youth justice system have experienced multiple ACEs is directly relevant to their expressive and receptive oral language skills, given the interpersonal space within which language is acquired, and the importance of warm, reliable, trusting relationships with primary caregivers in the early years for both secure attachment and early language skills (Cohen, 2001; Snow, 2009). ACEs exert two important influences in the lives of vulnerable young people: they elevate the risk of initial offending and also increase the risk of recidivism (Baglivio et al., 2014). This means that all therapeutic services (including SLT) need to be provided within a trauma-informed therapeutic model whereby behaviours such as difficulty establishing rapport with a clinician are seen as manifestations of learned functional responses to adults who repeatedly disappoint and/or create anxiety and hyper-arousal. This changes the question that clinicians need to address from "What is wrong with you?" to "What has happened to you?"

It is important to consider the impact of ACEs on early language acquisition. In their study of 100 young offending males completing custodial sentences, Snow and Powell (2011) reported higher rates of language disorder (around two-thirds) in young people who had experienced out-of-home care placements compared to those who had not. Lum, Powell, Timms and Snow (2015) completed a meta-analysis that establishes a clear relationship between child maltreatment and impaired expressive and receptive language skills. Hence it is reasonable to assume that, at least to some extent, language disorders seen in young offenders can be traced to early maltreatment experiences.

Clinicians working with young offenders require flexible and highly-developed therapeutic skills. It is challenging to measure and quantify progress in SLT interventions with this population, as a wider than usual number of factors needs to be considered in designing, delivering, and evaluating such services.

First, it is important to examine prevalence estimates of language disorder in youth offender samples as these are universally elevated, though they do vary widely between studies and jurisdictions.

Prevalence of language disorder in young offenders

In an epidemiological sense, if the prevalence and incidence of a condition are to be accurately measured and described, a robust definition of the condition is needed, together with agreed-upon criteria for determining its presence. Unfortunately, until very recently no such consensus has existed in this field and, as a consequence, prevalence estimates pertaining to language disorder in young male offenders range far too widely: from the 19.6% described in the US by Sanger, Creswell, Dworak, and Schultz (2000), to the 60% described by Bryan (2004) and Bryan, Freer, and Furlong (2007), with Australian estimates falling in between, and ranging from 36.7% (Snow, Woodward, Mathis, & Powell, 2015) to 52% (Snow & Powell, 2008). Such differences reflect methodological issues such as inclusion criteria, selection of measurement items, and identification of cut-off points, and possibly also differences in offending criteria in different countries. Although the degree of variation in prevalence estimates is above what would generally be considered within reasonable tolerance limits, all of these reported rates are well above those reported in community samples, which range from 5% (Larson & McKinley, 2003) to 7% (Tomblin et al., 1997) and 14% (McLeod & McKinnon, 2007). Unfortunately, few workers have systematically examined rates of language disorder in young female offenders; however, recent evidence (Snow et al., 2015) suggests that although such rates (approximately 25%) fall below those of young male offenders, they are elevated relative to those in community samples. Further research is thus needed on both quantitative and qualitative features of language profiles of young females in the justice system. It is also important to understand both the similarities and differences in risk trajectories for young female and male offenders, in the sense that some factors, such as level of parental monitoring, may be more important for females than males (Wong, Slotboom, & Bijleveld, 2010). The psychosocial and educational trajectories of at-risk girls need to be studied more closely, and with an explicit focus on oral language skills, so that needs which are shared with young males, as well as those that are gender-specific, can be characterized and addressed.

While adolescents with neurodevelopmental disorders such as autism, intellectual disability, and acquired brain injury are over-represented in youth justice statistics (Talbot, 2008; Williams et al., 2010), many studies have specifically excluded such groups because of the known impact of these disorders on receptive, expressive, and/or pragmatic language skills (e.g., Snow & Powell, 2004, 2008, 2011). Even in studies where such exclusions do not occur, it is probable that such young people self-exclude, based on their reluctance to engage in assessment tasks they anticipate being difficult. The important implication of such exclusions is, of course, that prevalence estimates based on their absence will significantly *under*-estimate the prevalence of language disorders in this population as a whole. While it might be argued that the presence of neurodevelopmental disorders such as those identified above would flag communication impairment for youth justice staff, in practice high levels of awareness cannot be assumed (Gregory & Bryan, 2011). There are good grounds, therefore, for consideration of universal language skills screening of adolescents entering custodial settings, as per recent recommendations by Snow et al. (2015). A counter-view, however, is that language disorder prevalence in such settings is so high as to warrant a 'universal precautions' approach to compromised communication skills (Snow, Bagley, & White, 2017). This issue requires further consideration and debate in the SLT and youth justice communities.

An important consideration with respect to the risk profiles of adolescents in the youth justice system is the notion of a 'school-to-prison pipeline' (Christle, Jolivette, & Nelson, 2005). This is created when young people (typically but not exclusively) from low-SES communities display both oppositional behaviour and learning difficulties, and are met with sometimes inflexible, coercive school disciplinary approaches that favour suspension and exclusion over more therapeutic, strengths-based approaches. Evidence indicates that young people at risk of school exclusion face increased likelihood of undiagnosed language disorders (e.g., Clegg, Stackhouse, Finch, Murphy, & Nichols, 2009; Ripley & Yuill, 2005). This means that they will experience many everyday difficulties understanding both academic and behavioural expectations, complying with instructions, and using oral and written language appropriately within the formal curriculum. Behaviour difficulties often mask underlying communication difficulties (Cohen, 2001; Snow et al., 2015), and a young person's responses may be incorrectly interpreted as rudeness, disinterest, and/or poor motivation. However, unless parents and teachers recognize this masking effect of language impairment regarding behaviour, disciplinary approaches that emphasize punitive consequences and exclusion only serve to further punish disadvantage and disability rather than finding ways of scaffolding a struggling learner's language skills. Somewhat perversely, it has been reported that students who under-perform academically may experience harsher punishments than those who are achieving educational benchmarks (Katsiyannis, Ryan, Zhang, & Spann, 2008). Sadly, as observed by Christle and Yell (2008), "Because only 15% of youths who have been incarcerated manage to graduate from high school … the line to education may be forever broken for most youths who are incarcerated" (p.157). Breaking vulnerable youths' connection with school therefore not only precludes academic achievement, but also reduces exposure to the prosocial attitudes, beliefs, and behaviours of non-offending peers.

All of this means, then, that serious efforts to disrupt the school-to-prison pipeline need to begin early in the trajectories of vulnerable students, so that appropriate supports are put in place at system and individual levels. Schools need to ensure that early-years teaching is informed by a strong understanding of the linguistic basis of the transition to literacy, and also by the application of evidence concerning the importance of systematic synthetic phonics teaching at the outset of reading instruction (Moats, 2014), in addition to promoting vocabulary and other oral language skills. It is also vital that children who do not attend school, or who access criminal justice or substance abuse services, are screened for language difficulties (Bryan, Garvani, Gregory, & Kilner, 2015). School staff should also be better equipped and supported to manage challenging behaviour, so that they can meet the learning needs of a wide range of students while maintaining a safe environment for all.

Providing communication support to young offenders

Forensic interviewing

When confronted with the stressful and high-stakes prospect of a police interview, most of us feel anxious and self-conscious regarding the adequacy of our verbal responses. Imagine, then, the compounding effect of this anxiety for adolescents in the youth justice system, many of whom will have inadequate receptive and expressive oral language skills to fully engage with the complex embedded statements, multi-element questions, direct and indirect questions, implicature, and idiomatic language (e.g., irony, sarcasm) that they are likely to encounter. Consider, too, the communicative consequences of difficulties processing such linguistic devices, in the context of a communicative exchange that is fundamentally asymmetrical regarding speaker rights. Speaker rights (Wilson, 1989) refers to the extent to which there are equitable opportunities to initiate and change topics, to correct apparent misunderstandings on the part of the communication partner and, perhaps most importantly, to decide that the interaction can end. Clearly, in the context of a police interview, none of these rights can be exercised by the young offender.

One of the key tasks of a young person who is being interviewed by police is to 'tell their story', i.e., to account for their actions by providing information in a logical, coherent, and complete manner. Evidence indicates, however, that young offenders display spoken narrative skills that are lacking in detail and essential content (Snow & Powell, 2004, 2008). This creates the risk that they provide narrative accounts of their actions which are judged by police as inadequate or improbable, and/or that they are judged as speakers to be lacking in authenticity and willingness to cooperate and hence incur harsher consequences than might otherwise have been the case. An additional threat to natural justice lies in the fact that adolescents with poor comprehension and/or expressive skills may be prone to acquiescence and suggestibility in the context of police interviews (Snow, Powell, & Sanger, 2012). There is a pressing need, therefore, for information about young offenders' oral language skills to be embedded into police training, along with guidelines about how to use best-practice interviewing techniques to elicit the young person's evidence. At-risk adolescents have contact with the police not only as suspects but also as victims and witnesses to crime, and a failure to employ appropriate interviewing techniques may obscure important facts that need further investigation and/ or need to be taken into account when determining next steps. In some jurisdictions, it is a statutory requirement that young people who have an intellectual disability are interviewed in the presence of an independent third person in order to ensure that coercion and/or unduly complex questions are not used by police as strategies to elicit a confession. In England and Wales, Northern Ireland, New Zealand, and some parts of Australia, Registered Intermediaries can be commissioned for vulnerable victims and witnesses to promote communication success during interviews or court cases (Plotnikoff & Wolfson, 2015). Alleged offenders, however, are generally not afforded this protection, and this imbalance needs to be redressed.

SLT interventions with youth offenders

Adopting a trauma-informed approach has already been advocated and accords well with therapeutic principles that underlie SLT intervention. Gregory and Bryan (2013) demonstrated that SLT intervention could be successfully delivered within custodial youth offender settings in both smaller, specialized environments and in large custodial environments with rapid through-put of offenders, including offenders categorized as dangerous. The service described by Bryan et al. integrated well and the SLTs became an important part of the multidisciplinary team. In a smaller establishment, communication screening of all entrants was feasible and enabled the care team to adapt interventions to the level of language demonstrated. In the larger establishment, referral processes were required to manage numbers, but gradually evolved into referral of any entrant who was recognized as vulnerable, failing in education, or not seeming to communicate with the induction officers who were skilled at making an initial assessment of need. Assessment of communication is complex and is normally not considered unless something is obviously wrong with expressive skills. Bryan et al. (2004) therefore developed a short set of screening questions with induction officers that focus on encouraging staff to reflect on their conversations with young offenders and whether these interactions seemed successful. The questions to the officers were:

1. Does he have a speech problem? yes □   no □

 (e.g., stammer or difficult to understand)

2. Does he have difficulty understanding what you say? yes □ no □

3. Are his responses minimal or limited? yes □   no □

Referral was triggered by the answer to any of the above being "yes". Clinicians judged these to be effective insofar as they gave officers confidence to refer. Almost no inappropriate referrals were made. However, some offenders with significant language difficulties were not recognized until later in their sentence, and some may have been missed altogether.

Subsequently, Crew and Gregory (2008) developed a communication screen that mirrors the approach used in the 'Asset' structured assessment tool used by UK Youth Offending Teams. Gregory and Bryan (2011) used this part of the assessment process within an SLT service in a community youth offending team. Staff were trained and supported to use the screen and reported favourably on its value (Bryan & Gregory, 2013). However, the

2011 study showed that this type of screening was insufficient to fully identify all adolescents with communication problems; further, in some cases self-report and questioning do not elicit the necessary information, particularly where young people are reluctant to admit to difficulties. The UK Youth Justice Board has recognized the need for more comprehensive assessment of developmental skills, including language and cognition, and so has developed the Comprehensive Health Assessment Tool (CHAT; Lennox et al., 2013) that can be used by a range of professionals. This is a welcome development and the tool is undergoing evaluation. It will be important to establish the level of knowledge and skills about language and cognition needed by assessors to administer it, as well as the role of professionals such as SLTs, psychologists, and support staff who conduct the assessments and evaluate the profiles.

Once a language need is demonstrated, SLT assessment using other instruments such as the Clinical Evaluation of Language Fundamentals, 4th edition (CELF-5; Wiig, Semel, & Secord, 2017) can be utilized based on the SLT's decision-making and hypothesis-testing approach, as for any client. While the evidence base for SLT intervention in prisons or community justice settings is limited, there is an emerging evidence base for the effectiveness of SLT for particular disorders such as stammering, and language interventions irrespective of where the client resides (Bryan et al., 2015).

Gregory and Bryan (2011) demonstrated positive outcomes in terms of improved scores on standardized language tests, and this finding was replicated by Snow and Woodward (2016), who also showed that personal goal setting and self-assessments by the young people were useful to augment documented improvements on standardized measures. However, the sustainability and 'real-world' translation of these improvements requires further research. It is also important for clinicians working with offenders to demonstrate the value of their involvement in terms of outcomes for the young person. Bryan's study (Bryan, 2004) identified outcomes in terms of achievement of SLT targets, but also the contribution of SLT to achievement of more general goals, such as attendance at educational programmes and engaging in more prosocial behaviour. This approach is more formally advocated in the Therapy Outcome Measures approach (Enderby et al., 2013). Such findings are also echoed in the positive responses of youth justice staff to the provision of SLT services to young people in both the UK (Bryan & Gregory, 2013) and Australia (Snow et al., 2017).

The high prevalence of language disorder in youth justice settings warrants formal SLT assessment on intake to determine the young person's particular strengths and difficulties. Snow et al. (2015) have proposed a modified Response to Intervention (RTI) framework to support the communication assessment and intervention planning for adolescents in youth justice settings. This builds on the widely-used RTI approach emanating from the US mainstream education system and comprising universal, small group and individual levels of intervention. It has a focus on oral language skills, prosocial behaviour and academic engagement/attainment, and offers a means of targeting and prioritizing services as well as using ongoing assessment data to monitor progress and response to the services provided. A challenge to the application and evaluation of such models, however, is the relatively brief duration of typical sentencing periods relative to the ground that these young people have already lost in mainstream education.

The following sections address the contribution of SLT to assessment and profiling of language levels in young offenders, their role in informing the multidisciplinary team on how low levels of language might impact on verbally mediated interventions, and how SLTs can advise on modifying language requirements and modes to make other interventions more accessible.

Restorative justice conferencing

Restorative Justice Conferencing (RJC) is an increasingly popular alternative to the adversarial and punitive measures traditionally employed with young offenders. It sits well with the general principle that system approaches to young offenders should be diversionary and therapeutic wherever possible, taking account of developmental needs and often complex trauma backgrounds (Chrzanowski & Wallis, 2011). This is a therapeutic jurisprudence approach that revolves around a conversation (facilitated by a trained convenor) between a young person who admits guilt (to either police or the courts, depending on the jurisdiction) and the victim or, in some cases, victim representatives. RJC seeks to more closely align the young person's values with those of the mainstream, and ultimately to reduce the risk of reoffending. As the name suggests, RJC is aimed at achieving mutual understanding, restoration and repair of relationships and a sense of community wellbeing rather than simply being concerned with punishment. However, by virtue of the fact that it is fundamentally a conversational process, RJC possibly stands to place unreasonable demands on the young person's receptive and expressive language skills, particularly where significant, yet undiagnosed, language difficulties exist.

One of the key measures of the success of a RJC is the extent to which victims feel that the young person has expressed remorse, and has done so with genuineness and authenticity (Hayes & Snow, 2013; Snow & Sanger, 2011). There is currently no empirical research of which we are aware that addresses the extent to which deficits in receptive and expressive language skills, difficulties understanding idiomatic language and reduced abstract language skills compromise a young person's capacity to fully engage in RJC. Extrapolating from the extensive international literature that identifies young offenders as a communicatively vulnerable group to the types of communication tasks inherent in RJC raises concerns, however. First, such conferences require the processing of sometimes emotionally-charged narratives of others. In addition to their linguistic complexity and sometimes nonlinear structures, such narratives typically also contain a range of emotions, such as anger, fear, resentment and distress. Evidence indicates that young offenders have difficulty identifying their own emotional states, a phenomenon referred to as *alexithymia* (Snow et al., 2015). Furthermore, the extent to which they are able to infer affective states in others in the context of RJCs is not known. In addition to processing the language of others, the young person must also say things that sound plausible and authentic to other parties in attendance, most notably the victim(s). In order to do so, they need to produce elaborate responses, at the very least sentences if not connected discourse, rather than one or two syllable responses. Unfortunately, however, evidence indicates that young offenders may resort to single-word utterances or nonspecific responses such as "maybe", or "I don't know" (Hayes & Snow, 2013). Failure to successfully engage in RJC may count against the young person in subsequent sentencing.

These concerns are not intended to signify lack of support for RJC, as this is an approach that has been found to show promise in changing the offending trajectories of some high-risk adolescents (Rodriguez, 2007). However, the fact that at least one in two young male offenders has clinically significant yet unidentified language disorders suggests a likely benefit from an assessment of their language skills as part of the assessment of suitability for RJC. Provision of explicit language support in the preparation, conduct and follow-up to high-stakes conferences could be provided by SLTs. It is to be hoped that, in the future, such expertise will be called upon to support the parties to the conference, and in so doing, support the conference itself.

Engagement in verbally-mediated psychological interventions

Many young offenders have complex criminogenic needs, i.e., biopsychosocial factors, that elevate their risk of offending and reoffending (Richards, 2011), and because of their developmental vulnerability need to be afforded therapeutic opportunities to address mental health problems (many of which are trauma-related), problematic substance abuse, academic/vocational struggles, and significant family tensions (see Andrews & Bonta, 2010, for a detailed description of the risk-needs-responsivity model of offender rehabilitation). In addition to the psychological needs listed above, Andrews and Bonta refer to the need to target procriminal attitudes (thoughts, values and sentiments supportive of criminal behaviour).

The obvious medium by which such difficulties and attitudes are addressed is an intervention to prevent reoffending, sometimes referred to as a 'talk therapy' (e.g., cognitive behaviour therapy [CBT]). Psychological therapies (and the assessments leading to these) require the young person to engage in 1:1 therapeutic encounters that require verbal accounts (e.g., narratives) of key events or experiences, and reflections on these using both cognitive and affective 'filters'. Taking part in psychological therapies such as CBT requires the ability to discuss thoughts and feelings and to speculate about those of others, using appropriately nuanced vocabulary. As such, it requires high-level receptive and expressive verbal skills, the ability to think in the abstract, and capacity to verbalize alternative explanations or cognitive re-frames.

Many psychological therapies and social skill interventions employ role-plays, e.g., to practise negotiation skills, to clarify the difference between assertive and aggressive responses, to rehearse verbal responses that might be needed in a job interview, and to practise giving and receiving feedback in socially acceptable ways. All of these tasks exact a high toll on verbal skills, but if underlying language competence is not considered, it may be that the young person's lacklustre efforts are misinterpreted as poor motivation to engage. It should be noted, too, that some young offenders are mandated by the court to take part in specialist psychological interventions, such as anger management and sex offender programmes, so careful account of verbal skills should be taken in order to maximize the clinical utility and therapeutic fit of such approaches, given the escalating sentences associated with reoffending for violent and/or sexual crimes.

There is a clear role, therefore, for SLTs to consult with mental health practitioners such as psychologists and social workers, on the basis of their assessment of the young person's expressive and receptive language skills, and to provide guidance as to likely impacts that may accrue in the context of psychological counselling.

Literacy interventions for adolescents completing custodial sentences

One of the largest barriers standing between adolescents exiting the youth justice system and prospects of open employment is their low literacy skills. Although a number of studies have reported low literacy skills in adult prison populations (e.g., Snowling, Adams, Bowyer-Crane, & Tobin, 2000) and in youth offender samples (e.g., Putnins, 1999; Vacca, 2008), there has been little-to-no explicit linking of the evidence concerning poor literacy skills with the evidence concerning poor oral language skills. Snowling et al. (2000) referred in their study to the prevalence of 'specific' reading difficulties in an adult offender sample; however, it is most likely that the difficulties experienced by this population were *non*-specific, given the complex biopsychosocial risks they face from early life as outlined earlier in this chapter.

While it is common for custodial settings to provide some form of educational/literacy programmes for young offenders (and mandatory for those below the school leaving age), this varies with respect to the skill base and experience of staff and the theoretical underpinnings of the intervention approach. There is little evidence that educational programmes in youth justice settings currently explicitly approach reading interventions from a linguistic perspective. It is known, however, that learners from more disadvantaged backgrounds benefit from explicit rather than indirect approaches to reading instruction (Foorman, Francis, Fletcher, & Schatschneider, 1998). There is a pressing need for research that examines the contribution of core language skills such as phonemic awareness, vocabulary, and comprehension, so that reading interventions for young offenders can directly address these subskills. Having everyday literacy skills may reduce the likelihood of recidivism through the promotion of engagement in the economic mainstream. SLT assessment can be used to guide education staff on the level of language skills that a young person has, and in assisting staff to modify delivery of the programme to ensure that the young person can participate effectively (Bryan & Gregory, 2013). A young person not engaging or failing in education should in particular be flagged for a language assessment.

Conclusions

A high proportion of adolescents who are involved in criminal justice systems will have language disorders, and these are often overlooked. Language difficulties are over-represented in low-SES communities and contribute to early educational disengagement, challenges engaging with justice processes, and accessing education, rehabilitation and restorative measures designed to prevent reoffending. Speech and language therapy expertise can assist in identifying language problems, in enabling other practitioners to modify delivery of verbally-mediated interventions to make them more accessible, and in providing direct intervention to address language difficulties. The evidence base for speech and language intervention is emerging, although more research is needed.

Reflective questions

1. How might knowledge of early trauma-exposure inform SLT case-formulation with young offenders?

2. What factors might make evaluation of intervention effectiveness particularly challenging in the youth offender setting?

3. What are the consequences of high levels of communication difficulties in young offenders for the development of policy to prevent and manage youth offending?

4. What can schools do to offset some of the challenges faced by young people facing multiple risks for early academic disengagement and possible anti-social behaviour?

References

Andrews, D.A. & Bonta, J. (2010). Rehabilitating criminal justice policy and practice. *Psychology, Public Policy, and Law, 16*(1), 39–55.

Australian Institute of Health and Welfare (2015). *Youth Justice in Australia 2013–14,* Bulletin No.127.Cat.no.AUS 188.Canberra: AIHW.

Baglivio, M.T., Epps, N., Swartz, K., Sayedul Huq, M., Sheer, A., & Hardt, N.S. (2014). The prevalence of Adverse Childhood Experiences (ACE) in the lives of juvenile offenders. *Journal of Juvenile Justice, 3*(2). Available at http://www.journalofjuvjustice.org/JOJJ0302/article01.htm Accessed June 5, 2015.

Bishop, D.V.M. (2014). Ten questions about terminology for children with unexplained language problems. *International Journal of Language and Communication Disorders, 49*(4), 381–415.

Bishop, D.V.M., Snowling, M.J., Thompson, P.A., Greenhalgh, T., and the CATALISE consortium. (2016). CATALISE: A multinational and multidisciplinary Delphi consensus study. Identifying language impairments in children. *PLoS ONE, 11*(7), e0158753. doi:10.1371/journal.pone.0158753

Bishop, D.V.M., Snowling, M.J., Thompson, P.A., Greenhalgh, T., and the CATALISE-2 consortium. (2017). Phase 2 of CATALISE: A multinational and multidisciplinary Delphi consensus study of problems with language development: Terminology. *Journal of Child Psychology and Psychiatry*. doi:10.1111/jcpp.12721

Bryan, K. (2004). Preliminary study of the prevalence of speech and language difficulties in young offenders. *International Journal of Language and Communication Disorders, 39*, 391–400.

Bryan, K. & Gregory, J. (2013). Perceptions of staff on embedding speech and language therapy within a youth offending team. *Child Language Teaching and Therapy, 29*, 359–371.

Bryan, K., Freer, J., & Furlong, C. (2007). Language and communication difficulties in juvenile offenders. *International Journal of Language and Communication Disorders, 42*(5), 505–520.

Bryan, K., Garvani, G., Gregory, J., & Kilner, K. (2015). Language difficulties and criminal justice: The need for earlier identification. *International Journal of Language and Communication Disorders, 50*, 763–775.

Christle, C.A. & Yell, M.L. (2008). Preventing youth incarceration through reading remediation: Issues and solutions. *Reading & Writing Quarterly: Overcoming Learning Difficulties, 24*(2), 148–176.

Christle, C.A., Jolivette, K., & Nelson, C.M. (2005). Breaking the school to prison pipeline: Identifying school risk and protective factors for youth delinquency. *Exceptionality, 13*(2), 69–88.

Chrzanowski, A. & Wallis, R. (2011). Understanding the youth justice system. In A. Stewart, T. Allard, & S. Dennison (Eds), *Evidence Based Policy and Practice in Youth Justice* (pp.7–27). Leichardt: Federation.

Clegg, J., Stackhouse, J., Finch, K., Murphy, C., & Nicholls, S. (2009). Language abilities of secondary age pupils at risk of school exclusion: A preliminary report. *Child Language Teaching and Therapy, 25*(1), 123–139.

Cohen, N.J. (2001). *Language Impairment and Psychopathology in Infants, Children and Adolescents.* Thousand Oaks, CA: Sage.

Crew, M. & Gregory, J. (2008). *Communication Screen.* Leeds: Leeds Community Healthcare Trust.

Dudley-Marling, K. & Lucas, K. (2009). Pathologizing the language and culture of poor children. *Language Arts, 86*(5), 362–370.

Enderby, P., John, A., & Petherham, B. (2013). *Therapy Outcomes Measures for Rehabilitation Professionals: Speech and Language Therapy, Physiotherapy, Occupational Therapy.* Chichester: John Wiley & Sons.

Foorman, B.R., Francis, D.J., Fletcher, J.M., & Schatschneider, C. (1998). The role of instruction in learning to read: Preventing reading failure in at-risk children. *Journal of Educational Psychology, 90*(1), 37–55.

Gregory, J. & Bryan, K. (2011). Speech and language therapy intervention with a group of persistent and prolific young offenders in a non-custodial setting with previously undiagnosed speech, language and communication difficulties. *International Journal of Language and Communication Disorders, 46*, 202–215.

Hart, B. & Risley, T. (1995). *Meaningful Differences in Everyday Parenting and Intellectual Development in Young American Children.* Baltimore: Brookes.

Hayes, H. & Snow, P. (2013). Oral language competence and restorative justice processes: Refining preparation and the measurement of conference outcomes. *Trends & Issues in Crime and Criminal Justice, 463*, 1–7.

Hoff, E. (2003). The specificity of environmental influence: Socioeconomic status affects early vocabulary development via maternal speech. *Child Development, 74*, 1368–1378.

Katsiyannis, A., Ryan, J.B., Zhang, D., & Spann, A. (2008). Juvenile delinquency and recidivism: The impact of academic achievement. *Reading & Writing Quarterly: Overcoming Learning Difficulties, 24*(2), 177–196.

Larson, V. & McKinley, N. (2003). Service delivery options for secondary students with language disorders. *Seminars in Speech and Language, 24*(3), 181–197.

Lennox, C., King, C., Chitabesan, P., Theodosiou, L., & Shaw, J. (2013). *The Development and Pilot of the Comprehensive Health Assessment Tool (CHAT): Young People in the Secure Estate.* Manchester: Offender Health Research Network.

Locke, A., Ginsborg, J., & Peers, I. (2002). Development and disadvantage: Implications for the early years and beyond. *International Journal of Language and Communication Disorders, 37*, 3–15.

Lum, J., Powell, M., Timms, L., & Snow, P. (2015). A meta-analysis of case-control studies investigating language in maltreated children. *Journal of Speech, Language and Hearing Research, 58*, 961–976.

McLeod, S. & McKinnnon, D.H. (2007). Prevalence of communication disorders compared with other learning needs in 14,500 primary and secondary school students. *International Journal of Language and Communication Disorders, 42*, 37–59.

Michaels, S. (2013). Déjà-vu all over again: What's wrong with Hart & Risley and a "linguistic deficit" framework in early childhood education? *LEARNing Landscapes, 7*(1), Autumn, 23–41.

Ministry of Justice. (2014). *Offender Management Statistics Annual Tables 2013.* London: Ministry of Justice.

Moats, L. (2014). What teachers don't know and why they aren't learning it: Addressing the need for content and pedagogy in teacher education. *Australian Journal of Learning Difficulties, 19*(2), 75–91.

Plotnikoff, J. & Wilson, R. (2015). *Intermediaries in the Criminal Justice System: Improving Communication for Vulnerable Witnesses and Defendants.* Bristol: Policy.

Putnins, A.L. (1999). Literacy, numeracy and non-verbal reasoning skills of South Australian young offenders. *Australian Journal of Education, 43*, 157–171.

Reilly, S., Tomblin, B., Law, J., McKean, C., Mensah, F.K., Morgan, A., Goldfeld, S., Nicholson, J.M., & Wake, M. (2014). Specific language impairment: A convenient label for whom? *International Journal of Language and Communication Disorders, 49*(4), 416–451.

Richards, K. (2011). What makes juvenile offenders different from adult offenders? *Trends & issues in Crime & Criminal Justice*, No. 409. Canberra: AIC.

Ripley, K. & Yuill, N. (2005). Patterns of language impairment and behaviour in boys excluded from school. *British Journal of Psychology, 75*, 37–50.

Rodriguez, N. (2007). Restorative justice at work: Examining the impact of restorative justice resolutions on juvenile recidivism. *Crime & Delinquency, 53*(3), 355–379.

Roy, P. & Chiat, S. (2013). Teasing apart disadvantage from disorder. The case of poor language. In C.R. Marshall (Ed.), *Current Issues in Developmental Disorders* (pp.125–150). London: Psychology Press.

Sanger, D., Creswell, J.W., Dworak, J., & Schultz, L. (2000). Cultural analysis of communication behaviors among juveniles in a correctional facility. *Journal of Communication Disorders, 33*, 31–57.

Schilling, E.A., Aseltine, R.H., & Gore, S. (2007). Adverse childhood experiences and mental health in young adults: A longitudinal survey. *BMC Public Health, 7*(30). doi:10.1186/1471-2458-7-30

Snow, P.C. (2009). Child maltreatment, mental health and oral language competence: Inviting Speech Language Pathology to the prevention table. *International Journal of Speech Language Pathology, 11*(12), 95–103.

Snow, P.C. & Powell, M.B. (2004). Developmental language disorders and adolescent risk: A public-health advocacy role for speech pathologists? *International Journal of Speech Language Pathology, 6*(4), 221–229.

Snow, P.C. & Powell, M.B. (2008). Oral language competence, social skills, and high risk boys: What are juvenile offenders trying to tell us? *Children and Society, 22*, 16–28.

Snow, P. & Powell, M. (2011). Oral language competence in incarcerated young offenders: Links with offending severity. *International Journal of Speech-Language Pathology, 13*(6), 480–489.

Snow, P.C. & Sanger, D.D. (2011). Restorative justice conferencing and the youth offender: Exploring the role of oral language competence. *International Journal of Language and Communication Disorders, 46*(3), 324–333.

Snow, P.C. & Woodward, M.N. (2016). Intervening to address communication difficulties in incarcerated youth: A Phase 1 Clinical Trial. *International Journal of Speech Language Pathology*. Released early online October 8, 2016.

Snow, P.C., Bagley, K., & White, D. (2017). Speech-language pathology intervention in a youth justice setting: Benefits perceived by staff extend beyond communication. *International Journal of Speech Language Pathology*. Released early online March 15, 2017.

Snow, P.C., Powell, M.B., & Sanger, D.D. (2012). Oral language competence, young speakers and the law. *Language, Speech & Hearing Services in Schools, 43,* 496–506.

Snow, P.C., Sanger, D.D., Caire, L., Eadie, P., & Dinslage, T. (2015). Improving communication outcomes for young offenders: A proposed Response to Intervention framework. *International Journal of Language and Communication Disorders, 50*(1), 1–13.

Snow, P.C., Woodward, M., Mathis, M., & Powell, M.B. (2015). Language functioning, mental health and alexithymia in incarcerated young offenders. *International Journal of Speech Language Pathology, 18*(1), 20–31.

Snowling, M.J., Adams, J.W., Bowyer-Crane, C., & Tobin, V. (2000). Levels of literacy among juvenile offenders: The incidence of specific reading disabilities. *Criminal Behaviour and Mental Health, 10*(4), 229–241.

Spencer, S., Clegg, J., & Stackhouse, J. (2012). Language and social disadvantage: A comparison of the language abilities of adolescents from two different socio-economic areas. *International Journal of Language & Communication Disorders, 47*(3), 274–284.

Stewart, A., Dennison, S., & Waterson, E. (2002). Pathways from child maltreatment to juvenile offending. *Trends and Issues in Crime and Criminal Justice,* No. 241, Canberra: AIC.

Talbot, J. (2010). Prisoners' voices: Experience of the criminal justice system by prisoners with learning disabilities. *Tizard Learning Disability Review, 15,* 33–41.

Tomblin, B., Records, N.L., Buckwalter, P., Zhang, X., Smith, E., & O'Brien, M. (1997). The prevalence of specific language impairment in kindergarten children. *Journal of Speech, Language and Hearing Research, 40,* 1245–1260.

Vacca, J.S. (2008). Crime can be prevented if schools teach juvenile offenders to read. *Children and Youth Services Review, 30,* 1055–1062.

Weisleder, A. & Fernald, A. (2013). Talking to children matters: Early language experience strengthens processing and builds vocabulary. *Psychological Science, 24*(11), 2143–2152.

Wiig, E., Semel, E., & Secord, W.A. (2017). *Clinical Evaluation of Language Fundamentals* (5th edition). London: Pearson.

Williams, W.H., Cordan, G., Mewse, J., Tonks, J., & Burgess, N.W. (2010). Self-reported traumatic brain injury in male young offenders: A risk factor for re-offending, poor mental health and violence? *Neuropsychological Rehabilitation, 20,* 801–812.

Willingham, D. (2012). Why does family wealth affect learning? *American Educator,* Spring, 33–39.

Wilson, J. (1989). *On the Boundaries of Conversation.* Oxford: Oxford University Press.

Wong, T.M.L., Slotboom, A., & Bijleveld, C.C.J.H. (2010). Risk factors for delinquency in adolescent and young adult females: A European review. *European Journal of Criminology, 7*(4), 266–284.

5 Teenagers' communication and their mental health

Judy Clegg

Learning outcomes

This chapter will enable readers to:

1. Describe the importance of adolescence in a young person's psychosocial adjustment and the implications of this for their wellbeing and mental health

2. Discuss specific challenges of adolescence for young people with SLCN and the impact of SLCN on meeting these challenges

3. Apply theoretical frameworks to understand the challenges of adolescence for young people with SLCN and how these can inform effective intervention and support.

Introduction

There is an increasing awareness and interest in the wellbeing and mental health of children, young people and adults with speech, language and communication needs (SLCN). Individuals with SLCN are known to be at risk of difficulties in their educational engagement and attainment, their employability, their friendships and relationships and their overall mental health and wellbeing. These individuals have complex needs, and although we know more about their needs in childhood we know much less about how these individuals manage the challenges of adolescence and negotiate their way through this transition phase into adult life. Adolescence is an important stage for wellbeing and mental health. However, the potential impact of SLCN on this stage is not well understood.

This chapter views SLCN as both primary and specific impairments and as part of other developmental disorders such as learning disability and autism spectrum disorders (ASD). The main focus of this chapter is exploring the challenges of adolescence for young people with SLCN and the implications of this for their psychosocial adjustment and wellbeing and mental health.

Adolescence

Adolescence is a fundamental transition stage between childhood and maturity. At the end of adolescence, society expects young people to be independent individuals who have developed sufficient maturity and responsibility to learn to drive, enter employment and be financially independent. Emotional turmoil, upheaval and storminess are historically associated with adolescence (Hall, 1904) but this has been substantially challenged over the years (Arnett, 1999; Offer & Shabshin, 1966, 1969). Nevertheless, adolescence is characterized by important changes in the young person's internal and external experiences. The dynamic interplay between these internal and external factors is considered crucial in the effective psychosocial adjustment necessary for entry into adult life.

Adolescence as a developmental stage

Internal or developmental changes are those that are intrinsic to the young person and include *biological changes, changes in brain development* and subsequent *functional* changes in cognition. In contrast, external or social changes are extrinsic to the young person and encapsulate the changes in the young person's environment as he/she moves into adolescence where there are substantial and influential changes in society's expectations of the young person.

With respect to internal changes, the main *biological* factor is the hormonal changes that occur with puberty. This is a time of rapid physical and sexual development with associated emotional development. *Biological* also encapsulates changes in brain development and structure, and is a recent theoretical development in how we understand adolescence. Research confirms the continuing development of brain structures such as the frontal lobes and the limbic system (see useful reviews by Blakemore & Choudry, 2006; Tamnes, Herting, Goddings, et al., 2017; Walker, 2002). The continuing development of these structures in adolescence is important as this is associated with further functional development in cognition. For example, increased activation of the prefrontal cortex is associated with higher level cognition and cognitive control needed for aspects of executive function such as attention and impulsivity control. Further development or maturation of the limbic system is associated with social cognition such as understanding the perspectives of others and being empathic. The resulting functional development then enables the young person to manage adolescence, for example making informed and effective decisions, controlling their own behaviour and managing the demands of complex peer relationships.

In addition to these cognitive changes, language and communication abilities are also considered as a further *functional* change where language and communication skills continue to develop in adolescence (Nippold, 2007). Although not surprising now, it was not long ago that we considered language and communication development to be complete by the end of childhood. It must be noted these changes are not yet linked to specific brain structures although it is plausible that the further maturation of the brain structures previously discussed could be involved. The important point is the continued brain development and neurodevelopmental change in adolescence with associated functional outcomes that impact on how the young person can negotiate the adolescent stage.

External factors are defined by changes in society's expectations of the young person as they leave childhood and enter adolescence. Responsibility shifts to the young person and away from the parent/carer. The young person is expected to manage the demands of complex peer groups and relationships and the structures that support the young child change in adolescence (for example, the change from primary school to secondary school).

It is the dynamic interplay between the internal developmental changes and the external social changes that are now considered. For example, the brain development and neurodevelopmental changes that result in more developed social cognition abilities are needed for the young person to engage in more complex peer groups. The changes in teaching style at secondary school are reliant on the young person's higher-level language development and so together these should enable the young person to be an effective learner. This dynamic interplay is essential to the young person managing the demands of adolescence. Language and communication ability is an integral component in this dynamic interplay.

The challenge is understanding the adolescent experience for young people who do not move through a trajectory of what we understand as typical adolescent development. Very little is known about the adolescence of young people who have developmental difficulties or disorders where SLCN are an integral component of their difficulties. Considering the internal and external factors within a demands and capacities framework offers a way to understand the challenges these adolescents may experience and why adolescence can be a risk factor for these individuals in their overall psychosocial adjustment, wellbeing and mental health as they move towards and enter adult life.

Adolescence and mental health

Research confirms an increase in mental health difficulties in the adolescence period for all teenagers. The increase is specifically associated with the adolescent period where there are significant changes in the rate and pattern of psychopathology (see Rutter, 2007, for an in-depth and very informative review).

Mental health is a positive term used to refer to a state of psychological wellbeing (Pilgrim, 2009). Psychological wellbeing has proved hard to define but broadly refers to a positive state of being which enables the person to engage effectively in their everyday life as he or she wishes to. A mental health difficulty is another term for mental disorder or psychopathology, which are medical/psychiatric terms to describe atypical behaviour and/or psychological patterns that cause distress and/or disability.

Mental health difficulties in adolescence usually have the same or similar symptomatology to those in adult life. A basic distinction is made between subjective symptoms and objective symptoms. Subjective symptoms are those that the person reports and are not easily observable, e.g., the person reports feeling sad or down. Objective symptoms are those that can be observed in the person, e.g., a reduction in the person's energy or a change in their everyday activity. These subjective and objective symptoms result in a functional disturbance or a significant change to the person and their everyday life and are then defined as a mental disorder or mental health difficulty, usually when any physical or medical causes have been excluded. A further historical distinction is made between neuroses and psychoses. Neuroses is a long-standing term used to describe mental health difficulties where the person's symptoms are considered understandable but are more excessive or severe than usual but the person maintains an insight into these symptoms and is aware of them. The term psychoses involves symptoms where the person loses contact with reality and the symptoms are not easily understandable, for example experiencing hallucinations and delusions. In psychoses, the person is considered not to have insight into their symptoms.

More common mental health difficulties include anxiety and depression. Anxiety is a normal phenomenon but when excessive and/or severe it is considered a mental health difficulty. Anxiety is a symptom of many mental health difficulties, for example depression. It is characterized by symptoms in three domains: apprehension (feeling tense, restless and finding it difficult to attend and concentrate); motor tension (being overly sensitive to noise and other stimuli and experiencing frequent headaches); and autonomic over-activity (these are the symptoms associated with the 'fight or flight' response such as sweating and feeling dizzy). Insight is maintained. Depression is a mood disorder and characterized by biological or somatic symptoms (disruption to sleep, weight loss, a slowness or increased motor movement), and symptoms of mood (sadness and a loss of interest and energy) and cognition (poor concentration and feelings of guilt, worthlessness, hopelessness and suicidal thought). Insight is usually maintained. Psychoses are a more complex mental health difficulty where the person is described as experiencing a loss of contact with reality. The person experiences hallucinations (seeing visions, hearing voices and smelling scents that no one else can) and delusions (believing something that no one else does) and experiencing thought disorder (disruptions to thinking that are not logical and are observed through the person's spoken language/talking). Insight is usually not maintained. It is beyond the scope of this chapter to give a detailed account of mental health difficulties, so the following accessible resources are recommended (Davies & Craig, 2009; Pilgrim 2009).

In the typically developing population, adolescence is associated with an increase in mental health difficulties such as depression, antisocial and subsequent criminal behaviour, schizophrenia and attempted suicide/suicide. There is a considerable increase in depression in adolescence, with females more affected than males, a pattern that is consistent beyond adolescence into adult life but not observed in childhood (Glowinski et al., 2003; Hankin et al., 1998). Convictions for criminal behaviour increase in adolescence and are understood as a consequence of earlier childhood physical aggression and defiant and oppositional behaviour (Colman et al., 2009; Moffitt et al., 2001). Attempted suicide rates increase in adolescence but are not maintained at such a rate in adult life (Kreitman, 1976). Although it is unusual to diagnose schizophrenia in children, these diagnoses increase in late adolescence (Gillberg et al., 1986). Rutter (2007) eloquently discusses the potential mechanisms or causal pathways to explain the complex interplay between biological, psychological and social factors that lead to this increase. For example, these include the hormonal changes leading to bodily changes, neurodevelopmental changes and the resulting psychological response to sexual changes and relationships within a context of increased social pressures brought about by academic expectations, social relationships and other stressors.

There is a 'prodromal' stage in adolescence considered as a precursor stage of serious mental illness, specifically psychoses as part of late adolescence-onset schizophrenia. This is a time in adolescence when the young person experiences vague or subtle symptoms of psychoses such as mild depressive feelings and an inability to manage everyday stressors. Research confirms associations between late adolescence-onset schizophrenia and earlier developmental disorders, specifically those involving significant impairments in cognition and language development. Research proposes that the neurodevelopment that typically takes place in adolescence is in some way impacted upon by the earlier unresolved neurodevelopmental disorders. Drug use and the adolescence life stressors are also implicated here. There are complex mechanisms or pathways operating here, so identifying a specific causal pathway is not feasible. However, research confirms adolescence as a sensitive period that increases susceptibility to mental health difficulties.

The process of diagnosis of mental health difficulties is challenged when the person is not able to fully describe their symptoms, particularly subjective symptoms such as feeling down or sad or worried or able to express verbally the hallucinations or delusions he/she may be experiencing. For young people with SLCN, it can be very challenging to accurately identify mental health difficulties when the process of diagnosis becomes more dependent on observing and identifying changes in their behaviour and everyday functioning rather than the adolescent being able to describe and explain their experiences and symptoms.

Teenagers with SLCN and their mental health

This section explores the specific issues of the adolescence of young people with developmental disorders, the specific challenges teenagers with SLCN can experience and the impact of SLCN on managing the challenges of adolescence.

Adolescence of young people with developmental disorders

Young people with developmental disorders are the children with labels of autism spectrum disorders (ASD), learning difficulties, primary or associated SLCN and others who have grown up into teenagers. Some will have attended special schools at primary school age and many will have attended mainstream provision with varying levels of support in place. A small proportion may never have fully engaged in any educational provision. SLCN continues to be an integral part of their overall needs. The same theoretical framework of internal and external factors is considered to understand their adolescent experience. The majority of these young people will experience the same internal and external changes but there may be specific groups who experience additional changes and challenges.

Internal factors

Most young people with developmental disorders will experience the *biological* process of puberty in the same trajectory as others. However, some young people with specific syndromes of learning difficulties do not have this experience. Noonan Syndrome is a genetic disorder and children with this disorder experience significant medical difficulties and significant delays in many aspects of their development. Hearing and speech is often affected as well as overall language and communication ability. Males with Noonan Syndrome have a delayed onset of puberty and often reduced pubertal growth leading to infertility in adult life (see van der Burgt, 2007, for a review). Klinefelter syndrome is a chromosomal disorder with a range of medical and associated developmental difficulties only affecting males. Young people with Klinefelter syndrome start puberty at the expected age but the process can be incomplete due to insufficient production of the hormone testosterone (see Groth, Skakkebaek, & Host, 2013, for a review). Turner Syndrome is a chromosomal disorder only affecting females with consequences for the process of puberty in adolescence. These young people have specific challenges around these internal changes as they are not experiencing puberty at the same onset and rate as others and this biological internal change will have significant implications for their adolescent experience (see Bondy, 2014, for a review). For those young people with developmental disorders who do experience a 'typical' biological process of puberty, the emotional aspects of puberty and sexuality are often challenging.

Neurodevelopmental changes in young people with developmental disorders are less well understood. Adolescence can be a developmental stage where the phenotype of learning difficulties changes (O'Brien, 2006). In Attention Deficit Hyperactivity Disorder (ADHD), the symptoms of hyperactivity can reduce in comparison to the inattentiveness and impulsivity (Hart, Lahey, et al., 1995; Resnick, 2005). In Fragile X Syndrome, the facial characteristics become more apparent in terms of how the young person looks (Hagerman, Turk, Schneider, et al., 2011). Such neurodevelopmental changes will impact on the challenges the adolescent will experience.

Language and communication ability as a *functional* cognitive change is important. Adolescence is considered a time when language and communication abilities slow down or plateau with little continued development. Language and communication development in Down syndrome plateaus at the end of childhood and early adolescence (Carr, 2011; Fidler & Daunhauer, 2011). In childhood, the strong communicative desire of children with Down syndrome is perceived as positive, yet in adolescence it is often viewed as problematic due to the 'over-friendliness', increasing these young people's vulnerability.

External factors

There are significant external or social changes for young people with developmental disorders. First of all, changes to the school system. Some individuals may continue in a special school system and others move away from a special school context to a mainstream one. As with all transitions there are significant changes, such as differences in institutional ethos, teaching style, school staff attitudes and expectations. Peer groups will become multiple and much more varied and expectations of the young person will change. Too much responsibility or too little responsibility can be assumed for the individual.

Ultimately, the dynamic interplay between the internal and external factors may cause particular issues for these young people where the demands of adolescence exceed the young person's capacities to manage the adolescence period effectively.

The specific challenges teenagers with SLCN can experience

Research studying the trajectories of children with SLCN into adolescence and adult life identifies SLCN as a risk factor for difficulties in emotional and behavioural functioning, psychosocial adjustment, wellbeing and mental health. Longitudinal studies are challenging to complete, so there are few of these studies following children up over the lifespan. The available studies focus on relatively small clinical populations and subsequently differ in terms of how the speech, language and communication difficulties of the original cohorts are identified and measured, the severity of the original speech, language and communication difficulties and how psychosocial adjustment, wellbeing and mental health are measured over time. Nevertheless, there is research evidence confirming the specific challenges this population experiences.

Teenagers and young adults with SLCN experience more bullying and have fewer friendships and relationships than their typically developing peers (Clegg, Ansorge, Donlan, & Stackhouse, 2012; Durkin & Conti-Ramsden, 2007; Knox & Conti-Ramsden, 2007; Mawhood, Howlin, & Rutter, 2000). Education is challenging with respect to securing appropriate educational provision and achieving within the school system with implications for educational outcomes (Clegg et al., 2012; Clegg, Hollis, Mawhood, & Rutter, 2005; Durkin, Simkin, Knox, & Conti-Ramsden, 2009). SLCN can prevent emotional wellbeing and effective psychosocial adjustment (Clegg et al., 2012; Conti-Ramsden & Botting, 2008). Adolescence is a developmental stage heavily influenced by childhood experiences. In a study of adults with persisting and severe SLCN who attended specialist residential provision, the adults and their parents expressed traumatic experiences of inappropriate educational provision in their early school careers and the negative impact of this on their children's emotional health and wellbeing despite being placed more appropriately in later childhood and adolescence (Clegg et al., 2012).

The impact of SLCN on managing the challenges of adolescence

How can we start to understand how SLCN fit into the frameworks we have discussed in terms of internal and external factors, and demands and capacities? Perhaps here we consider speech, language and communication development and ability as an internal factor linked to biological, neurodevelopmental and neurobiological changes but also an external factor in terms of the communication demands placed on the adolescent. This real case example aims to highlight the role language and communication can play.

Case example: Kaydie

Kaydie has recently turned 14 years of age. She has Turner Syndrome with associated hearing and communication needs and learning difficulties. As a consequence of the Turner Syndrome, Kaydie is very physically small for her age with people observing she is the height of a typical 6-year-old. She wears hearing aids and glasses. Kaydie is about to start some growth hormone treatment to initiate the onset of puberty. Kaydie is attending a mainstream school placement with support in an integrated resource. Kaydie has few friends and is often bullied due to how different she looks to her peers. Kaydie has two older siblings, 15 and 19 years of age, who regularly engage with social media. Kaydie also has a younger sibling. Kaydie is vulnerable around social media having previously posted a photograph of herself with no clothes on to one of her sister's friends on her sister's social media site. She has seen her older sister do this. The consequences of this were very difficult and safeguarding procedures put in place.

Due to various pressures in the family, Kaydie goes to respite foster care one weekend a month to enable her parents to spend quality time with her other siblings. At this foster care, there are two younger children who are 4 and 7 years of age. The placement is considered successful for a year but Kaydie becomes increasingly frustrated and requests not to go, saying the two children there are too 'babyish' for her. On one occasion, Kaydie takes her older sister's smart phone to the placement without the knowledge of her parents or the foster carers. Kaydie uses the smart phone to repeatedly text her older sister's friend with the same message saying, "hi ya missing you Kaydie". The friend is not empathic towards Kaydie, and by the end of the day she has posted via social media how 'stupid' and 'irritating' Kaydie is. This then leads to bullying at school the following week.

Kaydie wants to be part of her peer group but this is challenging due to Kaydie looking very different to them and not sharing the same experience of puberty as her peers do. She is expected to engage with much younger children on the foster care placement who developmentally may be at a similar level of communication and learning to her but her social needs are very different. Kaydie wants to be around her peers and engaging in teenage type activities and not going to the park or the soft play centre. The internal factors of her level of learning, not going through the physical process of puberty and so looking very different to her peers, her hearing, language and communication needs makes it difficult for her to understand and manage the external demands placed on her. Here, her desire to engage in teenage activities such as having a smart phone and engaging in social media and managing the expectations of the mainstream school placement is challenged.

Over a period of six months, the bullying intensifies and Kaydie starts to disengage from school. She becomes very anxious in the mornings complaining of stomach aches, feeling sick and being shaky. Her parents often keep her away from school, so her absences become concerning. At home, she becomes quiet and withdrawn and is very reluctant to leave the house. At a review appointment, a health professional starts to consider if Kaydie is struggling with anxiety and a low-level depression. This is based on changes to her behaviour as it is difficult for Kaydie to talk about and describe objectively how she is feeling.

Further to the internal and external changes, and demands and capacities, it is helpful to look to a more multifactorial model to explore and understand how SLCN are potentially involved in mental health difficulties.

Although sparse, research indicates that, for some children and young people with SLCN, the SLCN are in some way involved in the onset and maintenance of mental health difficulties in adolescence and adult life (Beitchman, Nair, Clegg, et al., 1986; Brownlie, Beitchman, Escobar, et al., 2004; Camarata & Gibson, 1999; Conti-Ramsden & Botting, 2008; Giddan, Milling, & Campbell, 1996; Yeh & O'Kearney, 2013). This is complex and there is no linear causal relationship between SLCN and mental health difficulties. There are no specific mental health difficulties that are clearly linked to specific types of SLCN. A wide range of mental health difficulties are reported in clinical studies of children and young people with SLCN ranging across ADHD, conduct disorders, social, emotional and behavioural difficulties, anxiety, and others. SLCN are often co-morbid with other developmental disorders where mental health difficulties feature.

From the above discussion, the complexity of the association between SLCN and mental health in adolescence is clear, highlighting how adolescents' development is multifactorial and interdependent. Therefore, a more dynamic approach is adopted whereby it is the interaction within development that needs to be more understood. A biopsychosocial or bioecological framework (Bronfenbrenner & Morris, 2006; Dodge & Petit, 2003) is informative here in identifying the role of within-child (biological), interpersonal (psychological) and environmental (social) factors in the association with an emphasis on the dynamic nature of how these factors interact at multiple levels through an adolescent's development.

A real case example is now used to illustrate these complexities.

Case example: Frank

Frank is 15 years of age and has a long-standing history of pervasive developmental disorders. He has diagnoses of language disorder, ASD, anxiety and psychoses with the labels of language disorder received in early childhood and the labels of ASD, anxiety disorder and psychoses in early adolescence. Frank was removed from his biological home before the age of 2 years and went to live with a family relative for a short period. This was not a successful placement and he has been in looked-after care in a series of foster care placements and then residential care for much of his life. He now lives in secure residential provision for young people with learning difficulties and mental health difficulties. Frank enjoys daily activities of some onsite school attendance, independent living skills such as supervised cooking and so on.

The professionals involved with Frank understand him as a very vulnerable young person. The diagnoses of language disorder, ASD, anxiety and psychoses are complex to understand in relation to Frank's everyday life. The challenge is understanding and differentiating the ASD behaviours from the psychoses symptoms. Frank is mostly nonverbal although he will sometimes say yes or no. He can use nonverbal means to communicate such as head nods for yes and no, pointing and showing others what he wants. Frank's behaviours of rocking, head banging and scratching his skin are understood as repetitive behaviours as part of his ASD diagnosis. However, these behaviours increase in both frequency and intensity and are accompanied by Frank withdrawing from others, so are now interpreted as part of Frank's anxiety. For example, when a new carer joins Frank's team or a relative comes to visit these behaviours increase.

At times, particularly in the past, Frank's behaviour has become very challenging: for example, trying to jump out of his bedroom window which is not on the ground floor; observed to be very agitated and scared when there is no clear cause or stimulus for this; being aggressive with others at times and refusing to eat and drink; and further withdrawal such as refusing to leave his bedroom. Here, the diagnosis of psychosis comes in where these behaviours are interpreted as Frank experiencing hallucinations and delusions. The introduction of antipsychotic medication significantly reduces these behaviours and Frank is able to engage in his usual activities. As Frank is nonverbal, there is no opportunity to observe changes to his language and/or any evidence of thought disorder so this complicates the diagnostic process.

A biopsychosocial model offers a framework to understand some of the complexity of Frank's needs. Taking the biological component first, research indicates that being a boy, early diagnosis of ASD and learning difficulties and a possible family history of learning difficulties in his biological parents all increase the risk of developing mental health difficulties in adolescence and adult life. The interpersonal component is very significant given Frank's early experiences of early and sustained neglect and reported physical abuse and removal from the biological home, subsequent foster placements and attachment difficulties and the impact of his ASD and delayed development in the attachment process. The environmental component is also significant here and refers to the social environment Frank has experienced, for example, residential provision, cared for by professionals, restrictions to his everyday life and opportunities.

The complexity is identifying and understanding the dynamic interactions between the biological, interpersonal and environmental not only in childhood but also in adolescence and the cumulative impact of this over time.

Frank is very vulnerable, and as he has moved through adolescence there are aspects of his development that have been considered. Frank has developed through the biological process of puberty at the usual onset and rate and he has been supported through this in terms of helping him to understand this from his own personal hygiene to his sexual understanding and behaviour. Frank is expected to become more independent and he will have to leave this provision when he is 18 years of age He has become more independent during this time and is able to go shopping, to the leisure centre, work in the onsite workshop and visit a family member, all with one-to-one support. Frank has experienced very challenging, and at times traumatic, events during his life. It is hypothesized that his response to this is expressed through his behaviour, which can be challenging, or a withdrawal from people. It has been imperative to constantly reinforce to Frank that he is safe in this provision and that he is kept safe. All of these aspects are considered within the context of Frank having ASD, learning difficulties, anxiety and psychoses. His care and provision has to meet his needs within this context of how he understands and relates to people, his ability to understand his environment, his anxiety where he will often have a high state of arousal and then times when he is experiencing psychoses.

The role of speech and language therapy was very much part of this multidisciplinary management of Frank. The overall aim of the SLT input was to enable Frank to be able to access and engage with all aspects of his provision. Communication is central to this and Frank and his carers and other professionals implemented an effective method of communication. At the core of this model is the role of a communication-friendly environment. All Frank's environments, whether in or outside the residential provision, are communication-friendly. Visual support is used consistently across environments and all staff are trained to simplify their language, understand Frank's nonverbal communication and identify behaviours that indicate increasing anxiety and psychoses. De-escalation techniques acknowledge Frank's limited communication as the language staff use with Frank during these times of agitation and aggression is simplified and again supported visually.

Summary and conclusions

This chapter has explored the complex associations between SLCN and psychosocial adjustment, wellbeing and mental health in adolescence. Theoretical frameworks of identifying the internal and external changes young people experience in adolescence as well as a biopsychosocial model has been applied to understand the adolescent experience of young people with SLCN as primary difficulties and as part of other developmental disorders. There is still much to learn about the impact of SLCN on the adolescent experience and how we can enable young people with SLCN to effectively meet the challenges of adolescence.

Reflective questions

1. Why is adolescence a particularly vulnerable time for mental health difficulties?

2. What support and/or intervention would you consider for Kaydie?

3. Can you apply a biopsychosocial model to a young person that you work with? How does this help to understand the potential complex and multifactorial relationships between their communication and mental health?

References

Arnett, J. (1999). Adolescent storm and stress reconsidered. *American Psychologist, 54*(5), 317-326.

Beitchman, J.H., Nair, R., Clegg, M., Ferguson, B., & Patel, P.G. (1986). Prevalence of psychiatric disorders in children with speech and language disorders. *Journal of the American Academy of Child and Adolescent Psychiatry, 40*, 75-82.

Blakemore, S.J. & Choudry, S. (2006). Development of the adolescent brain: Implications for executive function and social cognition. *Journal of Child Psychology & Psychiatry, 47*(3-4), 296-312.

Bondy, C. (2014). Recent developments in diagnosis and care for girls in Turner Syndrome. *Advances in Endocrinology*, Vol. 2014, Article ID 231089.

Bronfenbrenner, U. & Morris, P.A. (2006). The bioecological model of human development. In R.M. Lerner (Ed.), *Theoretical Models of Human Development. Volume 1 of the Handbook of Child Psychology, 6th ed.* (pp.993-1028). Hoboken, NJ: John Wiley & Sons.

Brownlie, E.B., Beitchman, J.H., Escobar, M., et al., (2004). Early language impairment and young adult delinquent and aggressive behavior. *Journal of the Abnormal Child Psychology, 32*, 453-467.

Camarata, S.M. & Gibson, T. (1999). Pragmatic language deficits in attention deficit hyperactivity disorder (ADHD). *Mental Retardation and Developmental Disabilities Research Review, 5*, 207-214.

Carr, J. (2011). Down Syndrome: Lifetime course and strategies for intervention. In P.A. Howlin, T. Charman, & M. Ghaziuddin (Eds), *The SAGE Handbook of Developmental Disorders*. London: Sage Publications.

Colman, I., Murray, J., Abbott, R.A., Maughan, B., Kuh, D., Croudace, T.J., & Jones, P.B. (2009). Outcomes of conduct problems in adolescence: 40 year follow-up of national cohort. *British Medical Journal, 338*, a2981.

Clegg, J., Ansorge, L., Donlan, C., & Stackhouse, J. (2012). Developmental communication impairments in adults: Outcomes and life experiences of the adults and their parents. *Language, Speech and Hearing Services in Schools, 43*(4), 521-535.

Clegg, J., Hollis, C., Mawhood, L., & Rutter, M. (2005), Developmental language disorders: A follow-up in later adult life: cognitive, language and psychosocial outcomes. *Journal of Child Psychology & Psychiatry, 46*, 128-149.

Conti-Ramsden, G. & Botting, N. (2008). Emotional health in adolescents with and without a history of specific language impairment (SLI). *Journal of Child Psychology & Psychiatry, 49*, 516-525.

Davies, T. & Craig, T. (Eds) (2009). *ABC of Mental Health, 2nd ed.* London: Wiley-Blackwell.

Dodge, K.A. & Petit, G.S., (2003). A biopsychosocial model of the development of chronic conduct problems in adolescence. *Developmental Psychology, 39*, 349-371.

Durkin, K. & Conti-Ramsden, G. (2007). Language, social behavior and the quality of friendships in adolescents with and without a history of specific language impairment. *Child Development, 78*, 1441-1457.

Durkin, K., Simkin, Z., Knoz, E., & Conti-Ramsden, G. (2009). Specific language impairment and school outcomes, II: Educational context, student satisfaction and post-compulsory progress. *International Journal of Language & Communication Disorders, 44*, 36-55.

Fidler, D.J. & Daunhauer, L. (2011). Down Syndrome: General overview. In P.A. Howlin, T. Charman, & M. Ghaziuddin (Eds), *The SAGE Handbook of Developmental Disorders*. London: Sage Publications.

Giddan, J.J., Milling, L., & Campbell, M.D., (1996). Unrecognised langage and speech deficits in preadolescent psychiatric inpatients. *American Jounral of Orthopsychiatry, 66*, 85-92.

Gillberg, C., Whalstrom, J., Forsman, A., Hellgren, L., & Gillberg, I.C. (1986). Teenage psychoses-epidemiology, classification and reduced optimality in the pre-, peri-, and neonatal periods. *Journal of Child Psychology & Psychiatry, 27*, 87-98.

Glowinski, A.L., Madden, P.A., Bucholz, K.K., Lynskey, M.T., & Heath, A.C. (2003). Genetic epidemiology of self-reported lifetime DSM-IV major depressive disorder in a population-based twin sample of female adolescents. *Journal of Child Psychology & Psychiatry, 44*, 988-996.

Groth, A.K., Skakkebaek, A., & Host, C. (2013). Klinefelter Syndrome. *Journal of Clinical Endocrinology & Metabolism, 98*(1), 20-30.

Hagerman, R.J., Turk, J., Schneider, A., & Hagerman, P.J. (2011). Fragile X syndrome – medical and genetic aspects. In P.A. Howlin, T. Charman, & M. Ghaziuddin (Eds). *The SAGE Handbook of Developmental Disorders*. London: Sage Publications.

Hall, G.S. (1904). Adolescence: Its psychology and its relations to physiology, anthropology, sociology, sex, crime, religion and education (Vols I & II). Englewood Cliffs, NJ: Prentice-Hall.

Hankin, B.L., Abramson, L.Y., Moffit, T.E., Silva, P.A., McGee, R., & Angell, K.E. (1998). Development of depression from preadolescence to young adulthood: Emerging gender differences in a 10-year longitudinal study. *Journal of Abnormal Psychology, 107*, 128-140.

Knox, E. & Conti-Ramsden, G. (2007). Bullying in young people with a history of specific language impairment (SLI). *Educational and Child Psychology, 24*, 130-141.

Kreitman, N. (1976). Age and parasuicide ('attempted suicide'). *Psychological Medicine, 6*, 113-121.

Mawhood, L., Howlin, P., & Rutter, M., (2000). Autism and developmental receptive language disorder: A follow-up comparison in early adult life. II: Social, behavioural and psychiatric outcomes. *Journal of Child Psychology & Psychiatry, 41*, 561-578.

Moffitt, T.E., Caspi, A., Rutter, M., & Silva, P.A. (2001). *Sex Differences in Anti-social Behavior: Conduct Disorder, Delinquency and Violence in the Dunedin Longitudinal Study*. Cambridge: Cambridge University Press.

Nippold. M., (2007). *Later Language Development: School Age Children, Adolescents and Young Adults, 3rd ed*. Austin, Texas: Pro-Ed.

O'Brien, G. (2006). Behavioural phenotypes: Causes and clinical implications. *Advances in Psychiatric Treatment, 12*, 338-348.

Offer, D. (1969). *The Psychological World of the Teenager*. London: Basic Books.

Offer, D. & Sabshin, M. (1966). *Normality: Theoretical and Clinical Concepts.* London: Basic Books.

Pilgrim, D. (2009). *Key Concepts in Mental Health.* London: Sage Publications.

Resnick, R.J. (2005). ADHD in teens and adults: They don't all outgrow it. *Journal of Clinical Psychology, 61*(5), 529-533.

Rutter, M., (2007). Psychopathological development across adolescence. *Journal of Youth & Adolescence, 36,* 101-110.

Tamnes, C.K., Herting, M.M., Goddings, A., et al. (2017). Development of the cerebral cortex across adolescence: A multi-sample study of interrelated longitudinal changes in cortical volume, surface area and thickness. *Journal of Neuroscience.* doi:10.1523/ JNEUROSCI.3302-16.2017

Van der Burgt, I. (2007). Noonan Syndrome. *Orphanet Journal of Rare Diseases, 2,* 4.

Walker, E.F. (2002). Adolescent neurodevelopment and psychopathology. *Current Directions in Psychological Science, 11*(1), 24-28.

Yeh, S.G. & O'Kearney, R. (2013). Emotional and behavioural outcomes in later childhood and adolescence for children with specific language impairments: Meta-analyses of controlled prospective studies. *Journal of Child Psychology & Psychiatry, 54,* 516-524.

Part II

Interventions for adolescents with language disorders

6 Interventions for grammar for adolescents with Developmental Language Disorder (DLD)

Susan Ebbels and Sarah Spencer

Learning outcomes

This chapter will enable readers to:

1. Present the rationale for delivering specialist interventions for grammar for adolescents with Developmental Language Disorder (DLD, often previously referred to as Specific Language Impairment, SLI)

2. Describe explicit approaches to grammar interventions (the SHAPE CODING™ system, the MetaTaal intervention programme and sentence-combining techniques) as well as principles of implicit grammar instruction

3. Summarize the evidence base for interventions aiming to increase comprehension and production of targeted grammatical structures for adolescents with DLD.

Introduction

This chapter presents information on interventions for grammar for adolescents with DLD. Many adolescents with DLD continue to have difficulties with both production and comprehension of many aspects of grammar, including verb morphology (e.g., van der Lely & Ullman, 2001), verb argument structure

(Ebbels, Dockrell, & van der Lely, 2012), sentences with more complicated structures such as passives (e.g., van der Lely, 1996) and some '*wh*'-questions (e.g., van der Lely & Battell, 2003), and with complex sentences involving embedded clauses where they produce shorter and less complex sentences when compared to peers without DLD (Bishop & Donlan, 2005; Marinellie, 2004; Nippold, Mansfield, Billow, & Tomblin, 2008, 2009; Scott & Windsor, 2000; Ward-Lonergan, Miles, & Anderson, 1999). These difficulties may well affect their ability to communicate clearly and efficiently, understand classroom instructions, curriculum content and academic texts. This could result in reduced social participation and academic achievement. Thus, it is important that adolescents are supported and provided with intervention to maximize their use and understanding of grammar.

Interventions for grammar ultimately aim to enable adolescents with DLD to understand and communicate more complex ideas using more effective language structures (Nippold et al., 2009). Such interventions often target features of complex syntax, although some adolescents with DLD may still have difficulties with aspects of grammar at the single clause level. A number of therapy approaches have been put forward to work on grammar, including explicit approaches such as: (a) the SHAPE CODING™ system developed at a specialist school and college in the UK; (b) The MetaTaal intervention programme, which was developed in the Netherlands and uses Lego® bricks to represent words; and (c) sentence-combining methods. Also, implicit approaches such as modelling and recasting, which have been shown to be effective for some groups of younger children, have been recommended for older children, perhaps in combination with more explicit methods (e.g., Eisenberg, 2013; Scott 2004). These approaches will now be described in Part I, before examining the evidence base for grammar interventions for adolescents with DLD in Part II.

Part I: Therapy approaches to supporting grammar

Explicit approaches to intervention for grammar

The SHAPE CODING™ system

The Shape Coding system is a meta-linguistic therapy approach which uses a combination of shapes, colours, arrows and lines to indicate phrases, parts of speech and morphology respectively (Ebbels, 2007). The Shape Coding system was developed by the first author of this chapter (SE) at Moor House School & College, a specialist centre in the UK for children with language disorders aged between 7 and 19 years. Within this context, there was a need for a visual system to support older children with language disorders with more complex syntactic structures than those usually targeted in younger children, such as *wh*-questions, passives, conjunctions, tense, aspect and noun-verb agreement (Ebbels, 2007). The Shape Coding system builds on other explicit approaches for teaching syntax to younger children using visual supports which colour code different parts of sentences (Colourful Semantics; Bryan, 1997; and the Colour Pattern Scheme; Lea, 1970), but aims to teach more complex aspects of language than is possible with these other systems and hence may be more useful for adolescents. It is not a prescriptive intervention programme, but rather a tool to help professionals make grammatical rules visual and explicit when providing grammatical intervention.

The Shape Coding system has four main components: (1) shapes (for phrases, such as Noun Phrase, Verb Phrase, Adjective Phrase) which are linked with questions such as 'who', 'what doing', 'what like' and 'how feel'; (2) colours (for parts of speech); (3) arrows (for verb tenses); and (4) single/double lines (for marking singular and plural).

Shapes

Each shape groups words into phrases which answer a question such as 'who', 'where', 'what doing' (see Figure 6.1).

- Ovals and rectangles are used for Noun Phrases (NPs) and answer the questions 'who' or 'what' (ovals are used for Noun Phrases which are external arguments, usually subjects in active sentences, while rectangles are used for Noun Phrases in all other positions, which 'belong' inside other shapes).

- Clouds are used for Adjective Phrases and answer the questions 'what like' or 'how feel'.

- Semi-circles answer the question 'where' and usually involve a Prepositional Phrase, including both a preposition and a Noun Phrase (coded in a rectangle, answering 'who' or 'what').

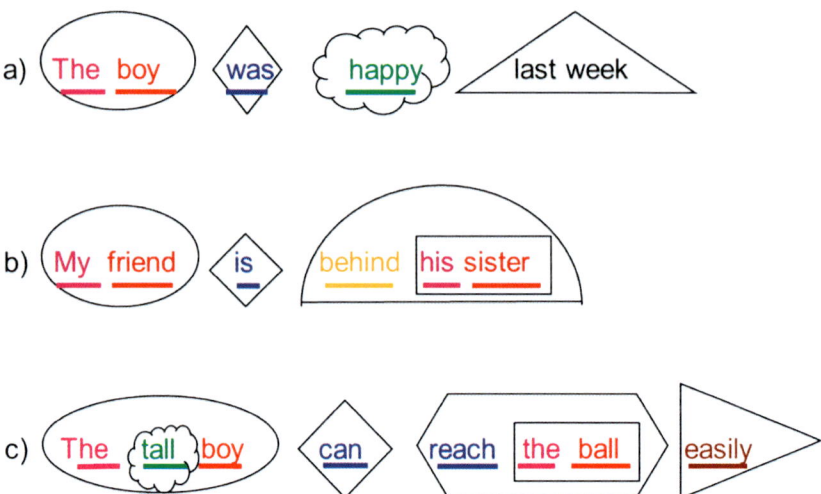

Figure 6.1 Examples of the Shape Coding system applied to simple sentences.

- Hexagons are used for Verb Phrases and answer the question 'what doing'.
- Diamonds are used for auxiliaries (e.g., *be*, *is*, *do*, *has*, *did*), copulas (e.g., *is*, *are*) and models (e.g., *can*, *could*, *will*, *would*, *may*). These are kept separate from the main verb, because they move to the front during question formation in English.
- Triangles answer the question 'when'.
- Flags answer the question 'how'.

While particular colour words are required in some shapes (e.g., a red word/ Noun is required in an oval/NP), in others, such as the shape for 'when', a range of words can appear. In most shapes, other words can also appear in addition to the one with the required part of speech. Colours may not always be used as this can be too confusing, especially when lots of words are included; in this case the words may just be shown in black and white. The sentences in Figure 6.1 are simple sentences, but the same patterns could also be used for complex sentences with each shape containing many words. Figure 6.2 shows the same basic patterns but applied to complex sentences. Here the colours are not used, nor the internal structure, as the aim is to show the overall meaning of the sentence. However, colours and additional internal shapes could be included, if desired.

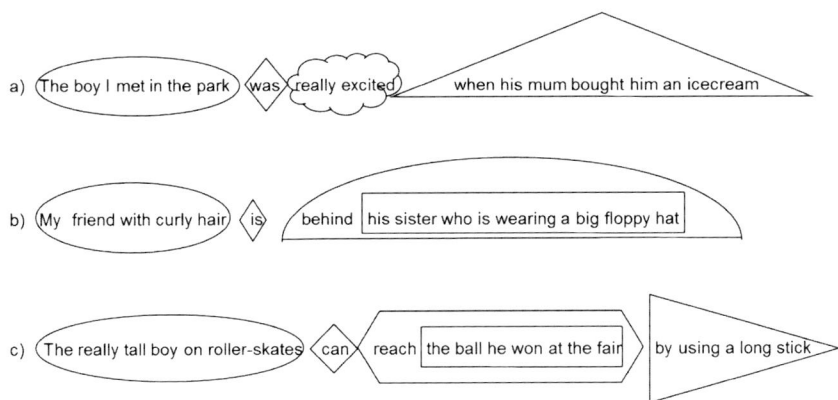

Figure 6.2 Examples of Shape Coding applied to complex sentences.

Colours

Colours are used for parts of speech and are associated with particular shapes.

- Red = Nouns and pronouns (e.g., *cat, table, boy, I, me*), required in ovals and rectangles (NPs).

- Pink = Determiners and possessive pronouns (e.g., *the, a, my*), may appear with 'red words' in ovals and rectangles (NPs).

- Blue = Verbs. This includes main verbs (e.g., *skip, smile*), required in hexagons (VPs) and also auxiliaries, copulas and modals (e.g., *be, is, are, do, did, has, can, could, will, would, may*) which appear in diamonds (and move to the front in English question formation).

- Green = Adjectives (e.g., *tall, happy*), required in clouds (APs).

- Yellow = Prepositions (e.g., *in, through, behind*), usually appear together with rectangles in semi-circles (PPs).

- Brown = Adverbs (e.g., *quickly, fast*), appear in flag.

- Purple = Coordinating conjunctions (e.g., *and, but, or*).

- Orange = Subordinating conjunctions (e.g., *because, when, if*).

Arrows

Verb morphology is indicated by underlining verbs (in blue) and using arrows (see Figure 6.3). Tensed verbs have vertical arrows: present tense verbs have the vertical arrow in the middle of the line, past tense verbs have arrows at the left-hand side of the line. The present participle has a zigzag under '*-ing*' to represent that it is continuous. Adolescents are taught that every sentence must have 'a down arrow' (i.e., a tensed verb).

Lines for singular and plural

Noun–verb agreement is shown in Shape Coding by using double lines under plural nouns and verbs and single lines under singular nouns and verbs (see Figure 6.4). This helps avoid errors such as 'the men is walking', as the noun and verb must match in terms of single or double lines. If there is a double line in the noun phrase (the red lines in the oval), the copula also requires a double line (the blue lines in the diamond). If there are two entities in the noun phrase oval (and hence two red lines in total, e.g., one under *man* and

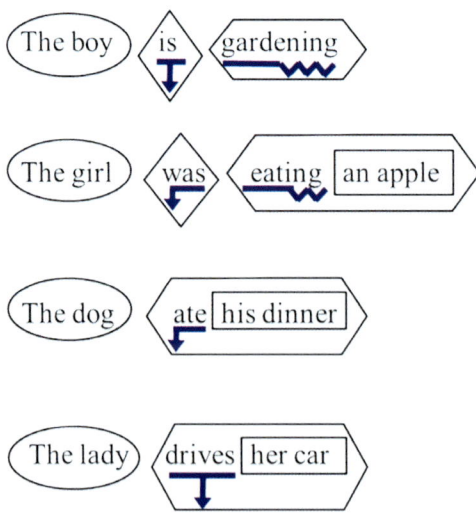

Figure 6.3 Example of Shape Coding applied for teaching verb tenses.

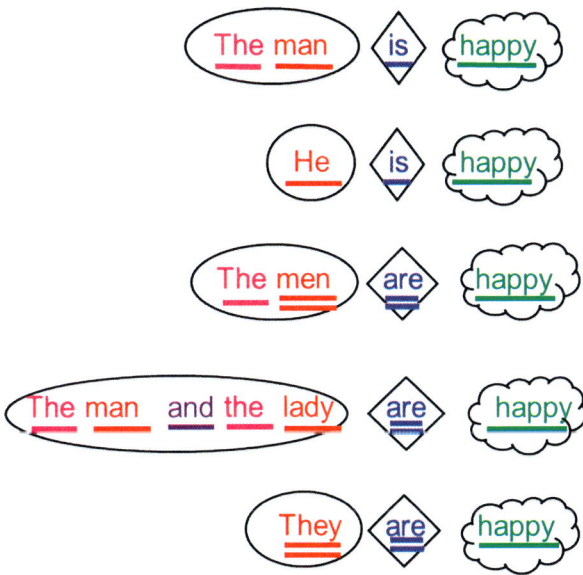

Figure 6.4 Examples of Shape Coding demonstrating noun–verb agreement.

one under *lady*) a double line is required under the verb. This can help prevent errors such as 'the man and the lady is walking' as the single line under 'is' doesn't match the two red lines in the oval.

The Shape Coding system is flexible and aims to be able to represent most English sentences visually (it could also be adapted for other languages). The system is also theoretically motivated, based on syntactic theory and fits well within theories of language disorders which stress the relative strength of declarative and visuo-spatial memories (Lum et al., 2012). The majority of evaluation studies of the Shape Coding system are small scale and have been conducted at Moor House School & College (see Part II for further information about these studies), which means that caution is required in generalizing results to children and adolescents attending other settings. However, preliminary analyses found no correlations between progress during interventions using the Shape Coding system and specificity of difficulties, nonverbal abilities or severity of language disorder, at least within the study participants, who all had severe language disorder (Ebbels et al., 2014) and therefore early findings suggest the method may be suitable for use with a range of adolescents with DLD.

The MetaTaal intervention programme

The MetaTaal intervention programme (developed for Dutch) uses Lego* bricks to represent words (Zwitserlood, Wijnen, van Weerdenburg, & Verhoeven, 2015). Differently shaped and coloured bricks are used to represent different word types. For example, red 2×3 bricks are used for verbs, green 1×2 bricks are used to represent determiners, blue 2×4 bricks are nouns. Zwitserlood et al. (2015) describe the programme within a paper evaluating its potential for increasing use and understanding of relative clauses (the evaluation is described in Part II below). The programme first introduces the concept that bricks can be used to represent words (a crib sheet with different bricks and words is provided, so there is no need to memorize the representations). Adolescents also identify different clause types and conjunctions in sentences. Then they are supported to build simple sentences (subject, verb, object) using the bricks, and next to add elements such as prepositional phrases, plural nouns and subject–verb agreement. The next step is to build coordinated sentences using an arched bridge brick (e.g., *the girl sat in the park and the girl read*), before creating truncated sentences by reducing the second main clause (e.g., *the girl sat in the park and read*). When the adolescent can create these 'bridging sentences', relative clauses are introduced (e.g., *the girl looks at the dog that chases the cat*). For these sentences, a bridge brick is put at right angles to the other bricks, so that the relative clause happens 'below' or at another level to the main clause (see Zwitserlood et al., 2015, for pictures). Conversations, short stories and pictures are used to elicit relative clauses during the intervention sessions. The use of bricks means that participants with poorer literacy skills can still access the intervention.

Sentence-combining

Sentence-combining includes a range of practical techniques for moving from simple sentences to compound and complex sentences, primarily in writing (Scott & Nelson, 2009). Nippold (2014b) recommends writing sentences on a computer and editing and combining them into complex sentences in partnership with the young person. The experience of creating complex sentences collaboratively means that adolescents have a model for how sentences can be information-rich and yet clear and efficient. In her approach to grammar interventions, Nippold recommends that this is combined with discussion around the topic, role playing, highlighting points of controversy, asking questions of peers. Reviews have reported this technique significantly improves the writing accuracy and quality of typically developing (TD) adolescents (e.g., Andrews et al., 2006; Graham & Perin, 2007). One study has recently been published investigating the effectiveness of a meta-linguistic method including sentence combining in adolescents with DLD (Balthazar & Scott, 2018). This is discussed in Part II below.

Implicit interaction strategies to support grammar

Research with young children with DLD has examined the role of implicit methods of intervention such as modelling and re-casting for targeting grammar, but the effectiveness of such strategies for supporting grammatical skills in adolescents has received little research attention (Ebbels, 2014).

Modelling

Modelling is a strategy that provides children with lots of examples of the targeted grammatical form. Modelling can be followed by asking the child to imitate the target or may be followed by evoked production, where the child is asked to follow the model with a new utterance applying the same rule as the model. Studies have suggested that modelling with evoked production potentially impacts on production of grammatical targets with primary school aged children (Courtright & Courtright, 1976; Weismer & Murray-Branch, 1989). However, further research is needed to investigate the effectiveness of modelling as a strategy for older children with DLD.

Recasting

When a child fails to use a target grammatical form or makes an error, an adult can immediately follow up with a corrected version (the recast). This can be done within activities which increase the likelihood of a child trying to use the grammatical form, including following modelling and evoked production (e.g., Gillam, Gillam, & Reece, 2012). While the evidence for recasting is strong (and includes a meta-analysis: Cleave, Becker, Curran, Van Horne, & Fey, 2015), the research evidence includes only young children. However, we hypothesize that recasting may have a positive impact on some adolescents' syntactic skills, particularly to increase and generalize use of recently-acquired forms. It seems sensible to ensure that teachers and family are aware of grammatical targets being worked on. If they are then given information on recasting strategies, they could provide opportunities for generalization of targeted grammatical forms into conversation and school work, though this would need to be carefully introduced and its effectiveness monitored.

Combination of explicit and implicit approaches

The combination of explicit instruction with modelling and recasting may be more effective than just one method alone, as suggested by Scott and Balthazar (2013). It is possible that the most effective intervention could use explicit methods to introduce new grammatical forms and concepts and then implicit methods, especially recasting, to focus on generalization (see Ebbels, 2014, for further discussion). Alternatively, the two approaches could be combined within each session, starting with explicit instruction and then moving to use of the new rule within an embedded activity or discourse (see Eisenberg, 2013). However, at present there is no evidence regarding how to best combine explicit and implicit methods for adolescents with DLD.

Part II Evidence-based practice to support grammar during adolescence

We now have some research evidence that grammar (and other) interventions for adolescents can be effective and this evidence base is growing (e.g., Ebbels, Wright, Brockbank, Godfrey, Harris, et al., 2017). This is particularly encouraging in a context of wider concern over the lack of robustly evaluated interventions for children and adolescents with DLD, and in particular those with receptive difficulties (Boyle, McCartney, O'Hare, & Law, 2010; Law et al., 2004). The following sections build on an earlier piece of work (Ebbels, 2014) which examines the effectiveness of grammar interventions for school-aged children. Here we look in more detail at interventions focusing on grammar for students with DLD in secondary schools.

As concerns intervention studies focusing on grammar with adolescents with DLD, we are aware of only eight studies, which are listed in the appendix (ordered by the strength of their design). With the exception of Bishop et al. (2006), which focused on implicit learning via a computer (which was not effective), all of these studies focus on explicit approaches to grammar interventions. The following sections first consider intervention for grammar at a single clause level (verb morphology, verb argument structure, coordinating conjunctions within a single clause, passives and *wh-* questions) and then above the single clause level (complement clauses, relative clauses and subordinate clauses introduced with subordinating conjunctions).

Verb morphology

Children with DLD frequently make errors with verb morphology, both in terms of tense and agreement. They often omit third person singular *-s* and past tense *-ed* inflections (Rice, Wexler, & Cleave, 1995) or copula and auxiliary *be* and *do* (Kamhi, 2014). In terms of agreement, children with DLD frequently make errors of singular/plural agreement (Leonard et al., 2003), for example using 'is' with a plural subject, e.g., 'the boys is cooking'. Difficulties with these areas have been found in younger adolescents with DLD (Bishop, 1994; van der Lely, 1997; van der Lely & Ullman, 2001). Even in adulthood, young adults with a previous diagnosis of specific language impairment have difficulties in grammatical awareness tasks involving verb tense and agreement (Poll, Betz, & Miller, 2010).

We know of only one study which has focused on improving use of verb morphology in adolescents with DLD (reported in Ebbels, 2007). This focused on the use of the past tense in written language. A group of adolescents received a term of intervention using the Shape Coding system taught as a class in English lessons delivered collaboratively by speech and language therapist (SLT) and teacher. After the intervention they used a greater proportion of verbs with the required past tense forms than before intervention. Within-group variation showed that three participants did not show progress, but for the two who had another period of paired intervention with the SLT following the initial class work, their scores also then improved.

Although the Shape Coding system is frequently used to teach the concepts of subject-verb agreement, no studies have yet been published on the effectiveness of this.

Verb argument structure

Verb argument structure contains information regarding the syntactic behaviour of verbs and acts as the interface between verb semantics and syntax. It includes information about which participants in an event are obligatorily expressed and the syntactic positions in which they should appear. The importance of verb argument structure is shown in the examples below:

1(a) *the man is devouring

1(b) *the lady is putting the cup

1(c) *the girl is filling the water in the cup

1(d) *the boy is pouring the cup with water

2(a) the man is eating

2(b) the lady is dropping the cup

2(c) the girl is pouring the water in the cup

2(d) the boy is filling the cup with water

The pairs of sentences in 1 and 2 (a–d) have identical syntactic structures, but the verbs in 1(a–d) cannot appear in these structures. The verbs in 1(a) and 1(b) both require additional participants in the event to be expressed in the syntax, either in the object position (1a) or in a prepositional phrase (1b). These participants are optionally expressed with the verbs in 2(a) and (b). The participants in the *pouring* and *filling* events of (c) and (d) are assigned to the incorrect syntactic positions in 1, but the correct positions in 2. These verbs differ in whether they focus on a change of location (*pouring* focuses on the change of location of *the water*) or change of state (where *filling* focuses on the change of state of *the cup*, from not full to full). Some verbs (called alternating verbs), can appear with more than one argument structure. For example, *wipe* can occur in a change of location (*the girl is wiping the crumbs off the table*) or a change of state construction (*the girl is wiping the table*) and *give* can occur in a change of location (*the girl gave the cat to the baby*), or the ditransitive dative construction (*the girl gave the baby the cat*).

Studies have shown that children and adolescents with DLD omit more obligatory arguments (e.g., 'he is giving the ball') than peers of the same age (Thordardottir & Weismer, 2002), younger children who have the same length utterances (Watkins & Rice, 1994) or children who have the same vocabulary knowledge (Ebbels, 2005). Adolescents with DLD also make more errors than age and vocabulary controls in production of change of state verbs such as *filling*, but not change of location verbs such as *pouring* (Ebbels et al., 2012).

Children with DLD have been found to have difficulties understanding sentences containing the ditransitive dative argument structure, e.g., *the girl gave the baby the cat*, which they sometimes misinterpret as if the sentence were *the girl gave the baby **to** the cat* (van der Lely & Harris, 1990). Studies have also found limited use of this construction both by children (Thordardottir & Weismer, 2002) and adolescents (Ebbels, 2005) with DLD, with a strong preference for the prepositional form, e.g., 'the girl gave the cat to the baby'.

In terms of intervention focused on verb argument structure, the ditransitive dative argument structure was the focus of a small study with just three adolescents (reported in Ebbels, 2007) using the Shape Coding system to target comprehension. For two, the intervention was highly effective, leading to a change from 0 to 100% on comprehension of this form. For the third adolescent, the intervention was not effective, perhaps due to his weak auditory memory and the need to remember the order of three participants for this structure.

A larger intervention study with 27 adolescents (aged 11-16 years) with DLD (Ebbels, van der Lely, & Dockrell, 2007) focused on another area of verb argument structure: production of change of state verbs (e.g., *fill*), change of location verbs (e.g., *pour*) and alternating verbs (e.g., *wipe*) which can use both change of state and location forms. This study compared two intervention approaches: one using the Shape Coding system (called semantic-syntactic therapy in the study) and the other focusing on verb semantics. The progress on verb argument structure of adolescents in the groups receiving each of these approaches was compared with that of a control group who received the same amount of intervention but on a control area (targeting inferencing skills, which was not expected to improve verb argument structure), thus controlling for nonspecific factors. In order to distinguish the effects of the two interventions, the semantic therapy concentrated on the detailed meaning of the verbs but did not include these verbs in a sentence. The semantic-syntactic therapy included work only on the broad meaning of the verbs, such as whether the focus is on something changing or moving, but then used the Shape Coding system to link these broad verb meanings to syntactic constructions.

Both of the targeted intervention groups made progress with improved linking of verb arguments to the correct syntactic position, therefore reducing errors such as *she is filling the water into the glass*, whereas those receiving the control therapy (using the Shape Coding system) made no progress. Results also showed generalization beyond the nine taught verbs to nontaught verbs and progress was maintained three months after the intervention ceased. The lack of progress of the control group and the lack of progress on a control measure of morphological errors provided evidence that the intervention was responsible for the participants' gains on verb argument structure. Therefore, the study showed that both semantic and syntactic-semantic (using the Shape

Coding system) interventions were effective in improving the overall accuracy of verb argument structure in adolescents with severe DLD. However, it was not possible to distinguish the effectiveness of the two interventions or the effectiveness of a combination of the two.

Passives

Passive sentences do not follow the typical pattern of active sentences where the first noun (the Subject) is typically the Agent of the verb. In passive sentences, the Subject is usually the Patient (i.e., the participant having the action of the verb done to them); this would usually appear in the Object position in an active sentence. For example, compare the active sentence *the girl hit the boy* (where the Patient, the one being hit, *the boy*, is in the Object position), with the passive sentence *the boy was hit by the girl* (where the Patient is in the Subject position). With passive sentences, the Agent need not be expressed, e.g., *the boy was hit*; indeed, this makes it a particularly useful construction for when the Agent is not known, or when the speaker does not wish to state who the Agent was.

Typically developing (TD) children begin to use passive sentences from 3 to 4 years of age (Budwig, 1990) and they comprehend passives with action verbs at about 80% accuracy by 5 years of age (Hirsch & Wexler, 2006). However, older children and adolescents with DLD can continue to have difficulties understanding passive sentences (Bishop, 1979; Marshall, Marinis, & van der Lely, 2006; van der Lely, 1996; van der Lely & Harris, 1990).

We know of only two intervention studies involving adolescents which included work on passives. Ebbels and van der Lely (2001) carried out a multiple-baseline design with four participants and showed that intervention using the Shape Coding system improved the production and comprehension of passive sentences in three out of four participants. Passives were also included in the study by Bishop et al. (2006), where computerized intervention with acoustically modified speech and implicit learning was not shown to be effective.

Wh- questions

Wh- questions are formed using words such as *who, which, where, when* or *how* to specify the information required. Some example sentences and possible questions appear below.

3 The tall girl is eating the chocolate ice cream quickly in the garden

(a) Who/which girl is eating the ice cream?

(b) What/which ice cream is the tall girl eating?

(c) How is the tall girl eating the ice cream?

(d) Where is the tall girl eating the ice cream?

(e) What is the tall girl eating the ice cream in?

4 The white cat is bigger than the brown dog

(a) What/which cat is bigger than the brown dog?

(b) What/which dog is the white cat bigger than?

In a question about the subject of the sentence, see examples 3(a) and 4(a) above, the word order of the statement is maintained. However, when the question is about another part of the sentence, the word order is changed, with both the *wh-* word (or full phrase in the case of *which*) and the auxiliary/copula appearing before the subject and not in the position of the phrase they replace, see examples 3(b–e) and 4(b). This could make these sentences harder to understand and use. In English, when no auxiliary is available (as in the past tense), '*do* support' also has to be used for all non-subject questions. For questions in the past tense, the past tense form of *do* ('did') is used and the main verb appears as a bare stem with no tense, see examples 5(a–c) below. This makes non-subject questions even more complex as shown in examples 5(b) and 5(c).

5 The tall girl ate the chocolate ice cream last week

(a) Who/which girl ate the ice cream?

(b) What/which ice cream did the tall girl eat?

(c) When did the tall girl eat the ice cream?

Studies have shown that some children and adolescents with DLD have difficulty comprehending non-subject *wh-* questions, such as 3(b–e), 4(b), 5(b–c), where the word order is different from the original statement (Ebbels, 2007; Ebbels & van der Lely, 2001; Friedmann & Novogrodsky, 2011; Marinis & van der Lely, 2007). They also make errors when forming *wh-* questions, particularly object questions (Connell, 1986; Ebbels & van der Lely, 2001; Leonard, 1995; van der Lely & Battell, 2003). Errors include lack of auxiliary inversion, difficulties with 'do support' (both addition of 'do/did' in subject questions and omission in object questions), and double tense errors in past tense object questions, where they use the past tense form for the main verb instead of the bare stem (e.g., 'What did they drank?').

We know of only one intervention study (with only four participants) which focused on this area with adolescents with DLD (using Shape Coding; Ebbels, 2007; Ebbels & van der Lely, 2001). The first part of the intervention was reported in Ebbels and van der Lely (2001) and focused on comprehension and use of subject and object questions. This showed that comprehension of *which* object questions, such as 3(b), improved for those participants who had difficulties understanding these before intervention. Production of *wh-* questions in the past tense was particularly difficult for the four participants pre-intervention with the percentage of questions produced accurately pre-intervention for object questions near zero. All four participants made significant progress with intervention on production of subject questions, although this was only maintained for one participant. For object questions, only two made significant progress, and this was not maintained, indicating that this was an area which was particularly challenging for the participants. The second part of the study (reported in Ebbels, 2007) focused on comprehension of *wh-* comparative questions (e.g., *what is bigger than a cat?* versus *what is a cat bigger than?*) with two of the original four participants from Ebbels and van der Lely (2001). Both participants had particular difficulties with comprehension of non-subject questions (as in 4(b)) pre-intervention, but showed significant progress with intervention.

Coordination

Coordination involves the linking of two clauses or phrases by a coordinating conjunction such as *and, or,* or *but.* When coordinating clauses, the second clause is fully independent with a subject and a verb, such as *the woman walked her dog and her friend put the kettle on.* Coordinating conjunctions can also join phrases within single clauses. This can be done with a variety of phrase types, e.g., Adjective Phrases: *the ball is <u>red and blue</u>*; Verb Phrases: *the girl will <u>run or walk</u>*; Noun Phrases: *<u>the boy and the girl</u> are happy*; or Prepositional Phrases: *the cup is <u>on the table but not on the saucer</u>.*

Coordinating conjunctions are frequently used in classroom instructions and conversation, and any difficulties with these could therefore impact on functional comprehension and communication. Ebbels et al. (2014) showed that intervention using the Shape Coding system delivered by each participant's usual SLT improved comprehension of coordinating conjunctions within single clauses by adolescents with severe language disorders following four hours of individual intervention focusing on the comprehension of the conjunctions *but not, neither nor, not only but also*.

An example of how the Shape Coding system was used to help comprehension is shown in Figure 6.5. Crosses are used under some conjunctions to show that the following phrase is negative. Crucially, the phrase *not only but also* does not have any crosses and thus has a similar meaning to *and*. Each step of the intervention protocol was worked on until the SLT judged it was understood by the participant, before moving on to the next step. Due to differing levels of comprehension of the conjunctions pre-intervention, not all participants completed the programme during the four hours available. Despite this, the intervention was shown to be effective; participants receiving intervention made significantly greater gains than the waiting control group, who then also made progress when they received the intervention. The original

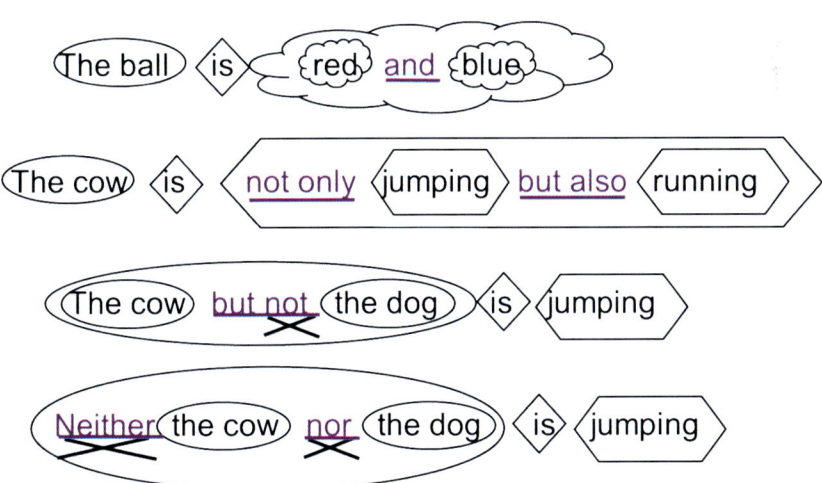

Figure 6.5 Examples of the Shape Coding system applied to coordinating conjunctions.

intervention group also maintained the progress they made for four months. There were also significant gains on a standardized test of grammar. However, progress didn't generalize to passives which have a different structure.

Complex sentences

Complex sentences involve two or more clauses with one clause functioning as the main clause and one (or more) functioning as subordinate clauses. Complex sentences can be formed by: (1) dependent clauses appearing as the subject or object of the sentence (known as complementation), e.g., *the woman thought it was sunny*; (2) with relative clauses modifying a noun, e.g., *the cat that is big pushed the dog*; or (3) by introducing subordinate clauses with subordinating conjunctions (also known as adverbial clauses), e.g., *I had a small hot chocolate, because it was cheaper*. Each of these is discussed in more detail in the sections below.

TD children begin to use early complex syntax very early, between 2-3 years (Diessel, 2004) and this develops in parallel with their acquisition of morpho-syntax at the single clause level, but then continues throughout adolescence (Frizelle, Thompson, McDonald, & Bishop, 2018).

Arndt and Schuele (2013) provide a table detailing studies showing that children with DLD have more difficulties than TD children with complex syntax, with more omissions of obligatory grammatical elements (e.g., *to* in infinitives, *that* in relative clauses), more limited range of complex syntax use with a more limited range of verbs and later emergence (between 3-4 years). Thus, these authors and others (e.g., Kamhi, 2014) argue that intervention should focus on production and comprehension of complex syntax from the preschool years onwards and should not wait for children to master basic clause structure and grammatical morphology (such as those areas discussed above) before targeting complex syntax.

Complement clauses

Complement clauses (also known as nominal clauses) are the earliest developing form of complex sentences (Diessel, 2004). These involve dependent clauses that serve as one of the arguments of the main clause verb, most commonly as the object (e.g., *the woman thought it was sunny*). Complement clauses occur most often with cognitive verbs referring to perception, desire and mental states and are often introduced by *that*, *whether* or *if* (e.g., *the woman hoped/noticed (that)/wondered whether/if her son was late*), communicative acts (e.g., *the girl said (that) she loves hot chocolate*) or states of being (e.g., *the girl let the hot chocolate go cold*). In all of these examples, the dependent complement clause is in the object position; however, it can also appear in the subject position (e.g., *that she liked hot chocolate bothered her dad* or *drinking hot chocolate can damage your teeth*). Complement clauses can also be introduced by a *wh-* word, which also has a role in the embedded clause (e.g., *I didn't understand what she was saying*).

The use of complement clauses starts young, in the third year of life (Diessel, 2004), with the range of uses increasing during childhood and adolescence (Nippold, Hesketh, Duthie, & Mansfield, 2005). A study of TD adolescents showed that those who use more meta-cognitive verbs also produce sentences which are longer and more complex (Sun & Nippold, 2012).

Adolescents with DLD have been shown to use fewer complement clauses than TD adolescents (Nippold et al., 2009). The study by Balthazar and Scott (2018) using sentence-combining techniques with adolescents with DLD included a focus on object complement clauses. However, they showed little effect on sentences including these, which they suggested could have been partly due to relatively high performance on these structures pre-intervention.

Relative clauses

A relative clause is a dependent clause that modifies and provides more information about a noun or noun phrase (the 'head' of the relative clauses) in an adjacent main clause. Relative clauses may modify the Subject of the main clause (e.g., *the cat that is big is pushing the dog*), or the Object (e.g., *the cat is pushing the dog that is big*). The relative clause may itself contain a Subject and an Object and the element of the main clause which is relativized, may be the Subject or Object of the relative clause (or indeed may take several other syntactic roles (Frizelle & Fletcher, 2015). De Villiers, Tager Flusberg, Hakuta, and Cohen (1979) give examples of each of these:

(1) *The cat (S) [that (S) bit the dog] chased the rat* (SS: Subject of main clause is Subject of relative clause)

(2) *The cat (S) [that (O) the dog bit __] chased the rat* (SO: Subject of main clause is Object of relative clause)

(3) *The cat bit the dog (O) [that (S) chased the rat]* (OS: Object of main clause is Subject of relative clause)

(4) *The cat bit the dog (O) [that (O) the rat chased ___]* (OO: Object of main clause is Object of relative clause)

When the Subject of the main clause is relativized, as in (1) and (2) above, the relative clause interrupts the main clause (these are often known as 'centre-embedded'). Where the Object of the main clause is relativized, as in (3) and (4) above, the relative clause appears after the end of the main clause (often known as 'right-branching'). Studies have found that TD children have more difficulties comprehending centre-embedded than right-branching relative clauses (Kidd & Bavin, 2002). Studies often distinguish between subject-relatives and object-relatives. Usually this refers to the role played in the relative clause where 'subject-relatives' follow the patterns in (1) and (3) and 'object-relatives' follow the pattern in (2) and (4).

Compared to complement clauses, relative clauses are infrequent in early child speech and particularly rare are centre-embedded relative clauses (like (1) and (2) above) that modify the Subject (Diessel, 2004). As concerns the internal syntax of the relative clause, subject-relatives are more common than object-relatives up until the age of 3;0, but by 4–5 years object-relatives are more frequently produced than subject-relatives (Diessel, 2004). However, development of use of relative clauses continues throughout childhood and increases significantly during adolescence (from age 13) and into adulthood (Nippold et al., 2005).

Relative clause comprehension and use is an area of difficulty for adolescents with DLD, particularly object-relatives (Friedmann & Novogrodsky, 2007; Novogrodsky & Friedmann, 2006; Riches, Loucas, Baird, Charman, & Simonoff, 2010). Two studies also found that adolescents with 'non-specific language impairment' (many of whom would probably now meet criteria for DLD) used fewer relative clauses in discourse and explanations than TD controls (Nippold et al., 2009; Nippold, Mansfield, Billow, & Tomblin, 2008).

A team in the Netherlands used the MetaTaal approach to teach production and comprehension of relative clauses to 12 participants with DLD aged between 9;3 and 12;8 years and found that the participants' ability to produce complex sentences containing relative clauses by combining short written sentences improved following twice weekly intervention for 5 weeks (Zwitserlood et al., 2015). Balthazar and Scott (2018) reported a similar finding after once or twice weekly intervention for 9 weeks using sentence-combining techniques. However, these findings appear to be limited to this specific task, as comprehension of relative clauses did not improve in Zwitserlood et al.'s (2015) study and use of complex sentences in written narratives did not improve in Balthazar and Scott's (2018) study.

A single case study has also been carried out in Hebrew (Levy & Friedmann, 2009) using methods similar to the Shape Coding system. This targeted comprehension and production of relative clauses (and topicalization) and measured progress on these and the related (but untreated area) of Object *wh-* questions. They found significant progress in comprehension, repetition, paraphrasing and production of object-relative clauses. They also found generalization to Object *wh-* questions.

A similar study has also been carried out investigating the effectiveness of the Shape Coding system for teaching comprehension of relative clauses. The results have not yet been fully analyzed or reported, but initial analyses indicate that, as in Zwitserlood et al. (2015), comprehension did not improve significantly. However, both studies tested comprehension using a choice of four pictures which Frizelle, O'Neill, and Bishop (2017) show is affected by factors other than syntactic competence. In particular, Frizelle and colleagues suggest that requiring children to rule out three alternative interpretations (presented in the distractor pictures) greatly increases the processing and working memory load and thus this assessment design increases the influence of non-syntactic factors. Therefore, the failure of both studies to show improved comprehension of relative clauses following intervention may be partly due to the design of the comprehension test. This could also account for why changes in production, but not comprehension, were found in the Zwitserlood et al. (2015) study.

Subordinate clauses introduced by subordinating conjunctions (adverbial clauses)

Subordinating conjunctions (such as *because, unless, if,* or *while*) can introduce subordinate clauses which are dependent on the main clause and often add information about time, purpose, conditionality, manner or place (often known as adverbial clauses). For example, *I had a small hot chocolate because it was cheaper.* Usually the main clause appears first, but the subordinate/adverbial clause can be pre-posed: *if you finish your peas, you can have pudding.*

Observational studies of typical development (e.g., Diessel, 2004) suggest that, by 3 years of age, a wide range of adverbial clauses are used appropriately and from 3 years onwards some adverbial clauses begin to be pre-posed, and the proportion increases until, by 5 years, a similar proportion is produced before and after the main clauses (although this does seem to vary with the conjunction used; Frizelle et al., 2018). From 8 years, use of adverbial clauses seems to be fairly stable. Indeed, Nippold et al. (2005) found that when giving explanations, the use of adverbial clauses by TD 8-year-olds was very similar to that of 44-year-old adults. However, for comprehension, experimental studies suggest that certain types of adverbial clauses are still not fully understood by 9 (Amidon, 1976) or even 11-year-olds (Murphy, Adams, Perovic, & Ebbels, in preparation).

As regards adolescents with DLD, Nippold et al. (2009) did not find that they differed from TD adolescents in their use of adverbial clauses in conversation or when giving explanations. However, given the poor performance of many children and adolescents on the Formulating Sentence subtest of the Clinical Evaluation of Language Fundamentals (Semel, Wiig, & Secord, 2006), which involves many adverbial clauses, and also the Concepts and Direction subtest which includes comprehension of adverbial clauses, this is often identified as a target by SLTs. Difficulties with use of adverbial clauses, such as those which encode causal information, could also have wider consequences than just for language production. Bishop and Donlan (2005) showed that the use of complex syntax was related to children's memory for events and suggested that children who do not encode causal information in a story may not form an integrated representation and the resulting series of fragmented details are more likely to be forgotten. Thus, limited use of complex syntax could have a potentially affect access to the school curriculum.

We are aware of only one published intervention study in this area at the time of writing (Balthazar & Scott, 2018). As with relative clauses, this study found progress in the ability to combine two written sentences into a complex sentence following sentence combining intervention, but no generalization to written narratives.

Conclusions

The goal of intervention programmes for grammar is to develop comprehension and production of a wider variety of sentence structures, reflecting the reality of academic demands during adolescence, which increases greatly in structural complexity. Indeed, Scott (2014) reported that only four out of 32 randomly chosen sentences in a seventh grade science book were not complex (i.e., contained only a single clause).

In this chapter, we have reviewed the evidence base for interventions for grammar with adolescents and have examined the key principles and therapeutic approaches used in intervention studies. There is increasing evidence that explicit interventions for grammar for adolescents with DLD such as the Shape Coding system, Metataal and sentence combining can be effective and result in improvements in production and, for the Shape Coding system, comprehension of grammar within a relatively short period of time. This is encouraging, particularly as earlier reviews (e.g., Cirrin & Gillam, 2008; Law, 2003) have found a lack of evidence for the effectiveness of speech and language therapy for adolescents with DLD.

While there is a growing body of evidence to support the implementation of interventions for grammar for adolescents with DLD, there is a need for much more information and research to inform clinical decisions. Future research should also investigate the implementation of intervention, including the ideal duration, frequency, distribution and amount of sessions for different grammatical targets, the relative efficacy of individual versus group sessions, the training needs of those delivering intervention (especially when delivered by non-SLTs), and the impact of working on multiple targets within one session or programme of intervention. While many questions remain, it is encouraging to see that the evidence base in this area in this area is growing and that it can be implemented to increase adolescents' use and understanding of grammar.

Reflective questions

1. Provide working descriptions/definitions of these terms:

(a) verb morphology

(b) relative clauses

(c) complex sentences

2. Think of a young person you know with DLD. How would you describe their grammar ability and difficulties?

3. There is now a growing body of evidence which demonstrates the impact of explicit grammar interventions for adolescents with DLD. How could you use this evidence base in your own work or study?

Appendix A

Studies targeting grammar in adolescents with DLD (adapted from Ebbels, 2014: pp.10–15)

Target	Reference	Number of participants	Age	Intervention programme	Delivery method	Design of evaluation	Duration of intervention	Outcome	Follow-up?	Progress generalized?
Production of verb argument structure	Ebbels et al., 2007	18 treatment and 9 controls	11;0–16;1	Shape Coding system	Direct 1:1	RCT design	1 × 30 minutes per week for 9 weeks. 4.5 hours in total	Both intervention groups improved significantly more than controls on verb argument structure. No progress on a control measure	After 3 months	To control verbs
Comprehension of coordinating conjunctions	Ebbels et al 2014	14 treatment (7 were waiting controls)	11;3–16;1	Shape Coding system	Direct 1:1	RCT: intervention vs. waiting control group	1 x 30 minutes per week for 8 weeks. 4 hours in total	Significant progress on targeted conjunctions	After 4 months	Yes to TROG-2 assessment, not to passives
Comprehension of reversible sentences (passives, comparatives and sentences including prepositions)	Bishop et al., 2006	24 (12 received treatment using modified speech, 12 treatment without modified speech) plus 9 controls	8–13 years	Acoustically modified versus unmodified speech	Computer 1:1	Two intervention groups plus control group; minimization method	1.5–7.25 hours	No differences between groups	n/a	n/a
Production of complex sentences (adverbials, object complement and relative clauses	Balthazar & Scott, 2018	30	10;10–14;11	Metalinguistic, including sentence combining	Direct 1:1	Multiple baseline	40-60 minutes once or twice a week for 9 weeks	Written sentence combining improved for adverbial and relative clauses for the majority of participants. No difference between the low and high dosage groups. No generalization to written narratives.	Not measured	Not to written narratives

Focus	Author	N	Age	System	Delivery	Design	Dosage	Outcome	Follow-up	Generalisation
Comprehension and production of wh-questions and passives formation	Ebbels & van der Lely, 2001	4	11–14 years	Shape Coding	Direct 1:1	4 case studies, multiple baseline design	2 × 30 minutes per week for 10 weeks for passives, 20 weeks for wh-questions	3/4 participants showed significant progress with comprehension and expression of passives. Two participants focussed on comprehension of wh-questions and made significant progress. All four focussed on production of wh-questions and made significant progress with Subject questions. 2/4 made significant progress with Object questions	At 30 weeks, progress maintained for 2/3 on passive comprehension and expression, 1/4 for production of wh-questions, 0/4 for production of Object questions.	Not measured
Comprehension of dative and wh-comparative questions	Ebbels, 2007	3	11;8 – 12;9 years	Shape Coding system	Direct 1:1	3 case studies, multiple baseline design	2 × 30 min per week for 10 weeks in total	2/3 children showed significant progress with dative, 2/2 progressed with wh-questions	Not measured	Not measured
Comprehension and production of relative clauses	Zwitserlood et al., 2015	12	9;3–12;8	MetaTaal	Direct 1:1	Single baseline	10 × 30 minutes twice a week for 5 weeks	Production of relative clauses via (written) sentence combining improved significantly with intervention. Elicited production (without written prompts) and comprehension of relative clauses did not improve.	After 3 months	Not measured
Use of past tense morphology in writing	Ebbels 2007	9	11–13 years	Shape Coding system	Direct group for 1:8, then 1:2 for two children	Pre- vs post-test score	1 hour per week for 16 weeks + approx. 4 hours for 2 children	6 children improved with group therapy; 2 improved only after additional paired therapy	Not measured	To spontaneous written work in class

References

Amidon, A. (1976). Children's understanding of sentences with contingent relations: Why are temporal and conditional connectives so difficult? *Journal of Experimental Child Psychology, 22*(3), 423-437.

Andrews, R., Torgerson, C., Beverton, S., Freeman, A., Locke, T., Low, G., Robinson, A., & Zhu, D. (2006). The effect of grammar teaching on writing development. *British Educational Research Journal, 32*(1), 39-55.

Arndt, K.B. & Schuele, C.M. (2013). Multiclausal utterances aren't just for big kids: A framework for analysis of complex syntax production in spoken language of preschool- and early school-age children. *Topics in Language Disorders, 33*(2), 125-139.

Bishop, D.V.M. (1979). Comprehension in developmental language disorders. *Developmental Medicine and Child Neurology, 21*, 225-238.

Bishop, D.V.M. (1994). Grammatical errors in Specific Language Impairment - Competence or performance limitations. *Applied Psycholinguistics, 15*(4), 507-550. Retrieved from <Go to ISI>://A1994QB51100004

Bishop, D. & Donlan, C. (2005). The role of syntax in encoding and recall of pictorial narratives: Evidence from specific language impairment. *British Journal of Developmental Psychology, 23*(1), 25-46.

Bishop, D.V.M., Adams, C.V., & Rosen, S. (2006). Resistance of grammatical impairment to computerized comprehension training in children specific and non-specific language impairments. *International Journal of Language & Communication Disorders, 41*(1), 19-40.

Boyle, J., McCartney, E., O'Hare, A., & Law, J. (2010). Intervention for mixed receptive–expressive language impairment: A review. *Developmental Medicine & Child Neurology, 52*(11), 994-999.

Bryan, A. (1997). Colourful semantics. In: S. Chiat, J. Law & J. Marshall (Eds), *Language Disorders in Children and Adults: Psycholinguistic Approaches to Therapy*. London: Whurr.

Budwig, N. (1990). The linguistic marking of nonprototypical agency: An exploration into children's use of passives. *Linguistics, 28*(6), 1221-1252.

Camarata, S.M., Nelson, K.E., & Camarata, M.N. (1994). Comparison of conversational-recasting and imitative procedures for training grammatical structures in children with specific language impairment. *Journal of Speech, Language, and Hearing Research, 37*(6), 1414-1423.

Cirrin, F.M. & Gillam, R.B. (2008). Language intervention practices for school-age children with spoken language disorders: A systematic review. *Language, Speech, and Hearing Services in Schools, 39*(1), S110-S137.

Cleave, P.L., Becker, S.D., Curran, M.K., Van Horne, A.J.O., & Fey, M.E. (2015). The efficacy of recasts in language intervention: A systematic review and meta-analysis. *American Journal of Speech-Language Pathology/American Speech-Language-Hearing Association, 24*(2), 237-255. Retrieved from MEDLINE:25654306

Connell, P.J. (1986). Acquisition of semantic role by language-disordered children: Differences between production and comprehension. *Journal of Speech and Hearing Research, 29*(3), 366-374. Retrieved from <Go to ISI>://A1986D959000008

Courtright, J.A. & Courtright, I.C. (1976). Imitative modeling as a theoretical base for instructing language-disordered children. *Journal of Speech, Language, and Hearing Research, 19*(4), 655-663.

Davies, P., Shanks, B., & Davies, K. (2004). Improving narrative skills in young children with delayed language development. *Educational Review, 56*(3), 271-286.

de Lopez, K.J., Olsen, L.S., & Chondrogianni, V. (2014). Annoying Danish relatives: Comprehension and production of relative clauses by Danish children with and without SLI. *Journal of Child Language, 41*(01), 51-83.

De Villiers, J.G., Tager Flusberg, H.B., Hakuta, K., & Cohen, M. (1979). Children's comprehension of relative clauses. *Journal of Psycholinguistic Research, 8*(5), 499-518.

Diessel, H. (2004). *The Acquisition of Complex Sentences.* New York: Cambridge University Press.

Ebbels, S.H. (2005). Argument structure in specific language impairment: From theory to therapy. (Unpublished doctoral dissertation), University College London, UK.

Ebbels, S.H. (2007). Teaching grammar to school-aged children with Specific Language Impairment using Shape Coding. *Child Language Teaching and Therapy, 23*(1), 67-93.

Ebbels, S. (2014). Effectiveness of intervention for grammar in school-aged children with primary language impairments: A review of the evidence. *Child Language Teaching and Therapy, 30*(1), 7-40.

Ebbels, S. & van der Lely, H. (2001). Meta-syntactic therapy using visual coding for children with severe persistent SLI. *International Journal of Language & Communication Disorders, 36*(supplement), 345-350. Retrieved from <Go to ISI>://000168604000062

Ebbels, S.H., van der Lely, H.K.J., & Dockrell, J.E. (2007). Intervention for verb argument structure in children with persistent SLI: A randomized control trial. *Journal of Speech Language and Hearing Research, 50*, 1330-1349.

Ebbels, S.H., Dockrell, J.E., & van der Lely, H.K.J. (2012). Production of change-of-state, change-of-location and alternating verbs: A comparison of children with specific language impairment and typically developing children. *Language and Cognitive Processes, 27*(9), 1312-1333. doi:10.1080/01690965.2011.605598

Ebbels, S. H., Wright, L., Brockbank, S., Godfrey, C., Harris, C., Leniston, H., Neary, K., Nicoll, H., Nicoll, L., Scott, J., & Marić, N. (2017). Effectiveness of 1:1 speech and language therapy for older children with (developmental) language disorder. *International Journal of Language & Communication Disorders, 52*(4), 528-539. doi:10.1111/1460-6984.12297

Eisenberg, S.L. (2013). Grammar intervention: Content and procedures for facilitating children's language development. *Topics in Language Disorders, 33*(2), 165-178. Retrieved from WOS:000318158800006

Fey, M.E. & Loeb, D.F. (2002). An evaluation of the facilitative effects of inverted yes-no questions on the acquisition of auxiliary verbs. *Journal of Speech, Language, and Hearing Research, 45*(1), 160-174.

Fey, M.E., Finestack, L.H., Gajewski, B.J., Popescu, M., & Lewine, J.D. (2010). A preliminary evaluation of Fast ForWord-Language as an adjuvant treatment in language intervention. *Journal of Speech, Language, and Hearing Research, 53*(2), 430-449.

Friedmann, N. & Novogrodsky, R. (2004). The acquisition of relative clause comprehension in Hebrew: A study of SLI and normal development. *Journal of Child Language, 31*(3), 661-681.

Friedmann, N. & Novogrodsky, R. (2007). Is the movement deficit in syntactic SLI related to traces or to thematic role transfer? *Brain and Language, 101*(1), 50-63. Retrieved from WOS:000246425400005

Friedmann, N. & Novogrodsky, R. (2011). Which questions are most difficult to understand? The comprehension of Wh questions in three subtypes of SLI. *Lingua, 121*(3), 367-382. Retrieved from WOS:000286545700004

Frizelle, P. & Fletcher, P. (2015). The role of memory in processing relative clauses in children with specific language impairment. *American Journal of Speech-Language Pathology/American Speech-Language-Hearing Association, 24*(1), 47-59. Retrieved from MEDLINE:25409883

Frizelle, P., O'Neill, C., & Bishop, D.V. (2017). Assessing understanding of relative clauses: A comparison of multiple-choice comprehension versus sentence repetition. *Journal of Child Language, 44*, 1435-1457.

Frizelle, P., Thompson, P.A., McDonald, D., & Bishop, D.V.M. (2018). Growth in syntactic complexity between four years and adulthood: Evidence from a narrative task. *Journal of Child Language*, 1-24. doi:10.1017/S0305000918000144

Gibson, E. (1998). Linguistic complexity: Locality of syntactic dependencies. *Cognition, 68*(1), 1-76.

Gillam, S.L., Gillam, R.B., & Reece, K. (2012). Language outcomes of contextualized and decontextualized language intervention: Results of an early efficacy study. *Language Speech and Hearing Services in Schools, 43*, 276-291.

Graham, S. & Perin, D. (2007). A meta-analysis of writing instruction for adolescent students. *Journal of Educational Psychology, 99*(3), 445.

Hirsch, C. & Wexler, K. (2006). Children's passives and their resulting interpretation. Paper presented at The Proceedings of the Inaugural Conference on Generative Approaches to Language Acquisition–North America. University of Connecticut Occasional Papers in Linguistics.

Kamhi, A.G. (2014). Improving clinical practices for children with language and learning disorders. *Language, Speech, and Hearing Services in Schools, 45*(2), 92-103.

Kidd, E. & Bavin, E.L. (2002). English-speaking children's comprehension of relative clauses: Evidence for general-cognitive and language-specific constraints on development. *Journal of Psycholinguistic Research, 31*(6), 599-617.

Law, J., Garrett, Z., & Nye, C. (2004). The efficacy of treatment for children with developmental speech and language delay/disorder: A meta-analysis. *Journal of Speech, Language, and Hearing Research, 47*(4), 924-943.

Lea, J. (1970). *The Colour Pattern Scheme: A Method of Remedial Language Teaching*. Oxted, Surrey: Moor House School.

Leonard, L.B. (1995). Functional categories in the grammars of children with Specific Language Impairment. *Journal of Speech and Hearing Research, 38,* 1270-1283.

Leonard, L.B. & Deevy, P. (2010). Tense and aspect in sentence interpretation by children with specific language impairment. *Journal of Child Language, 37*(2), 395-418.

Leonard, L.B., Deevy, P., Miller, C., Charest, M., Kurtz, R., & Rauf, L. (2003). The use of grammatical morphemes reflecting aspect and modality by children with specific language impairment. *Journal of Child Language, 30,* 769-795.

Levy, H. & Friedmann, N. (2009). Treatment of syntactic movement in syntactic SLI: A case study. *First Language, 29*(1), 15-50.

Marinellie, S.A. (2004). Complex syntax used by school-age children with specific language impairment (SLI) in child–adult conversation. *Journal of Communication Disorders, 37*(6), 517-533. doi:dx.doi.org/10.1016/j.jcomdis.2004.03.005

Marinis, T. & van der Lely, H.K. (2007). On-line processing of wh-questions in children with G-SLI and typically developing children. *International Journal of Language & Communication Disorders, 42*(5), 557-582. Retrieved from WOS:000249800200004

Marshall, C.R., Marinis, T., & van der Lely, H.K.J. (2006). Passive verb morphology: The effect of phonotactics on passive comprehension in typically developing and grammatical-SLI children. *Lingua, 117,* 1434-1447.

Murphy, C., Adams, S., Perovic, A., & Ebbels, S. (in preparation). School-aged children's comprehension and production of conjunctions.

Nippold, M.A. (2014a). *Language Sampling with Adolescents: Implications for Intervention.* San Diego: Plural Publishing.

Nippold, M.A. (2014b). Language intervention at the middle school: Complex talk reflects complex thought. *Language, Speech, and Hearing Services in Schools, 45*(2), 153-156.

Nippold, M.A., Frantz-Kaspar, M.W., Cramond, P.M., Kirk, C., Hayward-Mayhew, C., & MacKinnon, M. (2014). Conversational and narrative speaking in adolescents: Examining the use of complex syntax. *Journal of Speech, Language, and Hearing Research, 57*(3), 876-886.

Nippold, M.A., Hesketh, L.J., Duthie, J.K., & Mansfield, T.C. (2005). Conversational versus expository discourse: A study of syntactic development in children, adolescents, and adults. *Journal of Speech, Language, and Hearing Research, 48*(5), 1048-1064. doi:10.1044/1092-4388(2005/073)

Nippold, M.A., Mansfield, T.C., Billow, J.L., & Tomblin, J.B. (2008). Expository discourse in adolescents with language impairments: Examining syntactic development. *American Journal of Speech-Language Pathology, 17*(4), 356-366. doi:10.1044/1058-0360(2008/07-0049)

Nippold, M.A., Mansfield, T.C., Billow, J.L., & Tomblin, J. (2009). Syntactic development in adolescents with a history of language impairments: A follow-up investigation. *American Journal of Speech-Language Pathology, 18*(3), 241–251. Retrieved from WOS:000268697300005

Novogrodsky, R. & Friedmann, N. (2006). The production of relative clauses in syntactic SLI: A window to the nature of the impairment. *Advances in Speech Language Pathology, 8*(4), 364–375.

Petersen, D.B., Gillam, S.L., Spencer, T., & Gillam, R.B. (2010). The effects of literate narrative intervention on children with neurologically based language impairments: An early stage study. *Journal of Speech, Language, and Hearing Research, 53*(4), 961–981.

Poll, G.H., Betz, S.K., & Miller, C.A. (2010). Identification of clinical markers of specific language impairment in adults. *Journal of Speech, Language, and Hearing Research, 53*(2), 414–429.

Rice, M.L., Wexler, K., & Cleave, P.L. (1995). Specific Language Impairment as a period of extended optional infinitive. *Journal of Speech and Hearing Research, 38*(4), 850–863. Retrieved from <Go to ISI>://A1995RM86600011

Rice, M.L., Tomblin, J.B., Hoffman, L., Richman, W.A., & Marquis, J. (2004). Grammatical tense deficits in children with SLI and nonspecific language impairment relationships with nonverbal IQ over time. *Journal of Speech, Language, and Hearing Research, 47*(4), 816–834.

Rice, M.L., Taylor, C.L., & Zubrick, S.R. (2008). Language outcomes of 7-year-old children with or without a history of late language emergence at 24 months. *Journal of Speech, Language, and Hearing Research, 51*(2), 394–407.

Riches, N.G., Loucas, T., Baird, G., Charman, T., & Simonoff, E. (2010). Sentence repetition in adolescents with specific language impairments and autism: An investigation of complex syntax. *International Journal of Language & Communication Disorders, 45*(1), 47–60. doi:10.3109/13682820802647676

Saxton, M. (2000). Negative evidence and negative feedback: Immediate effects on the grammaticality of child speech. *First Language, 20*(60), 221–252.

Scott, C.M. (2014). One size does not fit all: Improving clinical practice in older children and adolescents with language and learning disorders. *Language Speech and Hearing Services in Schools, 45*(2), 145–152. Retrieved from WOS:000345680200009

Scott, C.M. & Balthazar, C.H. (2010). The grammar of information: Challenges for older students with language impairments. *Topics in Language Disorders, 30*(4), 288.

Scott, C.M. & Balthazar, C. (2013). The role of complex sentence knowledge in children with reading and writing difficulties. *Perspectives on Language and Literacy, 39*(3), 18–26. Retrieved from https://search.proquest.com/docview/1437302268?accountid=14511

Scott, C.M. & Nelson, N.W. (2009). Sentence combining: Assessment and intervention applications. *SIG 1 Perspectives on Language Learning and Education, 16*(1), 14–20.

Scott, C.M. & Windsor, J. (2000). General language performance measures in spoken and written narrative and expository discourse of school-age children with language learning disabilities. *Journal of Speech, Language, and Hearing Research, 43*(2), 324–339.

Semel, E., Wiig, E.H., & Secord, W.A. (2006). *CELF4. Clinical Evaluation of Language Fundamentals, 4th ed.* London: Pearson Assessment.

Sun, L. & Nippold, M.A. (2012). Narrative writing in children and adolescents: Examining the literate lexicon. *Language, Speech, and Hearing Services in Schools, 43*(1), 2-13.

Thordardottir, E.T. & Weismer, E. (2002). Verb argument structure weakness in specific language impairment in relation to age and utterance length. *Clinical Linguistics & Phonetics, 16*(4), 233-250. Retrieved from <Go to ISI>://000176917900001

van der Lely, H.K.J. (1996). Specifically language impaired and normally developing children: Verbal passive vs adjectival passive sentence interpretation. *Lingua, 98*(4), 243-272. Retrieved from <Go to ISI>://A1996UG12500002

van der Lely, H.K.J. (1997). Language and cognitive development in a grammatical SLI boy: Modularity and innateness. *Journal of Neurolinguistics, 10*(2-3), 75-107. Retrieved from <Go to ISI>://A1997XP99700003

van der Lely, H.K.J. & Battell, J. (2003). Wh-movement in children with Grammatical SLI: A test of the RDDR hypothesis. *Language, 79*, 153-181.

van der Lely, H.K.J. & Harris, M. (1990). Comprehension of reversible sentences in specifically language-impaired children. *Journal of Speech and Hearing Disorders, 55*, 101-117.

van der Lely, H.K.J. & Ullman, M.T. (2001). Past tense morphology in specifically language impaired and normally developing children. *Language and Cognitive Processes, 16*(2-3), 177-217. Retrieved from <Go to ISI>://000168711800003

Ward-Lonergan, J.M., Liles, B.Z., & Anderson, A.M. (1999). Verbal retelling abilities in adolescents with and without language-learning disabilities for social studies lectures. *Journal of Learning Disabilities, 32*(3), 213-223.

Weiler, B. (2013). Verb selection and past-tense morphology: Crystal's criteria revisited. *Topics in Language Disorders, 33*(2), 152-164.

Weismer, S.E. & Murray-Branch, J. (1989). Modeling versus modeling plus evoked production training: A comparison of two language intervention methods. *Journal of Speech and Hearing Disorders, 54*(2), 269-281.

Zwitserlood, R., Wijnen, F., Weerdenburg, M., & Verhoeven, L. (2015). 'MetaTaal': Enhancing complex syntax in children with specific language impairment - a metalinguistic and multimodal approach. *International Journal of Language & Communication Disorders, 50*(3), 273-297.

7 The power of storytelling during adolescence

Assessment and Intervention

Victoria Joffe

"Tell me the facts and I'll learn. Tell me the truth and I'll believe. But tell me a story and it will live in my heart forever." – Native American Proverb

---

Learning outcomes

This chapter will enable readers to:

- Describe and discuss the role of storytelling in adolescent development, and the powerful role it plays in language development, academic attainment, and social and emotional functioning

- Critique the current evidence base for the use of storytelling as an intervention in adolescents

- Employ a range of standardized and non-standardized measures to assess storytelling in older children and young people

- Incorporate storytelling in the teaching and therapy context at an individual, group and whole class level.

Introduction

Listening to and telling stories is much more a part of our lives than we might imagine. Narrative production or storytelling is pervasive in our daily lives, a universal habit common to us all. All cultures and societies draw upon storytelling in some way, and stories become part of our conversations, our memories, our future plans and aspirations (Meek, 1991). We use stories to connect and interact with others, to make friendships, to describe, explain, excuse, plan and express our thoughts, feelings and desires. Storytelling gives structure and meaning to our experiences and is a powerful means by which we organize and represent the world and make sense of it (Bruner, 1991; Meek, 1991; Naremore, Densmore, & Harman, 1995). Narratives (or stories), are viewed as an organized framework through which people can express themselves.

Individuals with speech, language and communication needs (SLCN) experience difficulties understanding and telling stories (Liles, 1993; Roth & Spekman, 1986; Wetherell, Botting, & Conti-Ramsden, 2007). As such, it is an excellent medium for learning and language development in the education, clinical, and social context for this population. There is a growing evidence base for incorporating storytelling as an intervention in therapeutic and educational contexts, and its use has been shown to be effective in enhancing language and communication in children and young people with SLCN (Davies, Shanks, & Davies, 2004; Joffe, 2006, 2011; Stringer, 2006; Swanson, Fey, Mills, & Hood, 2005). In addition to its value as a therapeutic tool, storytelling can also be used as a barometer of cognitive and linguistic skills, providing information on a student's cognitive abilities, and all elements of speech, language and communication. It therefore can play an important role in both the assessment and management of children and young people with SLCN.

The characteristics and types of narratives

Narration is one type of discourse and is more reflective of the everyday language that children and young people hear and use, mirroring more realistically the oral and written language expected in the classroom.

A narrative or story, in its broadest sense, is anything told or recounted, whether true or fictitious. Narratives consist of related events and are typically organized episodically, with the episodes linked temporally or causally (Naremore et al., 1995). The components within a story are logically related so that they are comprehended as related units rather than unrelated statements. Many stories are goal-directed narratives, in that they have a point and one can say what a story is about (Naremore et al., 1995). They have a definite structure to them: a story usually has a beginning, middle and end, with a coherent plot, different characters and some type of conflict, problem or main event, and resolution

(Stein & Glenn, 1979). These features, importantly, can differ markedly across different cultures and societies (McCabe & Rollins, 1994). African American children, for example, are reported to tell stories that combine events which have happened at different times and places into one narrative, referred to as Topic-Associating Narratives (Michaels, 1981). Japanese children and adults produce highly succinct narratives with minimal information, expecting the listener to fill in the gaps (Minami & McCabe, 1991).

Types of narrative

There are three main types of narratives: scripts, fictional, and non-fictional.

1. **Scripts**: A script is a general description of what usually happens in a routine event, for example, going to the dentist or attending a birthday party. Scripts "represent predictable sequences of events (helping) children make predictions and inferences" (Naremore et al., 1995, p.111). General event knowledge is an important prerequisite for the use of scripts (Hudson & Shapiro, 1991). They can act as a framework to describe routine events and can be used to help familiarize a student with an event to reduce unease and enhance awareness and comfort. For example, a script can be written about going to the hospital or sitting an examination.

2. **Fictional narrative**: Fictional narratives are made-up stories not based on facts, with the characters, plot, settings and events all created from the imagination of the narrator. The made-up story will usually draw on some knowledge of events occurring in the story either through general event or world knowledge, memory of an event or memory of another fictional story (Hudson & Shapiro, 1991). There are well-accepted internal organization rules, known as story grammar, which provide a common structure to fictional narratives. These components are referred to as the macrostructure of story. The number and type of components may differ depending on the specific story grammar framework being used (Mandler & Johnson, 1977; Rumelhart, 1975; Stein & Glenn, 1979), with most accounts including the following key components: setting (with characters, time and place); story episode/s where a goal is reached (including an initiating event, an attempt to deal with that event, and a consequence of that attempt); and the overall outcome (Naremore et al., 1995). The narrative may include internal

responses of the characters reflecting their thoughts and feelings. The episodes of the narrative are logically sequenced and connected causally and/or temporally.

3. **Non-fictional narrative**: Non-fictional narratives are stories based on facts. These may include an autobiography of a famous person, written by that person, or a biography, a story about the life of a famous person written by another person. Narrative non-fiction presents factual information in a narrative style using literary techniques including metaphor and characterization. Examples of narrative non-fiction include diaries or memoirs. A personal narrative is an example of a non-fictional narrative and is a story told by a person about a specific event/s that they have personally experienced.

Different narrative genres

The narrative has a range of different genres, with a similar theme or style, which appeal to different people depending on their interests. These different genres can be used to individualize programmes for young people and enhance overall interest and engagement. Fictional narrative genres include detective/crime, horror, fantasy, mystery, fairy tale, fable, romance, science fiction, historical fiction, classic, western, suspense/adventure, tragedy, action/adventure, satire, comedy and narrative poetry. Non-fictional genres include biography, autobiography, self-help, journalism, personal essay, memoir, laboratory report, personal narrative, travel/nature/science/sports/medical reports, and interview.

The importance of storytelling

Narratives form a bridge between oral and written language, and a transition between the language style of home and school (Westby, 1984, 1991). Narratives can serve many different functions for adolescents, and play an important role in communicative effectiveness, linguistic and cultural learning, educational success, social interaction and emotional wellbeing (Bliss, Covington, & McCabe, 1999; Kail, 2004; Petersen, Gillam, & Gillam, 2008). The sophistication of narratives has been reported to influence teachers' perceptions of their students' academic and intellectual abilities (Crais & Lorch, 1994), and they are rated by teachers as a high priority (Reed & Spicer, 2003). Moreover, storytelling has been found to play an important role in interpersonal interaction across many different societies (Peterson & McCabe, 1991). Storytelling provides students with an opportunity to practise and develop language, communication and language-related skills, including attention, listening, memory and social skills, all of which can enhance and facilitate students' access to the curriculum and improve social interactions. Narratives may also provide a more fertile ground for oral expression than conversational speech. Indeed, utterances tend to be longer in storytelling compared to ordinary conversation (Leadholm & Miller, 1992).

Narratives and educational achievement

Narratives are firmly embedded in the UK educational curriculum. Across the educational key stages 1–4 (ages 6–16), there is explicit mention of narratives, and an inclusion of the understanding and/or production of narratives across subjects (Department for Education, 2013). The importance of narratives in education is also evident in other countries, for example the USA (Nippold, Frantz-Kaspar, Crammond, et al., 2014).

Narrative ability has been shown to be a significant predictor of school performance, and a prognostic indicator of pervasive language disorder (Bishop & Adams, 1990; Bishop & Edmundson, 1987; Fazio, Naremore, & Connell, 1993; Paul, Hernandez, Taylor, & Johnson, 1996; Stothard, Snowling, Bishop, et al., 1998). Exposure to storytelling in the home and classroom has been reported to be an important determinant of literacy development (Wells, 1986); and children who are better storytellers are also more successful in reading (Reese, Suggate, Long, & Schaughency, 2010; Tabors, Snow, & Dickinson, 2001) and writing (Griffin, Hemphill, Camp, & Wolf, 2004).

Narratives and social and emotional development

Narratives have been shown to be significantly associated with social interactions and developing friendships (Dickinson, Wolf, & Stotsky, 1993) and play an important role in social and emotional development (Boudreau, 2008). Adolescents use narratives to explore and build social relationships by telling stories about themselves and others in order to help develop their own identify, self-esteem and emotional and social wellbeing (Schickedanz, Schickedanz, Forsyth, & Forsyth, 2001).

Narratives can also provide a window for how emotions are understood and expressed (Bohanek & Fivush, 2010). Personal narratives are important for social and psychological wellbeing because they allow opportunities to share personal events which form a major part of social interactions (Schank, 1990), and also relate to an individual's self-identity and self-determination (Westby & Culatta, 2016). "Adolescence is a critical period for the development of a healthy adult identity, and the ways in which adolescents narrate the emotional events of their lives provide a window into how they are creating sense and meaning of these events" (Bohanek & Fivush, 2010, p.376).

The skills underlying storytelling

Storytelling involves a number of complex cognitive and language skills, and an interaction between them (Naremore et al., 1995; Nippold, 2007). This can therefore prove challenging for some students. Listening to, understanding and telling stories draws upon all elements of language and communication (attention, listening, phonology, morphology, syntax, semantics, pragmatics), and cognitive functions, including an understanding of temporal and causal relationships, short- and long-term memory, and conceptualizing and interpreting internal states and goals. It also requires a general knowledge of events and awareness about the world around us, an ability to identify and link events in a coherent sequence, insight into people and typical social interactions, and some knowledge of the cultural conventions of storytelling (Liles, 1993; Peterson & McCabe, 1983). During adolescence, the more advanced skills of storytelling include character motivation, understanding and manipulating different perspectives of characters that may differ from each other or from the truth, thereby possessing a theory of mind, and inferential understanding. It may be necessary to have knowledge regarding social or cultural rules and norms, to persuade the reader or listener, and to use humour, metaphors, idioms and other figurative language in order to effectively tell a story (Cohen, 2001).

The development of storytelling across childhood and adolescence

There is a clear developmental sequence in narrative acquisition, with complex narratives emerging at around 12 years of age (Westby, 1984). For a description of narrative development in childhood, from 2-7 years of age, based on Piaget's (1959) stages of cognitive development, see Applebee (1978).

Narrative development, of course, does not stop in early childhood. Indeed, Nippold (2010) identifies a number of advances in narration that occur during adolescence, including the ability to recall events, organize complex information, consider and understand the emotional perspectives of others, and use complex syntax and vocabulary to express themselves with clarity and precision. Older children's narratives become longer, more complex and elaborate during the adolescent period, and one way this occurs is by increasing the complexity of episodes in a story. Hughes, McGillivray and Schmidek (1997) report four levels of episode complexity: (1) multiple episodes, where more than one complete episode (with initiating event, action, consequence, reaction) is included in the story; (2) complex episodes, refers to stories where obstacles challenge or complicate the solution or the character's plan for resolution; (3) embedded episodes, where one episode occurs within another episode in the story; and finally, (4) interactive episodes, where the narrative is told from two different perspectives. In order to describe this increase in complexity of narratives in older children, Applebee (1978) identified an additional four stages of narrative development following Piaget's (1959) concrete operational and formal operational stages of cognitive development:

I. 7–11 years: Children begin to summarize and categorize stories and are able to discuss features of the story, including the presence of literary devices.

II. 11–12 years: In early adolescence, children are producing more complex stories with multiple embedded structures.

III. 13–15 years: In the middle adolescent years, students become skilled at analyzing and evaluating stories.

IV. 16 years to adulthood: Individuals at this stage are capable of advanced analysis of a story, generalizing its meaning, and exploring their reaction to the story.

An alternative way of exploring the development of stories is using the story grammar framework, which reflects the underlying rules underpinning story structure. Several different story grammar frameworks have been proposed, but they all share the common features of including a beginning with a setting, a middle with episodes or actions, and an ending and resolution. A popular story grammar framework is one proposed by Stein and Glenn (1979) who suggest that all complete stories have a setting and one or more episodes. The setting will set out the context of the story, introducing the characters and describing the time and location. An episode will comprise of an initiating event, an internal response of the character/s, a plan, an attempt, a consequence and a reaction (Stein & Glenn, 1979). More than one episode is linked sequentially, causally or temporally (Roth, 1986).

While such story grammar frameworks do not fully describe all narratives, they provide a useful structure from which to assess an individual's ability to produce a narrative. During adolescence, students should be producing narratives containing all seven of these components.

High point analysis, which identifies six recurring and common narrative features in oral storytelling (namely: abstract, orientation, complicating action, resolution, evaluation, and coda), is another method of analyzing narratives, and can be used to assess the skills of the adolescent to include a more sophisticated climax or high point (Labov, 1972; McCabe, 1995). In high point analysis, narratives contain complicating actions (what happens), orientations (who, when, where), and evaluations (emotional references, judgements, perceptions). Complete narratives will also include a climax or high point, and a resolution (Peterson & McCabe, 1983). Older children can enhance their narratives by incorporating a more complex climax or several high points, including an introducer, an orientation, a complicating action, an evaluation, a resolution and a coda (McCabe, 1995).

Adolescence also brings enhancements to the microstructure of a story, which refers to the inclusion of the quantity, type and quality of linguistic forms. Westby (1998) identified four main linguistic elements that reflect further mastery of narrative production: conjunctions (excluding 'and' and 'then'), elaborated noun phrases, mental/cognitive and linguistic verbs, and adverbs.

It is apparent, then, that narrative development continues well into adolescence and even adulthood. It might be expected that Applebee's (1978) narrative stages will have been mastered by adolescence, but this is not the case with adolescents with speech, language and communication needs (SLCN) who show difficulties in the macrostructure and microstructure of narratives (Larson & McKinley, 2003).

Storytelling in children and young people with speech, language and communication needs

Considering the complex requirements of storytelling, it is unsurprising that individuals with SLCN have been found to have significant difficulties with interpreting and telling stories, in both the oral and written domains (Liles, 1993; Liles, Duffy, Merritt, & Purcell, 1995; Merritt & Liles, 1987, 1989; Roth & Spekman, 1986; van der Lely, 1997). The majority of studies exploring narrative production in individuals with SLCN include preschool or primary school-aged children (Bishop & Adams, 1992; Merrit & Liles, 1987; Miranda, McCabe, & Bliss, 1998; Roth & Spekman, 1986). Wetherell et al. (2007), however, investigated narrative production in adolescents with SLCN and age-matched controls and found that the SLCN group produced narratives with a greater number of tense and agreement, lexical subject omission and morpheme errors. When given more control over the style and content of their narratives (personal stories), young people with SLCN were better able to conceal their difficulties compared to a story generation task.

Snow and Powell (2005) have shown that young offenders aged between 13-19 years performed significantly more poorly than their peers at story production tasks. Whilst there were no significant differences between the number of story grammar components used, the young offenders were less able to express the character's plans, the direct consequences of actions and how resolutions were achieved. A recent study by Rollins (2014) comparing performance of 10 young adults (mean age=24.6 years) with high functioning autism on two narrative genres, a fictional and personal story, showed significantly poorer performance in narrative quality for the personal story, with particular difficulties with expression of mental states and story conclusion. She concluded that many high functioning young people with ASD experience difficulties expressing their feelings, and the ability to tell personal narratives is an important skill to develop in this group.

There is also a literature on the narrative development across different clinical groups of children with SLCN, including children with Down syndrome and with autism spectrum disorder (e.g., Botting, 2002; Norbury & Bishop, 2003; Liles et al., 1995; Norbury, Gemmell, & Paul, 2013). In summary, some of these studies report findings that show narratives can differentiate between clinical groups (Botting, 2002; Loveland, McEvoy, Tunali, & Kelley, 1990; Manolitsi & Botting, 2011). Narratives, therefore present an alternative to the sole use of standardized tests which are limited in the adolescent population.

Assessing storytelling in adolescents

Storytelling is one of the most ecological and practical ways of assessing communicative competence in typical and atypical populations (Botting, 2002).

Assessments using narratives provide a wealth of information on linguistic, cognitive and social skills, and are more engaging than standardized tests (Norbury & Bishop, 2003). They reflect more accurately everyday functional language use, and thereby present an important window into the young person's level of activity and participation (Westby & Washington, 2016).

Since narratives have such a clear developmental sequence, they can be used to compare typical and atypical groups, as well as to differentially diagnose within clinical groups. Narratives can also be employed to measure progress over time, and are therefore a valuable outcome measure for the clinician. The purposes of assessing narratives are numerous. Narrative assessments can inform us about the student's level of narrative ability. But they can do much more than this. Narratives, as part of an assessment battery, provide valuable information about the individual's speech, language and cognitive abilities, their social use of language and emotional wellbeing. Considering their appeal as a valid measure of communication, it is important to evaluate storytelling skills as a routine part of clinical assessment.

Narratives can be assessed through standardized and non-standardized assessments, and can be investigated at two levels:

1. Story Macrostructure, which assesses the ability to produce complex, well sequenced stories coherently, focusing on story grammar or story structure; and

2. Story Microstructure, which focuses on the structural language used at sentence-level evident in the narrative.

Standardized measures of oral narrative – norm referenced

The benefits of using a standardized test is that it is norm referenced and has standardization data. This is important as it provides you with information about the individual's performance relative to a normative sample. There are a number of standardized narrative tests for preschool and primary school-age children, but the choice is more limited for adolescents. Common standardized tests used with adolescents include:

1. *The Assessment of Comprehension and Expression 6–11* (Adams, Coke, Crutchley, et al., 2001) has a narrative subtest, with an age range from 6-11 years, and can therefore be used in early adolescence. It is a story retelling task with UK norms and provides a proposition score (macrostructure) and a total syntax/discourse score (microstructure).

2. *The Test of Narrative Language, 2nd ed.* (TNL) (Gillam & Peterson, 2017) measures narrative comprehension and production, both personal and fictional, for children age 4.11-15.11 years. The standardized sample is from the USA.

3. *The Expression, Reception and Recall of Narrative Instrument* (ERRNI) (Bishop, 2004) includes a storytelling, story recall and story comprehension task with an age range of 4 and above. Participants are asked to look at a sequence of pictures which tell a story and then to tell their own story using the pictures. Between 10-30 minutes later they are asked to retell their story. A set of comprehension questions is then given with the pictures in view. There are two matched stories allowing for retesting: a beach story and a fish story. UK norms are provided.

4. *The Clinical Evaluation of Language Fundamentals, 5th ed.* (CELF5) (Wiig, Semel, & Secord, 2013) includes an 'Understanding Spoken Paragraph' subtest measuring the ability to sustain attention and focus when listening to oral narratives of increasing length and complexity, and to create meaning and answer questions that require interpretation beyond the information provided in the text. The test can be used on individuals aged from 5 to 21 years, and has UK norms.

Non-standardized measures of narrative ability – criterion referenced

Standardized tests are not always appropriate for use with all individuals. The standardization sample, for example, can be very different to the individual being tested, and this puts into question the relevance of the normative data. Eliciting language samples through narrative provides an opportunity to measure an individual's language and communication in a more functional and fun way, and is suitable for bilingual students (Boerma, Leseman, Timmermeister, et al., 2016), and for those from different cultural and socio-economic backgrounds (Alt, Arizmendi, & DiLallo, 2016). The two types of assessments identify different aspects of performance, and support the practice of using a combination of the two in routine clinical practice to ensure a comprehensive assessment of strengths and areas of need (Ebert & Scott, 2014; Wetherell et al., 2007).

Procedures to elicit stories for assessment

Different types of narratives can be elicited using diverse materials and different levels of support. These choices will depend on the age of the student, their linguistic and cognitive abilities, and their level of engagement, as well as the primary aim of the narrative assessment. Story retell tasks can be better at identifying language difficulties because the student is constrained to tell a specific story (Merritt & Liles, 1989) and can also provide valuable information about attention and memory. Story generation is more difficult than story retell tasks because the story needs to be generated. It is also more reflective of spontaneous communication in everyday life. Given that personal narratives are easier to produce than fictional narratives (Hudson & Shapiro, 1991), a comprehensive assessment may need to include both types. An individualized plan for each person is required; for example, the level of structure or support provided can be varied depending on ability and age.

Narratives can be elicited from all different types of materials, and this selection can depend on the age and interests of the individual. A more challenging prompt, for perhaps older children, can include giving them a title, a beginning, or an ending, and asking them to tell a story around these prompts. For students more reticent to tell stories, or those with more significant speech, language or fluency difficulties, one can use story completion or 'cloze tasks' where a story is told to the individual who then has to fill in some missing words, phrases or sentences. Another useful activity to assess sequencing abilities, whilst also being a good warm-up activity for story production, is to mix up different parts of a story, either pictures or written sentences, and ask the student to order them into a coherent story. A series of popular wordless picture books by Mayer (1969, 1973, 1974), to elicit fictional stories, and guidance for elicitation (Berman & Slobin, 1994), are also available. These books consist of a series of illustrations that depict a story, and have been found to be effective with bilingual students (Berman & Slobin, 1994).

Once the story has been elicited, an analysis is then undertaken to provide detailed information on the individual's cognitive and linguistic functioning. Stories can be analyzed at the more global organizational level, the macrostructure; or at the sentence level, the microstructure. The type and level of analyses will depend on the abilities of the client and the main aims of the assessment.

Analyzing narrative skills at the macrostructure level

When assessing storytelling, one can use a developmental approach, such as Applebee's stages of development (1978) or a story grammar approach (Roth & Spekman, 1986). A developmental approach allows one to compare features of the client's production to the different levels of narrative leading up to the true narrative (Applebee, 1978). There is a wide variety of story grammar taxonomies that can be adopted to analyze the presence of common elements of a story (Merrit & Lilles, 1987; Stein & Glenn, 1979). All story grammars will have a setting where the character is introduced, and will describe the temporal and physical context in which the story takes place. Other required story grammar elements include a goal, and one or more episodes which contain an initiating event, an action, an outcome and an ending. The SALT (Systematic Analysis of Language Transcripts), a computerized approach to language sample analysis, includes a narrative coding scheme, the Narrative Structure Score, which is based on Stein and Glenn's (1979) story grammar framework, and provides guidelines on how to code story grammar and cohesion (Miller & Chapman, 2003). Standardized tests, for example the ERRNI and TNL, provide guidelines on transcription and scoring, and these can be adapted to other stories.

Westby (2005) proposes the use of a decision structure tree for assessing narrative organization, which incorporates a series of questions around whether the story has temporally and causally related events, goal-directed behaviour and other key story elements which then allow one to assign a stage of narrative development. For older children, macrostructure analyses can also include investigating the presence of a high point or climax to the story (McCabe, 1995) and the number of complex, multiple, embedded and interactive episodes (Hughes et al., 1997).

A second important aspect of story macrostructure for evaluation is story cohesion, which is the use of linguistic devices to connect sentences together to form an integrated story. Examples of cohesive devices include pronouns, conjunctions, conjunctive adverbs (for example, *nevertheless*, *however*), elliptical utterances (omitting utterance that are not required) and articles (*the*, *a*, *an*). Liles (1985) provides a detailed system for scoring cohesion, based on Halliday and Hasan's (1976) taxonomy.

Heilmann, Miller, Nockerts, and Dunaway (2010) have devised a comprehensive measure of narrative assessment, suitable for older children, 'The Narrative Scoring Scheme' which incorporates a Likert scale scoring approach for coding story elements, and evaluates seven narrative microstructure components: introduction, character development, mental states, referencing, conflict resolution, cohesion and conclusion. Story elements are coded as proficient (score of 5), emerging (score of 3), or minimal/immature (score of 1). Normative information generated from wordless picture books are included in the SALT manual (Miller, Andriacchi, & Nockerts, 2015).

Analyzing narrative skills at the microstructure level

Analyzing narratives at the microstructure levels allows for scrutiny of the semantics, vocabulary, syntax and grammar used. Measures that were found to be the strongest indicators of productivity and complexity included number of different words, total number of words, total number of T-units (the smallest grammatical sentence with a main clause and any subordinate clauses), average number of words per T-unit, and number and proportion of complex sentences (sentence containing a subordinate clause) (Justice, 2006). This grammatical information can be obtained from the SALT computer program (Miller & Chapman, 2003). Also available, is a coding manual devised by Norbury et al. (2013), providing an overall index of syntactic complexity. In the older child, microstructure analyses can include lexical diversity as well as the number of literary devices employed. Following Westby (1998), microstructure analyses for the young person can incorporate the number of subordinating conjunctions (example: however, although), elaborated noun phrases (example: 'the oozing green cupcake' or 'the angry boy in class 2'), mental (example: 'think', 'know') and linguistic (example: 'promise', 'report') verbs, and adverbs (example: 'angrily', 'cautiously'). The presence of dialogue can also be explored as a means of making a story more interesting and sophisticated.

The Index of Narrative Complexity tool combines analysis of both macrostructure and microstructure (Petersen et al., 2008). More recently, it has been revised into a measure, 'Monitoring Indicators of Scholarly Language (MISL)', designed to measure progress of the production of spontaneous narratives from simple descriptions to more advanced multi-episode narratives. The content of this tool, developed by Gillam, Gillam and Laing (2012), measures macrostructure (character, setting, initiating event, internal response, plan, attempt and consequence) and microstructure (coordinating and subordinating conjunctions, adverbs, metacognitive verbs, and elaborated noun phrases). A recent study showed it to have acceptable levels of psychometric properties for use as a progress monitoring tool, for aspects of narrative proficiency, demonstrating acceptable levels of internal consistency, reliability, inter-rater reliability and construct validity (Gillam, Gillam, Fargo, Olszewski, & Segura, 2016).

Storytelling as an evidence-based practice

Evidence exists for the effectiveness of narrative-based intervention for children with SLCN, with much of it pertaining to preschool and primary school-aged children. In a systematic review of narrative-based language intervention with children with SLCN from 1980, Petersen (2011) identified nine studies that met inclusion criteria, with the majority of them reporting moderate to large effect sizes for narrative macrostructure and microstructure. Only one of these nine studies included older children (Gillam, McFadden, & van Kleeck, 1995). Despite positive results, the author highlights the methodological limitations of the studies, including limited number of participants, little experimental control, and large variation in procedures and materials used. Conclusions drawn from this review were that narrative-based intervention is at an emerging stage of evidence and needs further investigation (Petersen, 2011). Nevertheless, effectiveness was reported across a range of service delivery models, including individual and group-based delivery, speech and language therapists and teaching and support staff involvement, as well as the total time and frequency of intervention, ranging from 40–50 minutes over 6–8 weeks in duration (Davies et al., 2004; Swanson et al., 2005).

There is some evidence for the effectiveness of narrative intervention in adolescence. Stringer (2006) explored the benefits of a narrative and social skills programme delivered in groups, twice weekly over five sessions (10 hours in total) to 12 secondary school-aged children with emotional and behavioural difficulties (mean age of 12.4 years). Significant improvements were made on standardized receptive and expressive language tests at the sentence level, but not on single word receptive and expressive vocabulary, or on an oral story comprehension task.

Joffe (2006) conducted a randomized control trial (RCT) with 54 adolescents (mean age: 12.8 years) with SLCN, exploring the effectiveness of a narrative and vocabulary intervention programme. Participants were randomized into two groups, to receive intervention delivered by student speech and language therapists, in small groups in mainstream secondary schools, for two 50-minute sessions a week over a 6-week period. One group received vocabulary intervention, the second, narrative intervention with a focus on story structure, story description and inferential understanding. Both groups made significant progress on receptive vocabulary, sentence recall and inferential understanding, as measured by standardized tests. Whilst these results suggest a generalization effect of intervention, there were no differential effects between the groups receiving narrative or vocabulary intervention.

Following on from this study, in one of the only large RCTs of secondary school students, Joffe, Rixon, Hirani and Hulme (submitted) explored the effectiveness of two language enrichment programmes, storytelling and vocabulary, delivered by teaching assistants in small groups in secondary schools. The intervention consisted of 18 sessions, of approximately 45 minutes each, over a 6-week period. A detailed manualized programme was provided and ongoing observations of the intervention were undertaken to ensure fidelity. A total of 21 teaching assistants from 21 secondary schools delivered the intervention to 358 secondary school students (mean age: 12.8 years) with SLCN. The students were randomly assigned to one of four intervention groups: storytelling, vocabulary enrichment, a combination of storytelling and vocabulary, and a delayed treatment group. The narrative intervention consisted of understanding and telling stories, with a focus on story structure and story description, using a story planner to facilitate learning. Different narrative genres were incorporated in the intervention, which was graded from first creating an awareness about the importance of storytelling, encouraging active listening of different stories, moving on to story retelling with sequence pictures, completing stories and filling in missing gaps, and building up to storytelling, from simple to more complex stories. The use of linguistic and paralinguistic features as dramatic effects in storytelling was also explored.

Standardized and non-standardized assessments were used to explore changes at post intervention. On the non-standardized measure of story grammar, the narrative and the combined group scored significantly better than the vocabulary group. The narrative group also scored significantly higher than the controls on a narrative awareness measure, assessing explicit knowledge of the role and components of narratives. The standardized narrative test (ERRNI; Bishop, 2004) did not differentiate between the three intervention groups; however, all three intervention groups showed significant improvements over time on the ERRNI's Initial Story Telling score compared to the control group.

Whilst there continues to be a need to strengthen the evidence base for narrative-based intervention, particularly during adolescence, the results are promising and these, together with the importance of narratives in language, educational and social and emotional development, make narratives a worthy addition to clinical and educational practice.

Storytelling as an intervention in adolescence

The inclusion of narratives in clinical practice provides opportunities for developing a more functional approach to intervention. Westby and Washington (2016) identify narratives as a route to working at the level of activity and participation, rather than just a focus on impairment, and therefore can support the application of the World Health Organisation's guidelines for the International Classification of Functioning, Disability and Health (WHO, 2001). Narratives offer great flexibility and diversity and present a multitude of opportunities through which to enhance language, communication and social interactions. Narratives can be elicited and facilitated in both the clinical and education contexts, and with individuals, pairs and groups of people, across the lifespan, and by a range of teaching, therapy and support staff. The inclusion of narratives as a therapeutic and educational target can therefore be implemented across a range of service delivery models.

By profiling the language and cognitive skills that are required for storytelling, and mapping requirements against current abilities, by drawing on the range of standardized and non-standardized narrative assessments available, strengths and specific areas of need can be identified and addressed. Narrative-based intervention can therefore offer a situation-specific, functional approach to language intervention which targets the skills needed to communicate a particular story effectively, in the context of a student's level of language and cognitive development. Working on storytelling provides opportunities to practise and develop language, paralinguistic language, metalinguistics, communication and other language and cognitive related skills, including attention, listening, memory and social skills, all of which can be incorporated as therapy targets, facilitating access to the education curriculum and improving social interactions.

Where to begin? Like any story, start at the beginning

One of the best ways to improve storytelling skills is to listen to stories. Therefore, for group members not ready to tell stories there are a range of listening tasks that can be given. It is important that each participant is encouraged to start wherever they feel most comfortable. Story production doesn't have to mean telling a story on one's own. Stories can be built and developed in a group, with each group member contributing one idea or a character. Emphasis is placed on the key features of active listening and storytelling, and the act of storytelling is viewed as an interactional process. Larson and McKinley (2003) identify critical listening as an essential component in the classroom, where adolescents are required to go beyond literal understanding to interpreting abstract meaning, the inferred intention and evaluate the effectiveness of the message.

The use of story types and genres in intervention

Scripts, fictional and non-fictional narratives all have an important role to play in narrative-based intervention. Scripts can be used to help individuals plan and prepare for routine events, like exams and job interviews. Scripts support the development of prediction and inferences (Naremore et al., 1995), and assist the young person to prepare for important life events. Scripts are also helpful to learn and revise some curricular content, for example experiments in Science and cooking in Home Economics.

Personal stories can be used to enhance social and emotional wellbeing (Boudreau, 2008), and help develop self-confidence and self-identity (Westby & Cullata, 2016). They also promote self-regulation and problem solving, and support the executive functions of planning and reflection (Westby & Culatta, 2016). Children naturally use more personal narratives in social interactions than other narratives (Preece, 1987), and these can be less challenging for the young person as the content is known to them. An activity in the Narrative Intervention Programme, which draws upon personal stories, invites young people to share their past, present and future autobiographies, and facilitates an awareness of culture, heritage, family, self-reflection and realistic future goal planning (Joffe, 2011). One young man changed his future story from an unrealistic dream to an achievable aspiration after sharing his story with the group (Joffe, 2013). Other non-fictional narratives from the History or Geography curricula can serve as a valuable means to a greater understanding of world events (Mello, 2001).

Fictional stories encourage productivity (Leadholm & Miller, 1992) and are often a good place to start with people reticent to share personal stories. Fictional stories are also important vehicles for exploration of emotions and actions experienced by young people. For example, the picture in Figure 7.1 was used to produce fictional stories exploring the themes of belonging, isolation and bullying (Joffe, 2011). Through characters from stories that are shared, appropriate behaviours and responses to common and difficult social situations can be modelled and explored. Through rehearsal and exploration of different story endings, problem solving, predicting, planning, and resilience can be learned.

Drawing on all available story genres can encourage engagement and enjoyment in the narrative process. Fables, for example, are an interesting narrative genre with a strong cultural heritage (Nippold, 2007). They are short imaginative stories which end with a proverbial statement or moral (Nippold, 2007, p.209), and as adolescence is a time when moral reasoning becomes more prevalent, fables can be highly engaging and appropriate for older children (Nippold, Frantz-Kaspar, Crammond, et al., 2014). During adolescence, individuals typically exhibit interests in specific areas, developing individualistic learning and what Nippold (1995) refers to as "linguistic individualism" (p.307). This individuality can be encouraged and shared through different story genres, whether this be science fiction, romance or mystery. Songs often have their own narrative and can be a great resource to use in adolescence to encourage an interest in storytelling. Limericks can also be great fun, and their humour can be appealing to this age group (Joffe, 2011). Across all these different narrative types and genres, important aspects of cognition, language, communication and paralinguistic features can be targeted.

Using stories to enhance cognition, language and communication

Storytelling provides rich opportunities to draw attention to and practise some important language-related skills, including attention, listening, eye contact and turn taking. Working at a conversational level, in a small group or classroom setting, provides instant feedback for storytelling techniques, and opportunities for modelling effective methods. The importance of, for example, attention, eye contact or listening, becomes even more salient when you, as the storyteller, are relying on the group to show these behaviours. Providing opportunities for group members to take turns at building a story creates greater awareness of the importance of turn taking in effective communication. If needed at the start of the intervention, a physical object, like a microphone, can be used to indicate more explicitly whose turn it is. Story retelling is useful to practise short- and long-term memory, using visual aids for support initially.

Identifying the different structural components in a range of different

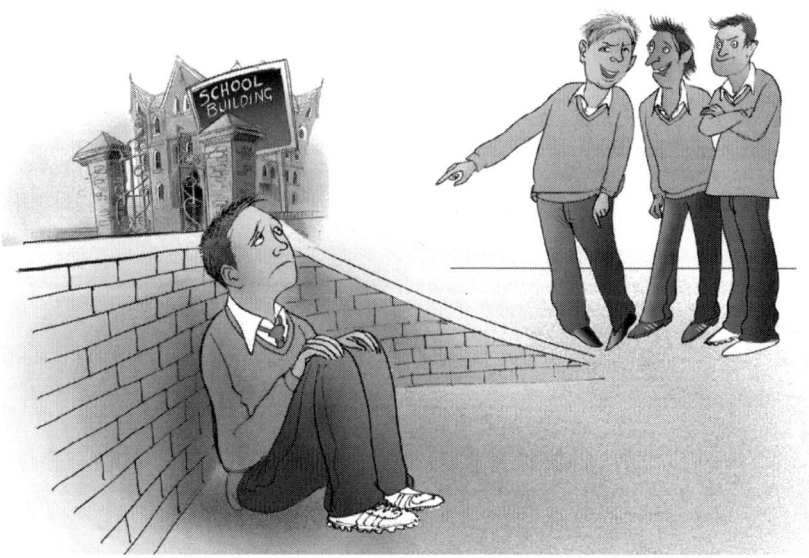

Figure 7.1. Picture elicitation of fictional stories from the Narrative Intervention Programme (Joffe, 2011).

stories supports the learning of a story framework that can underpin the telling and writing of stories in the classroom and in social settings. Using a set story grammar framework, for example Stein and Glenn's (1979) story grammar approach, provides valuable structure and cohesion to the oral and written productions of young people. Visual support, in the form of a story planner as shown in Figure 7.2, is helpful at making the different story components explicit, and can be displayed on the young person's desk throughout lessons, and used at home when preparing homework. Initially, greater focus can be given to the more concrete aspects of the story, for example the setting, and events. When the students become more skilled at storytelling, focus can then shift to more abstract elements, including the themes, motivation of characters and moral of the story (Westby, 1991). With experience, students can take turns telling the same story from the perspectives of the different characters, or providing different endings for the same story (Larson & McKinley, 2003).

Storytelling can also encourage a greater awareness and use of inferential understanding and figurative language. Providing young people with examples of a range of literary devices in stories - for example metaphor, personification,

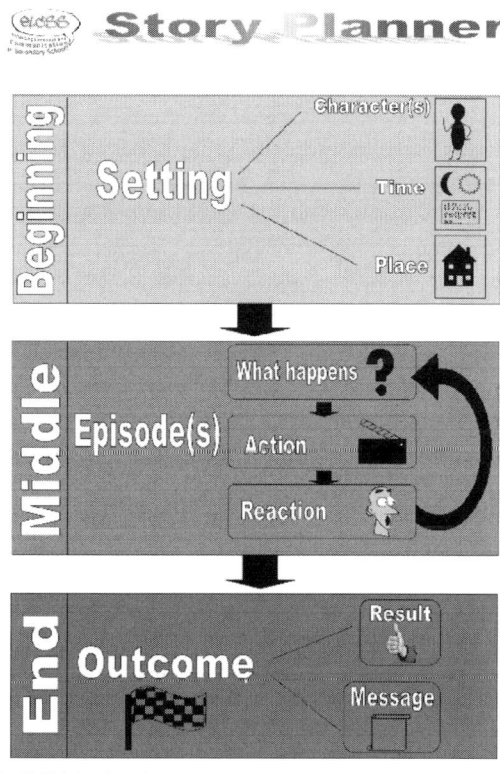

Figure 7.2 Story planner from the Narrative Intervention Programme (Joffe, 2011).

hyperbole – and exploring with the students their impact on the listener and the power they have to create images that go beyond the words produced, facilitates their understanding and appreciation of such devices, and encourages their use in their own narratives.

Supporting young people to understand double meanings and inferences is crucial, considering the important role that inferential language plays in the secondary school context (Nippold, 2007). Adolescents can be challenged, through stories and probing questions, to consider more deeply the words heard in a story, or even the words that are unspoken, and go beyond the literal interpretation. Encouraging students to ask questions and consider the characters' plans, motivations, feelings and goals, their interactions with each other, and how this might differ from what they would expect, or from their own behaviour and feelings, will assist in developing more advanced story comprehension skills (Westby, 2005).

Stories present a valuable vehicle for enhancing all areas of language. Speech, voice and fluency can be targeted at the more functional conversational level using narratives. Storytelling can highlight for students the power and fun of language through the use of characterizations and rich, complex and diverse language. Stories with detailed and interesting characters can help develop rich and new vocabulary. Similarly, narratives can be the vehicle for modelling correct use of and practising morphology and syntax, including tense markers, pronoun use, and inclusion of coordinating and subordinating conjunctions, extended noun phrases and complex sentences.

The area of paralinguistic language, including body language, gestures, facial expressions, tone and pitch of the voice, become prominent during the storytelling process when exploring different means to making a story more exciting and engaging, and can be an important therapy target. Stories provide opportunities through characterization and dialogue to vary paralinguistic language, for example pitch, rate, volume, and explore the impact this has on overall understanding.

General principles for intervention with adolescents

In order to get maximum participation from the older age group, it is important to make explicit the aims and learning objectives and, wherever possible, involve the young person in generating them and evaluating them at the end of the intervention programme (Joffe, 2011).

The benefits of storytelling may not be obvious to the student, and time spent on exploring the advantages of storytelling will be worthwhile. Ensuring the aims and content of the intervention are relevant to the client will maximize participation and motivation. Choosing content around the interests of the young person, and stories and themes that are being covered in the school curriculum, or are high profile in current affairs or in popular culture, guarantees that the intervention has relevance. Adolescence marks the move from concrete to formal operational thought (Piaget, 1959), providing the means for more abstract and logical thinking about complex issues. This can herald an interest in social, political and religious affairs (Santrock 1996; Schickedanz et al., 2001), an interest that should be encouraged and explored through current and relevant literature. This will help support the transfer and generalization of newly-learned skills to other settings.

Narrative group work can be valuable in this older age group, taking into account their focus on peers and socialization, and group members can be supported to provide constructive feedback and support to each other. This supports the development of self-regulation and self-appraisal, essential executive function skills developing in adolescence (Nippold, 2007). Storytelling intervention focusing on macrostructure and microstructure demands working at a metalinguistic and metacognitive level, which can be challenging for young people with SLCN, despite this being a requirement for academic attainment in secondary school (Nippold, 2007). Westby (1991) cites metanarrative skills as essential for developing an understanding of more complex embedded narratives typical during adolescence. A significant amount of practice should be given to support a more 'meta' way of thinking. Research from Blakemore and Choudhury (2006) suggests that during adolescence significant brain reorganization takes place in the frontal lobe where these executive functions occur, and this period is therefore a fertile ground from which to develop and train metacognition. This can take the form of a range of activities encouraging reflection on the language being used to tell a story, as well as discussion about the impact that different stories may have. Questions can be asked that encourage more metacognitive and metalinguistic thinking, for example, "Why do you think the character reacted in that way?", or "What specific words in the beginning of the story led you to believe the character was kind?"

Conclusion

Stories are a common feature of our lives and are associated with cognitive, language and communication levels, educational attainment and general psychosocial functioning. This chapter highlights their importance in adolescence, both as a tool for enhancing oral and written language as well as a means for developing self-esteem, confidence and enhancing psychosocial skills. Storytelling has a clear developmental progression, and develops from early childhood into adolescence. The inclusion of stories in assessment provides a functional and ecological dimension, and a window of cognitive, language and socio-emotional functioning. Narratives can play a role in identifying children with SLCN, and differentiating between different clinical groups. Storytelling can be used in flexible and creative ways to enhance a young person's educational attainment, language and social relationships. Stories occur across all societies and cultures, and can therefore be employed with students speaking different languages, and from different cultures and socio-economic backgrounds. Narratives should be used more frequently in clinical practice, both in the assessment and management of the adolescent. It is never too late to encourage a love for storytelling.

Reflective questions

1. Reflect on a challenge you have faced in your life and how sharing your story with others may have shaped its outcome or resolution.

2. How would you go about convincing a young person about the importance of stories to his overall development?

3. Think about a young person with whom you work who has social communication difficulties. How do you think you could use storytelling to support their social use of language?

4. Consider some strategies that you would use to elicit stories from a group of young people reluctant to express themselves.

5. How would you best assess storytelling with a young person with English as an additional language, exploring story structure and language features?

References

Adams, C., Coke, R., Crutchley, A., Hesketh, A., & Reeves, D. (2001) *Assessment of Comprehension and Expression 6-11*. London: NFER-Nelson.

Alt, M., Arizmendi, G.D., & DiLallo, J.N. (2016). The role of socioeconomic status in the narrative story retells of school-aged English language learners. *Language, Speech, and Hearing Services in Schools, 47*(4), 313-323.

Applebee, A. (1978). *The Child's Concept of a Story*. Chicago: University of Chicago Press.

Berman, R.A. & Slobin, D.I. (1994). *Relating Events in Narrative: A Crosslinguistic Developmental Study*. Hillsdale, NJ: Erlbaum,

Bishop, D.V.M. (2004). *Expression, Reception and Recall of Narrative Instrument: ERRNI*. London: Pearson.

Bishop, D.V.M. & Adams, C. (1990). A prospective study of the relationship between specific language impairment, phonological disorders and reading retardation. *Journal of Child Psychology and Psychiatry, 31*(7), 1027-1050.

Bishop, D.V.M. & Adams, C. (1992). Comprehension problems in children with specific language impairment: Literal and inferential meaning. *Journal of Speech and Hearing Research, 35*(1), 119-129.

Bishop, D.V.M. & Edmundson, A. (1987) Language-impaired 4-year-olds: Distinguishing transient from persistent impairment. *Journal of Speech and Hearing Disorders, 52,* 156–173.

Blakemore, S.J. & Choudhury, S. (2006). Development of the adolescent brain: Implications for executive function and social cognition. *Journal of Child Psychiatry and Psychology, 47*(3-4), 296-312.

Bliss, L.S., Covington, Z., & McCabe, A. (1999). Assessing the narratives of African American children. *Contemporary Issues in Communication Science and Disorders, 26,* 160-167.

Blom, E. & Boerma, T. (2016). Why do children with language impairment have difficulties with narrative macrostructure? *Research in Developmental Disabilities, 55,* 301-311.

Boerma, T., Leseman, P., Timmermeister, M., Wijnen, F., & Blom, E. (2016). Narrative abilities of monolingual and bilingual children with and without language impairment: Implications for clinical practice. *International Journal of Language & Communication Disorders, 51*(6), 626-638.

Bohanek, J.G. & Fivush, R. (2010). Personal narratives, well-being, and gender in adolescence. *Cognitive Development, 25*(4), 368-379.

Botting, N. (2002) Narrative as a tool for the assessment of linguistic and pragmatic impairments. *Journal of Child, Language, Teaching and Therapy, 18*(1), 1–21.

Boudreau, D. (2008). Narrative abilities. Advances in research and implications for clinical practice. *Topics in Language Disorders, 28*(2), 99–114.

Bruner, J. (1991). The narrative construction of reality. *Critical Inquiry, 18*(1), 1-21.

Cohen, N.J. (2001). *Language Impairment and Psychopathology in Infants, Children, and Adolescents.* London: Sage.

Crais, E.R. & Lorch, N. (1994). Oral narratives in school-age children. *Topics in Language Disorders, 14*(3), 13-28.

Davies, P., Shanks, B., & Davies, K. (2004) Improving narrative skills in young children with delayed language development. *Educational Review, 56*(3), 271–286.

Department for Education (2013). *The National Curriculum in England Framework Document.* London: Crown Copyright. Retrieved 10 February 2017 from https://www.gov.uk/government/uploads/system/uploads/attachment_data/file/381344/Master_final_national_curriculum_28_Nov.pdf.

Dickinson, D., Wolf, M., & Stotsky, S. (1993). Words move: The interwoven development of oral and written language. In J.B. Gleason (Ed.), *The Development of Language, 3rd ed.* (pp.369-420). Boston: Allyn & Bacon.

Ebert, K.D. & Scott, C.M. (2014). Relationships between narrative language samples and norm-referenced test scores in language assessments of school-aged children. *Language, Speech and Hearing Services in Schools, 45,* 337-350.

Fazio, B., Naremore, R., & Connell, P. (1993) Tracking children from poverty at risk for specific language impairment: A 3-year longitudinal study. *Journal of Speech and Hearing Research, 39*(3), 611–624.

Gillam, R.B. & Peterson, N.A. (2017). *TNL-2: Test of Narrative Language, 2nd ed*. Austin, TX: Pro-Ed Publications.

Gillam, S., Gillam, R.B., & Laing, C. (2012). *Supporting Knowledge in Language and Literacy (SKILL)*. Narrative Intervention Curriculum. Utah State University.

Gillam, S.L., Gillam, R.B., Fargo, J., Olszewski, A. & Segura, H, (2016). Monitoring Indicators of Scholarly Language (MISL): A Progress-monitoring Instrument for Measuring Narrative Discourse Skills. ComD Faculty Publications. Paper 494. Retrieved 8th August 2017 from http://digitalcommons.usu.edu/comd_facpub/494

Gillam, R.B., McFadden, T.U., & van Kleeck, A. (1995). Improving the narrative abilities of children with language disorders: Whole language and language skills approaches. In M. Fey, J. Windsor & J. Reichle (Eds), *Communication Intervention for School-aged Children* (pp.145–182). Baltimore, MD: Paul H. Brookes.

Griffin, T.M., Hemphill, L., Camp, L., & Wolf, D.P. (2004). Oral discourse in the preschool years and later literacy skills. *First Language, 24*(2), 123–147.

Halliday, M.A.K. & Hasan, R. (1976). *Cohesion in English*. London: Longman.

Heilmann, J., Miller, J.F., Nockerts, A., & Dunaway, C. (2010). Properties of the narrative scoring scheme using narrative retells in young school-age children. *American Journal of Speech-Language Pathology, 19*, 154–166.

Hudson, J.A. & Shapiro, L.R. (1991). From knowing to telling: The development of children's scripts, stories, and personal narratives. In: A. McCabe & C. Peterson (Eds), *Developing Narrative Structure* (pp.89–136). Hillsdale, NJ: Lawrence Erlbaum Associates.

Hughes, D.L., McGillivray, L., & Schmidek, M. (1997). *Guide to Narrative Language: Procedures for Assessment*. Eau Claire, WI: Thinking Publications.

Joffe, V.L. (2011). *Narrative Intervention Programme*. Milton Keynes, UK: Speechmark.

Joffe, V.L. (2006). Enhancing language and communication in language-impaired secondary school-aged children. In J. Ginsborg & J. Clegg (Eds), *Language and Social Disadvantage* (pp.207-216). London: John Wiley & Sons.

Joffe, V.L. (2013). Using narratives to enhance language and communication in secondary school students. In N. Grove (Ed.), *Using Storytelling to Support Children and Adults with Special Needs* (pp.55–63). London: David Fulton.

Joffe, V.L., Rixon, L., Hirani, S., & Hulme, C. (submitted). Improving storytelling and vocabulary in secondary school students with language and communication difficulties: A randomized control intervention study. *International Journal of Language and Communication Disorders*.

Justice, L. (2006). Evidence-based practice, response to intervention and the prevention of reading difficulties. *Language, Speech and Hearing Services in Schools, 37*(4), 284–297.

Kail, M. (2004). On-line grammaticality judgments in French children and adults: A crosslinguistic perspective. *Journal of Child Language, 31*(3), 713–737.

Labov, W. (1972). *Language in the Inner City*. Pittsburgh, PA: University of Pennsylvania Press.

Larson, V.L. & McKinley, N.L. (2003). *Communication Solutions for Older Students. Assessment and Intervention Strategies.* Eau Claire, WI: Thinking Publications.

Leadholm, B. & Miller J. (1992). *Language Sample Analysis: The Wisconsin Guide.* Madison, WI: Wisconsin Department of Public Instruction.

Liles, B.Z. (1985). Cohesion in the narratives of normal and disordered children. *Journal of Speech and Hearing Research, 28,* 123–133.

Liles, B.Z. (1993). Narrative discourse in children with language disorders and children with normal language: A critical review of the literature. *Journal of Speech and Hearing Research, 36,* 868–882.

Liles, B.Z., Duffy, R.J., Merritt, D.D., & Purcell, S.L. (1995). Measurement of narrative discourse ability in children with language disorders. *Journal of Speech and Hearing Research, 38,* 415–425.

Loveland, K.A., McEvoy, R.E., Tunali, B., & Kelley, M.L. (1990). Narrative story telling in autism and Down's syndrome. *British Journal of Developmental Psychology, 8,* 9–23.

Mandler, J.M. & Johnson, N.S. (1977). Remembrance of things parsed: Story structure and recall. *Cognitive Psychology, 9*(1), 111–151.

Manolitsi, M. & Botting, N. (2011). Language abilities in children with autism and language impairment: Using narrative as an additional source of clinical information. *Child Language Teaching and Therapy, 27*(1), 39–55.

Mayer, M. (1969). *Frog, Where Are You?* New York: Dial Press.

Mayer, M. (1973). *Frog On His Own.* New York: Dial Press.

Mayer, M. (1974). *Frog Goes to Dinner.* New York: Dial Press.

McCabe, A. (1995). Evaluating narrative discourse skills. In K. Cole, P. Dale & T. Thal (Eds), *Assessment of Communication and Language* (pp.121-141). Baltimore, MD: Paul H. Brookes.

McCabe, A. & Rollins, P.R. (1994). Assessment of preschool narrative skills. *American Journal of Speech-Language Pathology, 3*(1), 45-56.

Meek, M. (1991). *On Being Literate.* London: Bodley Head.

Mello, R. (2001). The power of storytelling: How oral narrative influences children's relationships in classrooms. *International Journal of Education and the Arts, 2*(1). Retrieved 25 February 2015 from http://www.ijea.org/v2n1

Merritt, D.D. & Liles, B.Z. (1987). Story grammar ability in children with and without language disorder: Story generation, story retelling and story comprehension. *Journal of Speech and Hearing Research, 30,* 539-552.

Merritt, D.D. & Liles, B.Z. (1989). Narrative analysis: Clinical applications of story generation and story retelling. *Journal of Speech and Hearing Disorders, 54*(3), 438-447.

Michaels, S. (1981). "Sharing time": Children's narrative styles and differential access to literacy. *Language in Society, 10*(3), 423-442.

Miller, J.F. & Chapman, R. (2003). *SALT: Systematic Analysis of Language Transcripts.* Madison, WI: University of Wisconsin-Madison.

Miller, J.F., Andriacchi, K., & Nockerts, A. (2015). *Assessing Language Production using SALT Software. A Clinician's Guide to Language Sample Analysis, 2nd ed.* Middleton, WI: SALT Software LLC.

Minami, M. & McCabe, A. (1991). Haiku as a discourse regulation device: A stanza analysis of Japanese children's personal narratives. *Language in Society, 20*(4), 577–599.

Miranda, A.A, McCabe, A., & Bliss, L.S. (1998). Jumping around and leaving things out: A profile of narrative abilities of children with specific language impairment. *Applied Psycholinguistics, 19,* 647–667.

Naremore, R., Densmore, A., & Harman, D. (1995) *Language Intervention with School-Aged Children: Conversation, Narrative and Text.* San Diego: Singular.

Nippold, M.A. (2007). *Later Language Development: School-age Children, Adolescents, and Young Adults.* Austin, Texas: Pro-Ed.

Nippold, M.A. (2010). *Language Sampling with Adolescents.* San Diego: Plural.

Nippold, M.A. (1995). School-aged children and adolescents: Norms for word definition. An introduction. *Language, Speech and Hearing Services in Schools, 26,* 307–308.

Nippold, M., Frantz-Kaspar, M.W., Crammond, P.M., Kirk, C., Hayward-Mayhew, C., & MacKinnon, M. (2014). Conversational and narrative speaking in adolescents: Examining the use of complex syntax. *Journal of Speech, Language and Hearing Research, 57,* 876–886.

Norbury, C.F. & Bishop, D,V,M. (2003). Narrative skills of children with communication impairments. *International Journal of Language and Communication Disorders, 38*(3), 287–313.

Norbury, C., Gemmell, T., & Paul, R. (2013). Pragmatics abilities in narrative production: A cross-disorder comparison. *Journal of Child Language, 40,* 1–26.

Paul, R., Hernandez, R., Taylor, L., & Johnson, K. (1996). Narrative development in late talkers: Early school age. *Journal of Speech, Language, and Hearing Research, 39*(6), 1295–1303.

Petersen, D.B. (2011). A systematic review of narrative-based language intervention with children who have language impairment. *Communication Disorders Quarterly, 32*(4), 207–220.

Petersen, D.B., Gillam, S.L., & Gillam, R.B. (2008). Emerging procedures in narrative assessment. The index of narrative complexity. *Topics in Language Disorders, 28*(2), 115–130.

Peterson, C. & McCabe, A. (1983). *Developmental Psycholinguistics: Three Ways of Looking at a Child's Narrative.* New York: Macmillan.

Peterson, C. & McCabe, A. (1991). Linking children's connective use and narrative macrostructure. In A. McCabe & C. Petersen (Eds), *Developing Narrative Structure* (pp.29–53). Hillsdale, NJ: Erlbaum.

Piaget, J. (1959). *The Language and Thought of the Child.* London: Routledge & Kegan Paul.

Preece, A. (1987). The range of narrative forms conversationally produced by young children. *Journal of Child Language, 14,* 273–295.

Reed, V.A. & Spicer, L. (2003). The relative importance of selected communication skills for adolescents' interactions with their teachers: High school teachers' opinions. *Language, Speech, and Hearing Services in Schools, 34*(4), 343–357.

Reese, E., Suggate, S., Long, J., & Schaughency, E. (2010). Children's oral narrative and reading skills in the first three years of reading instruction. *Reading & Writing: An Interdisciplinary Journal, 23*, 627–644.

Rollins, P.R. (2014). Narrative skills in young adults with high-functioning autism spectrum disorders. *Communication Disorders Quarterly, 36*(1), 21–28.

Roth, F.P. (1986). Oral narrative abilities of learning-disabled students. *Topics in Language Disorders, 7*(1), 21–30.

Roth, F.P. & Spekman, N.J. (1986) Narrative discourse: Spontaneously generated stories of learning-disabled and normally achieving students. *Journal of Speech and Hearing Disorders, 51*, 8–23.

Rumelhart, D.E. (1975). Notes on a schema for stories. Representation and understanding. *Studies in Cognitive Science, 211*(236), 45.

Santrock, J.W. (1996). *Adolescence: An Introduction, 6th ed.* Madison, WI: Brown & Benchmark.

Schank, R. (1990). *Tell Me a Story: Narrative and Intelligence.* Evanston, IL: Northwestern University Press.

Schickedanz, J.A., Schickedanz, D.I., Forsyth, P.D., & Forsyth, G.A. (2001). *Understanding Children and Adolescents, 4th ed.* Boston, MA: Allyn & Bacon.

Snow, P.C. & Powell, M.B. (2005). What's the story? An exploration of narrative language abilities in male juvenile offenders. *Psychology, Crime & Law, 11*(3), 239–253.

Stein, N. & Glenn, C. (1979). An analysis of story comprehension in elementary school children. In R.O. Freedle (Ed.), *New Directions in Discourse Processing* (Vol 2, pp.53–120). Norwood, NJ: Ablex.

Stringer, H. (2006) Facilitating narrative and social skills in secondary school students with language and behaviour difficulties. In J. Ginsborg & J. Clegg (Eds), *Language and Social Disadvantage* (pp.199–206). London: John Wiley & Sons.

Stothard, S.E., Snowling, M.J., Bishop, D.VM., Chipchase, B.B., & Kaplan, C.A. (1998). Language-impaired preschoolers: A follow-up into adolescence. *Journal of Speech, Language, and Hearing Research, 41*(2), 407–418.

Swanson, L., Fey, M., Mills, C., & Hood, L. (2005). Use of narrative based language intervention with children who have specific language impairment. *American Journal of Speech-Language Pathology, 14*, 131–143.

Tabors, P.O., Snow, C.E., & Dickinson, D.K. (2001). Homes and schools together: Supporting language and literacy development. In D.K. Dickinson & P.O. Tabors (Eds), *Beginning Literacy with Language: Young Children Learning at Home and School* (pp.313–334). Baltimore, MD: Brookes.

van der Lely, H.J.K. (1997). Narrative discourse in grammatical specific language impaired children: A modular deficit? *Journal of Child Language, 24*, 221–256.

Wells, G. (1986). *The Meaning Makers: Children Learning Language and Using Language to Learn*. Portsmouth, NH: Heinemann Educational Books.

Westby, C.E. (1984). Development of narrative language abilities. In G.P. Wallach & K.G. Butler (Eds), *Language Learning Disabilities in School-aged Children* (pp.103–127). Baltimore: Williams & Wilkins.

Westby, C.E. (1991). Learning to talk – talking to learn. Oral-literate language differences. In C. Simon (Ed.), *Communication Skills and Classroom Success: Assessment and Therapy Methodologies for Language and Learning Disabled Students* (pp.334–357). Eau Claire, WI: Thinking Publications.

Westby, C.E. (1998). Communication refinement in school age and adolescence. In W. Hayes & B. Shulman (Eds), *Communication Development: Foundations, Processes and Clinical Applications* (pp.511–560). Baltimore: Williams & Wilkins.

Westby, C.E. (2005). Assessing and remediating text comprehension problems. In H. Catts & A. Kamhi (Eds), *Language and Reading Disabilities* (pp.157–232). Boston: Allyn & Bacon.

Westby, C.E. & Culatta, B. (2016). Telling tales: Personal event narratives and life stories. *Language, Speech, and Hearing Services in Schools*, *47*(4), 260–282.

Westby, C.E. & Washington, K.N. (2016). Using the international classification of functioning, disability and health in assessment and intervention of school-aged children with language impairments. *Language, Speech and Hearing Services in Schools*, *48*, 137–152.

Wetherell, D., Botting, N., & Conti-Ramsden, G. (2007). Narrative in adolescent SLI: A comparison with peers across two different narrative genres. *International Journal of Language and Communication Disorders*, *42*(5), 583–605.

World Health Organisation (2001). *International Classification of Functioning, Disability and Health (ICF)*. Geneva: World Health Organisation. Retrieved 23 June 2017 from http://apps.who.int/iris/bitstream/10665/42407/1/9241545429.pdf

Wiig, E.H., Semel, E., & Secord, W.A. (2013). *Clinical Evaluation of Language Fundamentals, Fifth Edition (CELF-5)*. London: Pearson.

8 Vocabulary enhancement in teenagers with language difficulties

Hilary Lowe and Victoria L. Joffe

Learning outcomes

This chapter will enable readers to:

- Develop a critical awareness of the importance of vocabulary in adolescence and its impact on language, academic attainment and psychosocial functioning in adolescence and adulthood

- Describe the nature of vocabulary deficits in the adolescent population

- Evaluate evidence-based interventions at the universal, targeted, and specialist levels for supporting students who have these difficulties

- Identify key factors to consider when choosing an appropriate model of intervention delivery in the classroom, group or individual context.

Introduction

It is estimated that between 6 and 17 years of age, children acquire 3000 words per year (Clark, 1995), which equates to eight or nine new words a day. Acquiring new vocabulary poses a particular challenge for children with language disorder, and this continues to be the case for older children with language disorder. Rice and Hoffman (2015) examined the receptive vocabulary of 240 children with language disorder in comparison to 279 typically developing children aged

2:6, and reassessed them annually until they were 21 years of age. Those with language disorder had lower receptive vocabulary scores than their typically developing peers throughout this age range. As vocabulary knowledge is a key aspect of language and literacy, crucial for accessing the curriculum and academic success (Snowling, Muter, & Carroll, 2007), children with language disorder are thus placed at a disadvantage throughout their schooling.

Word learning

Early word learning in the first few months and years of life has been widely researched. In order to learn a new word, a network of connections needs to be built up: semantic (meaning), grammatical, and phonological (sound) (Leonard, 1998). In order to learn the meaning of a word, children need to identify a recurring phonological form from the stream of speech, and map that phonological form onto the meaning of the word (Bishop, 1997). In order to use a word expressively, children need to retrieve the phonological form that they have previously mapped onto the meaning of that word, and access the motor program required to produce the word (Stackhouse & Wells, 1997). In the first years of life, word learning becomes very efficient such that children can learn a meaning of a word, and can use it, with very few exposures; a phenomenon known as fast-mapping (Clark, 1993). Efficient word learners have intact cognitive skills, executive functions, and motivation to communicate. Young children make use of contextual cues to assist them in the mapping process, such as social, perceptual, semantic or intonational cues. For example, to map the word 'dinner' onto the object, a young child is following the caregiver's eye-gaze (social); seeing and smelling the food she is looking at and placing in front of him (perceptual); linking this word with other words the caregiver is using – "Here's your spoon for your dinner" – (semantic); and perhaps associating the sing-song tone of voice she might be using with a happy and routine event (intonational).

The fast-mapping process of young children is usually applied to the learning of labels for objects, and these are typically high frequency and concrete, for example, 'dog', 'spoon' and 'table'. The words children need to learn and use as they get older, however, become less concrete and more abstract, and include, for example, 'welfare', 'victory' and 'democracy'; therefore, the way in which children learn new words changes over time. As typically developing children get older, they are more likely to acquire new words through contextual abstraction rather than direct teaching (Nippold, 2007); however, they also need direct definitional instruction in order to generalize that learning to other contexts (Best, Dockrell, & Braisby, 2006). Children learn to map words onto actions, attributes, and concepts. Increased sophistication of cognitive and executive function skills is required as word learning increases in complexity. Adolescents can operate at a greater level of abstraction and metalinguistic awareness, and achieve more complex levels of attention, memory and processing skill (Ravid, 2004; van Kleeck, 1984). Furthermore, word learning is not an 'all-or-nothing' phenomenon (Beck, McKeown, & Kucan, 2002, p.9). Each individual's lexicon contains words with varying depths of knowledge: we know the vague meaning of some words but would have difficulty explaining what they mean; we might understand some words if we heard or read them, but would never use them expressively ourselves; and we may know a single meaning of some words but may not be aware of polysemous meanings which those words can have in different contexts.

Literacy also begins to play a larger role in word learning in older children. During the school years, language and literacy "enjoy a symbiotic relationship" (Nippold, 1988, p.29). With proficient literacy skills, children and adolescents can absorb new vocabulary through reading, such that spoken and written language develop hand in hand. Older children make use of their prior knowledge, and embed meanings of words within their knowledge of the semantic domain (Dockrell, Braisby, & Best, 2007). Newly-encountered words are compared and contrasted with words already in the lexicon in order to adjust and establish semantic boundaries (Nippold, 1988).

Vocabulary acquisition in children and adolescents with language disorder

Children with language disorder have difficulties with aspects of these fundamental building blocks required for word learning. This does not result in a complete inability to learn words, but reduced efficiency. Rice, Oetting, Marquis, et al. (1994) suggest that there is a minimal input constraint on the frequency of word exposure, and that if this is overcome children with specific language impairment have the capacity to learn new words. However, although they do acquire a breadth of vocabulary, their depth of understanding can still be limited (McGregor, Oleson, Bahnsen, & Duff, 2013). Children with language disorders find it harder to generalize meanings of words to new contexts, e.g., *dangerous* (dangerous dog and dangerous car), and to understand the subtle connotations of words with similar meaning, e.g., *frustrated* and *irritated*.

They are also less able to develop understanding of the figurative application of concrete words, e.g., *sweet* (sweet-natured man), *hard* (hard-hearted) (Dockrell & Messer, 2004).

Some children and young people present with a specific word-finding difficulty in which they have difficulty retrieving a known word. Kail and Leonard (1986) investigated the word-finding ability of children with language impairment compared to age-matched typically developing children aged 8:11–12:11 years. They found that the children with language disorder were slower to name items and named fewer items. These authors proposed that word retrieval difficulties are a result of word storage inadequacies leading to sparse semantic representations. With the mechanisms of word learning vulnerable from the very start, sparse semantic representations limit the foundation on which new vocabulary knowledge is built, thus vocabulary building continues to be a challenge.

Some researchers propose that word storage inadequacies are largely semantic in nature (Lahey & Edwards, 1999; McGregor, Newman, Reilly, & Capone, 2002); others that there is a weakness of phonological short-term memory or phonological processing, resulting in inaccurate phonological representations (Constable, Stackhouse, & Wells, 1997; Gathercole & Baddeley, 1990). The naming errors which children make are often used as evidence for the underlying nature of the difficulty. For example, 'broccoli' for *celery*, and 'colander' for *funnel* may be indicative of an underlying semantic impairment with the error word sharing many semantic properties with the target word. Similarly, a phonological weakness may account for the following substitutions, [hektagɒn] for *hexagon* and [pɔtentɪf] for *percentage*, with some small but key phonological differences between the error and target words. The heterogeneity of children's language disorder has long been established, and it can therefore be expected that the nature of vocabulary difficulties will vary across children, and in line with the individual's particular constellation of language and cognitive abilities.

Furthermore, there are often limitations in literacy development (McArthur, Hogben, Edwards, et al., 2000), affecting the acquisition of new vocabulary knowledge through reading, which in turn impacts upon reading comprehension and further literacy development (Stanovich, 1986). Thus, children with language disorder are less able to glean word knowledge from the written word, less likely to be able to derive the meaning of new vocabulary from context (Cain, Oakhill, & Lemmon, 2004), and less able to benefit from literacy-based approaches. Therefore, specific direct intervention to enhance vocabulary development is required.

Factors to consider in choosing an intervention

In devising appropriate intervention, the individual's linguistic and cognitive profile needs to be taken into account, as well as other intrinsic factors such as their motivation and ability to engage with intervention. Viewing the student in the context of their social and educational circumstances also plays an important part in the decision-making.

Which words to teach

A widely-advocated approach to vocabulary teaching is that of Beck, McKeown, and Kucan (2002, 2013), who promote the concept of robust vocabulary instruction. Robust vocabulary instruction involves explicit discussion of words when exploring literary texts in the classroom. The rationale is that there are simply too many words to teach individually, and therefore the aim is to create an interest in wanting to know what new words mean, to foster asking questions for clarification, and to encourage exploring and discussing personalized contexts in which one might use a word. There is an emphasis on using contextual cues from the adjacent text, and on using morphological cues within the word. This is essentially a literacy-based semantic approach which engenders independent word learning.

Beck and colleagues describe a three-tier approach to vocabulary (examples taken from Beck et al., 2013, p.16):

Tier 1: Basic, everyday words which most children will have acquired prior to school entry, e.g., *baby, happy.*

Tier 2: Words which are of high frequency within the vocabulary of mature language users, and can be used across a variety of contexts, e.g., *maintain, fortunate, perform.*

Tier 3: Low frequency words which will probably only be encountered in a topic-specific context, e.g., *isotope, peninsula.*

Robust vocabulary instruction focuses on the teaching of Tier 2 words: words which are crucial to the understanding of the text and are of maximum functionality. Beck and colleagues suggest that a rule of thumb for identifying a

Tier 2 word is whether it is a more advanced word for a concept which a child can already express, e.g., *fortunate* for *lucky*. In this way, children are given opportunities for building on prior knowledge, and adding to and enriching their existing lexicon. Robust vocabulary instruction in this form is often the remit of the English teacher, whereby literary appreciation is the content of the lesson; however, the concept of Tier 2 words as cross-curricular words can be encountered across many subjects. Tier 2 words often need to be taught before Tier 3 (subject-specific) words can be understood; for example, in explaining what *assassination* means, the student also needs to understand *political* and *motive*. Tier 2 also includes the words of instruction, sometimes known as command words or exam words. These are often verbs, such as *illustrate, evaluate, predict*.

Another approach, considering the high number of subject-specific words in each topic which are required in order to succeed in any given subject, is to focus on Tier 3 words from the curriculum. At secondary school, in each topic, typically taught over three to six weeks, up to 15 or 20 words may be identified as key words for that topic. This is beyond the reach of some young people with language disorder. One idea to address this is to use the concept of a vocabulary dartboard. In the centre of the dartboard, the teacher who is planning the topic decides on perhaps six or eight essential key words which all students need to learn, followed by a number of words which are desirable for most students to learn, and on the outside of the dartboard are the words which it might be nice for some students to learn. This approach is known variably as 'essential, desirable, might be nice'; 'all, most, some'; or 'must, should, could'. Those who are working with the student then know which words are the most important to target in vocabulary support. Collaboration between therapy providers and teachers is essential if therapy is going to include instruction in subject-specific words. A collaborative approach between teaching and therapy practitioners has been shown to be an effective way of addressing adolescents' language needs (Lowe & Joffe, 2017; Starling, Munro, Togher, & Arciuli, 2012).

A harmonization of these two approaches can be achieved by incorporating the principles of robust vocabulary instruction into the teaching of subject-specific words. The key ingredient – fostering independent word learning – can be central to both a Tier 2 approach and a Tier 3 approach: encouraging an interest in words, building on prior knowledge and adding to the child's existing lexicon, developing metalinguistic awareness, making using of contextual and morphological cues, and linking with literacy to develop the literate lexicon.

What to include in specific word-learning intervention

Self-awareness and motivation

Even before intervention starts, in order to exploit and develop metalinguistic awareness, it is useful for students to carry out a self-rating assessment to gauge their baseline knowledge of the words (Lubliner & Smetana, 2005). This can also provide a motivation for students. Motivation needs to be addressed in a different way than with younger children, who are easily motivated by games and intrinsic rewards (Joffe, 2011). A self-rating assessment provides a mechanism by which the students themselves identify which words they need to learn. Elks and McLachlan (2008) have devised a word-learning score task for this purpose, based on the depth of word knowledge scale developed by Dale (1965).

How this is used in practice will depend on whether it is done on a one-to-one basis with more in-depth discussion, or individually in class with the students rating themselves independently. Either way, it hooks them into learning (Watson, 1995) by raising their awareness of their own word knowledge and identifying for them which words they need to learn.

Semantic and phonological intervention

For children and adolescents with language disorder, a linguistic ingredient needs to be explicitly added depending on the source of their word-learning difficulty. To address semantic weaknesses, a closer focus on semantic organization can be targeted, and to address phonological weaknesses greater emphasis can be placed on the word's phonological representation through phonological awareness activities which encourage explicit exploration of the sound structure of words (for example, producing words that rhyme). In an online survey of 39 teachers and 104 speech and language therapists, carried out by the first author as part of her PhD research, practitioners were asked which strategies they used to teach new words, and which they felt were the most effective. Many teachers and speech and language therapists (SLTs) felt that a combination approach works best. This may be because a multifaceted approach addresses the unique constellation of skills in each individual, by not only developing skills in which there is a deficit but also building on strengths, as well as explicitly highlighting semantic and phonological features of the word for the student. A combination of phonological-semantic activities benefits those with phonological weaknesses but semantic strengths, as well as those with semantic weaknesses but phonological strengths (Lahey & Edwards, 1999).

Semantic representation

Semantic feature analysis includes discussion about function, location, attributes, category, and personalization of the word to the students' own experience. Semantic representations and organization can be strengthened by the use of a word map. Elks and McLachlan (2008) and Joffe (2011) are amongst those who have devised word maps with the adolescent population in mind. The essence of a word map is that it allows students to explore semantic features of the word and connect these with the word's phonological form. A word map can be used when new concepts are introduced, and forms the basis for discussion about what the word means. It provides multiple opportunities for the word to be modelled, thereby overcoming the minimal input constraint (Rice et al., 1994). The word map can be used across many different settings: in the classroom; in smaller groups as well as on a one-to-one basis; and at home, it can also form the basis of an easy shared activity between parents and their child.

Phonological processing

As well as providing a framework for exploring the semantic features of a concept, the word map has spaces to explore the phonological form of the word. This includes phonological awareness tasks such as initial sound, syllable, and rhyme. This provides opportunities for students to say the word aloud, which is crucial (Braisby, Dockrell, & Best, 2001). Word production activates the motor planning function of the speech processing system (the motor planning function is responsible for planning the neuromuscular activity required to articulate a word), and further strengthens the phonological representation of the word (Stackhouse & Wells, 1997). Using the word in a sentence brings phonology and semantics together and is an important longer-term goal of intervention.

Another simple activity providing opportunities to raise awareness of the phonological features of a word is Sound and Meaning Bingo (Lowe & Joffe, 2017). Topic words are written on the board and students choose a given number of them to write in their own grid. Bingo is an activity used by many teachers, usually delivered semantically only by giving definition clues. Sound and Meaning Bingo adds the phonological element to the clues given. Examples of clues for 'kinetic' might be: "It begins with k (phonological clue) and means movement energy (semantic clue)" or "It rhymes with frenetic (phonological) and is the type of energy created by a rolling ball (semantic)".

These activities necessitate frequent repetition of the word, slowing down speech rate and segmentation of the word to highlight phonological features of the word. Making the phonological features more salient supports speech processing and phonological short-term memory deficits. (Ellis Weismer & Hesketh, 1998).

The evidence for phonological-semantic intervention

Several small-scale studies have provided evidence of successful phonological-semantic intervention with primary school-age children with language disorder, all comparing progress in treated words versus control words. Easton, Sheach, and Easton (1997), for example, found that four 10-year-old children made progress in naming after 10 twice-weekly group therapy sessions in a specialist language setting. Parsons, Law and Gascoigne (2005) reported that two children aged 8:10 and 9:5 made progress in comprehension of maths words after 18 2–3-weekly individual therapy sessions. In a study by St John and Vance (2014), 18 5–6-year-old children were found to make progress in phonological and semantic knowledge and naming of 10 curriculum words, after daily small group sessions delivered by the teacher over three to four weeks. Motsch and Marks (2015) have added to the evidence provided by these small studies in a randomized controlled trial (RCT) of 153 8–9-year-old children using a group programme called Lexicon Pirate.

Joffe (2006) applied a small group model to the older age group, with speech and language therapy students delivering the vocabulary intervention. Fifty-four 10–15-year-old children made significant improvements on receptive vocabulary, recalling sentences, naming and idiomatic comprehension at the post-intervention testing point. Using a similar small group model but with intervention delivered by teaching assistants, Joffe (2017) conducted a RCT with 358 12-year-olds in mainstream secondary schools. Participants showed significant improvement in their understanding of idioms compared to a control group after three sessions of intervention per week over six weeks (18 sessions in total). Lowe and Joffe (2017) have shown the feasibility of a phonological-semantic approach delivered by the teacher in the classroom, integral to curriculum delivery in a mainstream secondary-school setting.

Derivation of meaning from context

Introducing new words in a context by reading aloud a passage contributes to a natural incentive for needing to know what words mean (Miller & Gildea, 1987), and provides the practitioner with opportunities to model what to do when s/he comes across a new word (Lubliner & Smetana, 2005). Beck et al. (2013) explain that direct instruction in how to derive meaning from context is necessary for children to develop independent word-learning skills. This allows students to develop their ability to use syntactic information to build knowledge about a word's meaning (Chiat, 2000). Joffe (2011) promotes the concept of being a word detective. Word detective strategies include:

- looking at the morphology of the word to gain clues from the root word, prefixes, and suffixes

- looking at the context to gain clues from the surrounding sentences

- asking a friend, teacher, or parent to seek clarification

- looking it up in a dictionary or on the internet.

Literacy

For adolescents, literacy needs to be incorporated seamlessly into intervention, but without detracting from the listening and speaking focus. This can be achieved simply by accompanying the spoken word with the written word: introducing new words in a written context; observing the written word in discussion about morphology; and writing the word and rhyming words on the word map.

Linking to prior knowledge

Dockrell et al. (2007) illustrate the importance of building on existing knowledge when introducing new concepts, and this needs to be complemented by comparing and contrasting new words with words already in the child's lexicon (Nippold, 1988). This can be addressed by an approach which fosters the generation of the student's own definitions rather than mere learning definitions by rote. This allows students to personalize their knowledge of the word in relation to their own experiences. The use of vocabulary books has been shown to be effective in young adult second language learners (Walters & Bozkurt, 2009), and has also been used by Beck et al. (2013). Each student

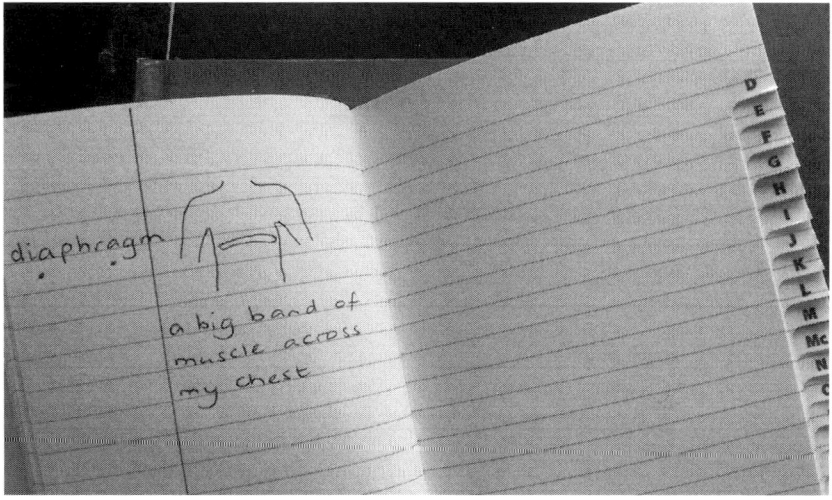

Figure 8.1 A vocabulary book entry.

is given their own vocabulary book. In this they write the word, place a dot under each syllable, and draw or write their own definition of what the word means (Figure 8.1).

A more user-friendly version of this might be to include key topic words on one sheet for the students to keep in their subject folders or exercise books.

Visual support

It is also helpful to utilize the visual modality: displaying each topic word with a visual image; drawing the concept; illustrating the word map as pictorially as possible (Pressley, Levin, & McDaniel, 1987; Steele & Mills, 2011). Using the highly literal visual depictions of idioms, for example, the picture of 'it's raining cats and dogs' as part of Joffe's (2011) Vocabulary Enrichment Intervention Programme (Figure 8.2) provided the students with support in developing a better understanding of idioms, and was one of the most enjoyable activities as reported by the participants.

The activities described above create an all-round package which builds on strengths as well as supporting weaknesses, addressing the individual needs of each student. Now we come to a more practical consideration: *how* to implement intervention?

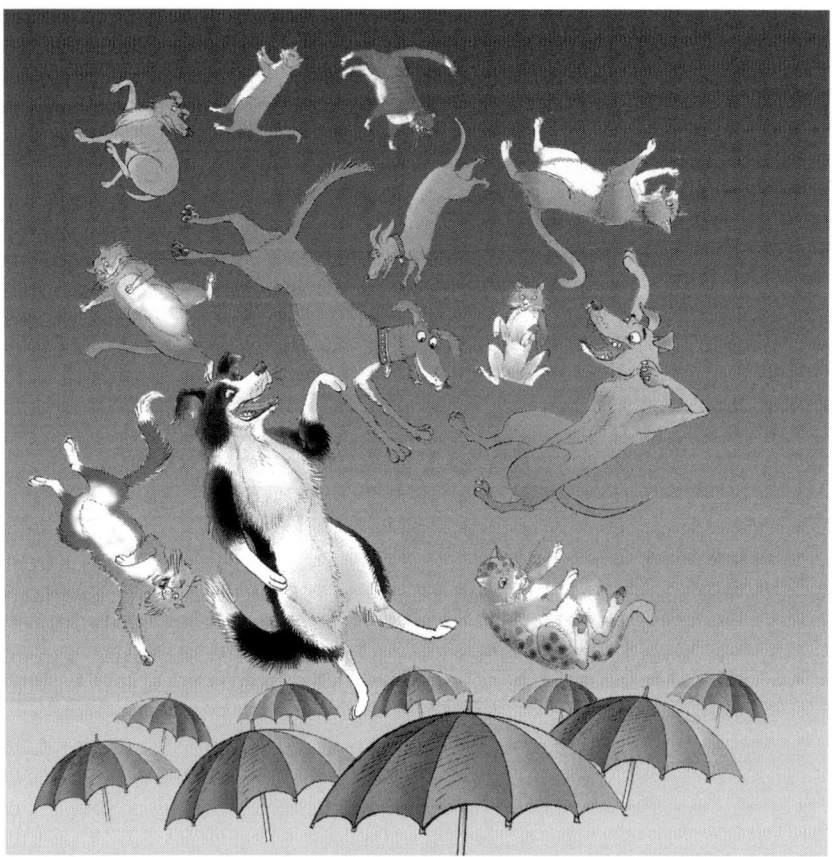

Figure 8.2 'It's raining cats and dogs' (Joffe, 2011).

Universal, targeted and specialist approaches to intervention

The Royal College of Speech and Language Therapists (RCSLT) recommends a framework of workforce management which accounts for the role of the speech and language therapist in universal, targeted and specialist provision. Universal services are services which are available to all children within mainstream provision. Targeted services are for children identified as being at risk, for example in association with social disadvantage, or children with transient speech or language difficulties. Specialist services are for children with significant and complex speech and language difficulties which require ongoing or intensive intervention. The balanced system model (Gascoigne, 2015) provides a way of illustrating how speech and language therapy resources could be deployed across these three levels. It shows a greater amount of speech and language therapy resource (specialist workforce) being used per child at targeted level than at universal level, and an even greater amount of speech and language therapy time per child at specialist level. These levels broadly equate to the waves model of intervention within the UK educational system (Department for Children, Schools, and Families, 2008). Wave 1 (universal) = "Quality First Teaching" for all students; Wave 2 (targeted) = small group time-limited additional intervention for students just below national expectations; Wave 3 (specialist) = individual or small group intervention with a trained and supported teaching assistant or specialist teacher.

In some cases, a universal model of speech and language therapy delivery has been adopted as the only service delivery model viable within a context of limited staffing resources, but the role of the SLT at the universal level can have an important function which goes much further than this. Working at the universal level may have a particular pertinence to the adolescent population due to the nature of the secondary school curriculum and student preferences. The timetabling of individual focused support time for one-to-one intervention in secondary schools is a challenge (Ehren, 2002), and remaining in the classroom rather than being withdrawn for individual tuition is preferable for many. Klingner, Vaughn, Schumm, Cohen, and Forgan (1998) found that 37.5% of a cohort of 32 9–11-year-old children with learning disability (known as specific learning difficulty or dyslexia in the UK) preferred an inclusion model of support. This percentage may be even higher during the teenage years, when peer acceptance becomes of paramount importance (Whitmire, 2000). Indeed, when looking at student preferences for ways to learn and remember new words, Lowe and Joffe (2017) reported that 60% of a cohort of 15 13–14-year-old students identified word games as a whole-class activity as their preferential word learning approach. Reasons they gave for this included: being fun; builds confidence; students can help each other; and no-one is left out. Again, collaborative partnership working may allow the development of an integrated model of service delivery which operates at universal, targeted, and specialist levels, according to the needs of the student, the school and the therapy service.

Evidence exists for the success of universal, targeted, and specialist models of vocabulary intervention with adolescents. Snow, Lawrence and White (2009) implemented a school-wide universal intervention of cross-curricular words with 697 11–14-year-olds for the duration of one academic year. The participating students, many of whom had low vocabulary levels in association with social disadvantage and second-language learning, made progress on word knowledge and, furthermore, vocabulary improvement was found to predict scores on the Massachusetts Comprehensive Assessment System, a curriculum assessment used in the USA. The studies above by Joffe (2006, 2017) illustrate successful targeted intervention for students with language needs. Ebbels, Nicoll, Clark et al. (2012) conducted a randomized control trial of individual therapy with 9–15-year-old students who had specific word-retrieval difficulty in a specialist language school. Knowledge of the words included in therapy was not assessed but, rather, progress in the use of word-finding strategies was measured through standardized assessment. Generalization of therapy to single-word naming on standardized assessment was found, though not at discourse level.

One further model to consider is a team teaching approach, in which therapists work in the classroom with the teacher, delivering intervention through modelling and team teaching. Throneburg, Calvert, Sturm et al. (2000) found this to be a successful model in younger children, and it has been successfully applied to the secondary school setting: Topping, Armstrong, Bayley et al. (2011) described the implementation of 'Listen-EAR', a programme focused on adaptation of teacher language and the development of active listening skills in students.

The decision as to which model to adopt rests on a combination of factors, illustrated in Table 8.1. Creative thinking and partnership working between schools and speech and language therapists can result in innovative and successful intervention models, adapted to the needs of the student, school, and therapy service.

Conclusion

This chapter highlights for readers the range of evidence-based service provision models that can be used to enhance vocabulary in adolescence, and the factors that need to be taken into account when considering which model of intervention is most appropriate, including the nature and severity of the vocabulary and/or language deficit as well as the nature and type of school and

Table 8.1 Factors for consideration when selecting universal, targeted and specialist models of intervention.

Factors for consideration	Universal	Targeted	Specialist
Student needs	Can address the needs of a wide range of students not just those individually identified	Can meet the needs of individual students with similar profiles in a group	Can be tailored exactly to student's language needs
Staffing resources	Places higher demand on the teacher. Teacher and Speech and Language Therapist (SLT) time required for collaborative planning	Higher demand on Teaching Assistant (TA) time if they deliver programme. SLT time required for training or setting up programme	Higher demand on SLT time but less demand on teacher or TA time
Student preference	Students may not wish to be singled out and want to learn with their peers	Has the advantage of peer support	Students may enjoy the individual attention
Applicability to curriculum	Can be directly applicable to and embedded into the curriculum	Can be a combination of curriculum relevance and wider word learning, for example social and emotional areas	Can be a highly tailored combination of curriculum relevance and wider word learning, for example social and emotional
Staff expertise	Uses the professional knowledge of the teacher in collaboration with the SLT	Usually involves TA training	Uses the professional knowledge of the SLT. Therapy may be adjusted according to clinical judgement

classroom, availability of resources and the level of knowledge and expertise of teaching and therapy staff.

Reflective questions for readers

Think of a young person with whom you work who has a vocabulary deficit:

1. Is this difficulty specific to vocabulary, or is there a more generalized language difficulty?

2. Does the vocabulary deficit incorporate difficulties with comprehension, expression, or both?

3. Does the young person have a specific word-finding difficulty in addition to a reduced vocabulary?

4. Which is more appropriate for this young person – a semantic or phonological-semantic approach, or both?

5. What does it mean to be an independent word learner, and how can you best facilitate this in young people?

References

Beck, I., McKeown, M., & Kucan, L. (2002). *Bringing Words to Life: Robust Vocabulary Instruction*. New York: Guilford Press.

Beck, I., McKeown, M., & Kucan, L. (2013). *Bringing Words to Life: Robust Vocabulary Instruction, 2nd ed.* New York: Guilford Press.

Best, R.M., Dockrell, J.E., & Braisby, N. (2006). Lexical acquisition in elementary science classes. *Journal of Educational Psychology, 98*(4), 824–838. http://doi.org/10.1037/0022-0663.98.4.824

Bishop, D.V.M. (1997). *Uncommon Understanding.* Hove: Psychology Press.

Braisby, N., Dockrell, J., & Best, R. (2001). Children's acquisition of science terms: Does fast mapping work? In M.B. Almgren, A. Ezeizabarrena, M.J. Idiazabal, & I. MacWhinney (Eds), *Research on Child Language Acquisition: Proceedings of the 8th Conference of the International Association for the Study of Child Language* (pp.1066–1087). Somerville, MA: Cascadilla Press.

Cain, K., Oakhill, J.V., & Lemmon, K. (2004). Individual differences in the inference of word meanings from context: The influence of reading comprehension, vocabulary knowledge, and memory capacity. *Journal of Educational Psychology, 96*(4), 671–681. http://dx.doi.org/10.1037/0022-0663.96.4.671"10.1037/0022-0663.96.4.671

Chiat, S. (2000). *Understanding Children with Language Problems*. Cambridge: Cambridge University Press.

Clark, E. (1993). *The Lexicon in Acquisition*. Cambridge: Cambridge University Press.

Clark, E. (1995). Later lexical development and word formation. In P. Fletcher & B. MacWhinney (Eds), *The Handbook of Child Language* (pp.293–312). Oxford: Blackwell.

Constable, A., Stackhouse, J., & Wells, B. (1997). Developmental word-finding difficulties and phonological processing: The case of the missing handcuffs. *Applied Psycholinguistics*, *18*(4), 507–536. http://doi.org/10.1017/S0142716400010961

Dale, E. (1965). Vocabulary measurement: Techniques and major findings. *Elementary English*, *42*(8), 895–948. https://www.jstor.org/stable/i40067354

Department for Children, Schools and Families (2008). *Personalised Learning: A Practical Guide*. London: DCSF Publications.

Dockrell, J.E., Braisby, N., & Best, R.M. (2007). Children's acquisition of science terms: Simple exposure is insufficient. *Learning and Instruction*, *17*(6), 577–594. http://doi.org/10.1016/j.learninstruc.2007.09.005

Dockrell, J. & Messer, D. (2004). Lexical acquisition in the early school years. In R.A. Berman (Ed.), *Language Development across Childhood and Adolescence* (pp.35–52). Amsterdam: John Benjamins.

Easton, C., Sheach, S., & Easton, S. (1997). Teaching vocabulary to children with wordfinding impairment using a combined semantic and phonological approach: An efficacy study. *Child Language Teaching and Therapy*, *13*, 125–142. https://doi.org/10.1177/026565909701300202

Ebbels, S.H., Nicoll, H., Clark, B., Eachus, B., Gallagher, A.L., Horniman, K., … Turner, G. (2012). Effectiveness of semantic therapy for word-finding difficulties in pupils with persistent language impairments: A randomized control trial. *International Journal of Language & Communication Disorders*, *47*(1), 35–51. http://doi.org/10.1111/j.1460-6984.2011.00073.x

Ehren, B. (2002). Speech-Language Pathologists contributing significantly to the academic success of high school students: A vision for professional growth. *Topics in Language Disorders*, *22*(2), 60–80. http://doi: 10.1097/00011363-200201000-00005

Elks, L. & McLachlan, H. (2008). *Secondary Language Builders: Speech and Language Support for 11–16s*. St Mabyn: Elklan.

Ellis Weismer, S. & Hesketh, L (1998). The impact of emphatic stress on novel word learning by children with specific language impairment. *Journal of Speech, Language & Hearing Research*, *41*(6) 1444–1458.

Gascoigne, M. (2015). The balanced system. MGA. Retrieved from www.mgaconsulting.org.uk/balanced-system/

Gathercole, S. & Baddeley, A. (1990). The role of phonological memory in vocabulary acquisition: A study of young children learning new names. *British Journal of Psychology*, *81*(4), 439–454.

Joffe, V.L. (2011). *Vocabulary Enrichment Intervention Programme*. Milton Keynes: Speechmark.

Joffe, V.L. (2006). Enhancing language and communication in language-impaired secondary school-aged children. In J. Clegg & J. Ginsborg (Eds), *Language and Social Disadvantage: Theory into Practice* (pp.207–216). Chichester: John Wiley & Sons.

Joffe, V.L. (2017). Enhancing vocabulary and independent word learning skills in adolescents with language disorder. Paper presentation at the International Association for the Study of Child Language (IASCL) conference, July, Lyon, France.

Kail, R. & Leonard, L. (1986). Word-finding abilities in language-impaired children. *ASHA Monographs, 25*.

Klingner, J., Vaughn, S., Schumm, J., Cohen, P., & Forgan, J. (1998). Inclusion or pull-out: Which do students prefer? *Journal of Learning Disabilities, 31*(2), 148. https://doi.org/10.1177/002221949803100205

Lahey, M. & Edwards, J. (1999). Naming errors of children with Specific Language Impairment. *Journal of Speech, Language, and Hearing Research, 42*, 195–205. http://doi: 10.1044/jslhr.4201.195

Leonard, L. (1998). *Children with Specific Language Impairment*. Cambridge, MA: MIT Press.

Lowe, H. & Joffe, V. (2017). Exploring the feasibility of a classroom-based vocabulary intervention for mainstream secondary school students with language disorder. *Support for Learning, 32*(2), 110–128. https://doi.org/10.1111/1467-9604.12157

Lubliner, S. & Smetana, L. (2005). The effects of comprehensive vocabulary instruction on title I students' metacognitive word-learning skills and reading comprehension. *Journal of Literacy Research, 37*(2), 163–200. http://doi.org/10.1207/s15548430jlr3702_3

McArthur, G.M., Hogben, J.H., Edwards, V.T., Heath, S.M., & Mengler, E.D. (2000). On the 'specifics' of specific reading disability and specific language impairment. *Journal of Child Psychology and Psychiatry and Allied Disciplines, 41*(7), 869–874. http://doi.org/10.1017/S0021963099006186

McGregor, K.K., Newman, R.M., Reilly, R.M., & Capone, N.C. (2002). Semantic representation and naming in children with specific language impairment. *Journal of Speech, Language, and Hearing Research, 45*(5), 998–1015. http://doi.org/10.1044/1092-4388(2002/081)

McGregor K.K., Oleson, J., Bahnsen, A., & Duff, D. (2013). Children with developmental language impairment have vocabulary deficits characterized by limited breadth and depth. *International Journal of Language & Communication Disorders, 48*(3), 307–319. http://doi.org/10.1111/1460-6984.12008

Miller, G. & Gildea, P. (1987). How children learn words. *Scientific American, 257*(3), 86–91. https://www.jstor.org/stable/24979482

Motsch, H.-J. & Marks, D.-K. (2015). Efficacy of the Lexicon Pirate strategy therapy for improving lexical learning in school-age children: A randomized controlled trial. *Child Language Teaching & Therapy, 31*(2), 237–255. http://doi.org/10.1177/0265659014564678

Nippold, M.A. (1988). *Later Language Development*. Boston/Toronto/San Diego: Little, Brown and Company.

Nippold, M.A. (2007). *Later Language Development: School-age Children, Adolescents, and Young Adults, 3rd ed.* Austin, TX: Pro-Ed.

Parsons, S., Law, J., & Gascoigne, M. (2005). Teaching receptive vocabulary to children with specific language impairment: A curriculum-based approach. *Child Language Teaching and Therapy*, *21*(1), 39–59. https://doi.org/10.1191/0265659005ct280oa

Pressley, M., Levin, J., & McDaniel, M. (1987). Remembering versus inferring what a word means: Mnemonic and contextual approaches. In M. McKeown & M. Curtis (Eds), *The Nature of Vocabulary Acquisition* (pp.107–127). London: Lawrence Erlbaum Associates.

Ravid, D. (2004). Derivational morphology revisited. In R. Berman (Ed.), *Language Development across Childhood and Adolescence* (pp.53–81). Amsterdam, PA: John Benjamins Publishing Co.

Rice, M.L., Oetting, J.B., Marquis, J., Bode, J., & Pae, S. (1994). Frequency of input effects on word comprehension of children with specific language impairment. *Journal of Speech and Hearing Research*, *37*(1), 106–122. http://doi.org/10.1044/jshr.3701.106

Rice L.M. & Hoffman, L. (2015). Predicting vocabulary growth in children with and without specific language impairment: A longitudinal study from 2;6 to 21 years of age. *Journal of Speech, Language & Hearing Research*, *58*(2), 345–359. http://doi.org/10.1044/2015

Snow, C.E., Lawrence, J.F., & White, C.E. (2009). Generating knowledge of academic language among urban middle school students. *Journal of Research on Educational Effectiveness*, *2*(4), 4,325–4,344. doi: 10.1080/19345740903167042."

Snowling, M.J., Muter, V., & Carroll, J.M. (2007). Children at family risk of dyslexia: A follow-up in adolescence. *Journal of Child Psychology and Psychiatry*, *48*, 609–618. http://doi.org/10.1111/j.1469-7610.2006.01725.x

St. John, P. & Vance, M. (2014). Evaluation of a principled approach to vocabulary learning in mainstream classes. *Child Language Teaching & Therapy*, *30*(3), 255–271. https://doi.org/10.1177/0265659013516474

Stackhouse, J. & Wells, B. (1997). *Children's Speech and Literacy Impairment*. London: Whurr.

Stanovich, K.E. (1986). Matthew effects in reading: Some consequences of individual differences in the acquisition of literacy. *Reading Research Quarterly*, *21*(4), 360–407. http://doi.org/10.1598/RRQ.21.4.1

Starling, J., Munro, N., Togher, L., & Arciuli, J. (2012). Training secondary school teachers in instructional language modification techniques to support adolescents with language impairment: A randomized controlled trial. *Language, Speech and Hearing Services in Schools*, *43*(4), 474–495. https://doi.org/10.1044/0161-1461(2012/11-0066

Steele, S. & Mills, M. (2011). Vocabulary intervention for school-age children with language impairment: A review of evidence and good practice. *Child Language Teaching & Therapy*, *27*(3), 354–370. http://doi.org/10.1177/0265659011412247

Throneburg, R.N., Calvert, L.K., Sturm, J.J., Paramboukas, A.A., & Paul, P.J. (2000). A comparison of service delivery models: Effects on curricular vocabulary skills in the school setting. *American Journal of Speech-Language Pathology*, *9*(1), 10–20. http://doi:10.1044/1058-0360.0901.10

Topping, C., Armstrong, S., Bayley, K., Goss, J., McLean, L., & Rowe, K. (2011). Great expectations: Can training programmes to embed speaking and listening skills within general teaching practice deliver on their promises for young people with SLCN? In: *Lost for Words: Lost for Life Conference*. London: City University London.

van Kleeck, A. (1984). Metalinguistic skills: Cutting across spoken and written language and problem-solving abilities. In G.P. Wallach & K. Butler (Eds), *Language Learning Disabilities in School-age Children* (pp.128–153). Baltimore/London: Williams and Wilkins.

Walters, J. & Bozkurt, N. (2009). The effect of keeping vocabulary notebooks on vocabulary acquisition. *Language Teaching Research, 13*(4), 403–423. http://doi.org/10.1177/1362168809341509

Watson, C. (1995). *Making Hanen Happen*. Toronto: Hanen Centre Publications.

Whitmire, K. (2000). Adolescence as a developmental phase: A tutorial. *Topics in Language Disorders, 20*(2), 1–14.

9 Breaking out of school

Two intervention programmes to support social communication skills for teenagers preparing to leave school

Rachel Mathrick and Courtenay Norbury

Learning outcomes

This chapter will enable readers to:

- Justify the need to support young people's language and communication skills as they make the transition from school towards adulthood

- Describe two intervention programmes which were designed and delivered to young people with SLCN: the first targets verbal and nonverbal interview skills, and the second uses song lyrics to develop skills in using contextual cues to identify and understand non-literal and figurative language

- Report on the impact of the intervention programmes for adolescents with persistent SLCN, as measured using functional, bespoke outcome measures.

Introduction

This chapter is based on work by Speech and Language Therapists (SLTs) who work at St Catherine's – a specialist residential school and sixth form college for children and young adults with speech, language and communication needs (SLCN). We work in a multidisciplinary team alongside occupational therapists, residential care staff, specialist teachers and learning support assistants to deliver a differentiated curriculum within school, alongside a life skills programme that is integrated into our curriculum. Our school population includes young people with a wide range of clinical diagnoses, including Autistic Spectrum Disorder (ASD), social and pragmatic communication disorders, and those with more specific language impairments (SLI), now identified as DLD developmental language disorder (Bishop 2017). In this chapter, we use the all-inclusive term SLCN to refer to these young people's difficulties.

At St Catherine's, we work with students in a holistic way to facilitate communication and empower them. Leaving school is the biggest change in a young person's life. To prepare them for this transition, they need support with curriculum-relevant language in order to achieve the best qualifications they can, as academic underachievement contributes to poorer employment outcomes for children with SLCN (Carroll & Dockrell, 2010; Clegg, Hollis, Mawhood, & Rutter, 2005). However, they also need to develop social communication skills so that when they leave school they can successfully navigate a complex social world and participate fully in social, leisure, and employment opportunities. There is also emerging evidence that difficulties with social communication and pragmatic aspects of language are a risk factor for developing mental health difficulties (Mok, Pickles, Durkin, & Conti-Ramsden, 2014; Yew & O'Kearney, 2013). Therefore, interventions to support social communication skills are required within a wider programme of interventions targeting structural language skills such as vocabulary and grammar.

While there is increasing research evidence that intervention significantly improves structural language skills for young people with SLCN (see Ebbels, 2014, for a review), very little research has evaluated the impact of interventions for social communication and pragmatic communication difficulties. We therefore developed two new programmes to support functional pragmatic and social communication skills:

1. A new interview skills training package designed to improve social communication behaviours critical for successful employment interviews (Mathrick & Meagher, 2012). We called this programme

'Breaking into Employment'.

2. A further programme targeted at using context to identify and understand non-literal language. We used song lyrics as a format for discussion of non-literal meaning. This programme is called 'Breaking into Society'.

This chapter focuses on two areas of practice, and for each programme we provide a rationale, an outline of the intervention programme, outcome measures, and provisional information about the evaluation of the impact of the interventions.

Breaking into Employment: Targeting interview skills for gaining employment

Rationale for supporting interview skills

Individuals with SLCN have poorer employment outcomes than their typically developing peers. Conti-Ramsden and Durkin (2012) showed this by interviewing 50 young people with SLI and 50 typically developing peers about their experiences of education and employment post 16-years, and found significantly more young people with SLI *not* in education, training or employment at age 19 relative to peers. Shattuck, Narendorf, Cooper et al. (2012) used national survey data in the USA to investigate post-education outcomes for young people with ASD. They reported that those with ASD were less likely than peers with other developmental disorders (including SLI and learning disabilities) to participate in further education (e.g., college or vocational training), or paid employment. Those with poorer functional skills and from more economically disadvantaged families were at greater risk of poor post-education outcomes.

Social communication difficulties are common in people with persistent SLCN and are associated with negative social, academic and vocational outcomes (Rao, Beidel, & Murray, 2007). Social communication is defined by Norbury (2014) as the: "understanding of speaker intentions and the verbal and nonverbal cues that signal those intentions, as well as the child's interpretation of the environmental context, societal norms and expectations and how these coalesce with structural aspects of language (e.g., vocabulary, syntax and phonology) to achieve successful communication" (p.204). Difficulties in any of the areas mentioned in the definition are likely to have an impact on performance during job interviews, and may present a barrier to employment. Training to develop interview skills has been recommended in order to bridge the gap between the worlds of education and work (Conti-Ramsden, Botting, & Durkin, 2008). There is a very little research in this area; however, early research suggested that improvement in interview skills following training is possible across a diverse range of participant groups (Grinnell & Lieberman, 1977; Hall, Sheldon-Wildgen, & Sherman, 1980; Kelly, Wildman, & Berler, 1980). More recently, Strickland, Coles, and Southern (2013) reported that an interview skills training package delivered in a virtual environment yielded significant improvements in verbal responses to interview questions for adolescents with ASD relative to the no-treatment comparison group. The programme was less successful at improving nonverbal social communication skills such as posture, eye contact, and facial expression. This could reflect the treatment environment; it was more difficult for the interviewer avatar to demonstrate subtle nonverbal cues and harder for the interviewee avatar to replicate them. Thus improving nonverbal communication skills remains an important consideration in intervention and research.

Interview skills intervention programme

The interview skills manualized training package (Mathrick & Meagher, 2012) was delivered to 34 young people in groups of 10-12 participants aged 17-18-year-olds with persistent SLCN over a three-year period. The intervention included 15-18 hours of direct intervention in groups, administered by two specialist speech and language therapists as part of the school curriculum. Role-play was used to target the following skills:

Nonverbal skills: including appropriate handshake, posture, eye-gaze, smiling, thinking facial expressions, and confident body language. Visual prompt cards are used to remind the young people of what they need to do to demonstrate appropriate communication behaviour.

Verbal skills: including planning answers to a range of possible interview questions (e.g., qualification, providing reasons for applying for the particular job, and recounting personal strengths, challenges and support needed). Therapists modelled concise responses and appropriate examples.

Memory prompts: (e.g., 'Mind Maps'™, Buzan, 1974) developed and available for use during the interview. The students learned to use this resource appropriately, politely asking to use their notes, and looking at the notes to help them remember what to say, but then making eye contact with the interviewer when they answered.

Outcomes: Measuring the impact of the interview skills programme

Students completed three interviews so that we could compare performance over time. They completed a baseline interview ('Time 1'), a pre-treatment interview ('Time 2') and a post-treatment interview ('Time 3'). The baseline period allowed us to identify potential practice effects, so that we could be sure that any changes in performance were due to the intervention programme (rather than the students just getting older and therefore more skilled, or improving due to practising the interview task itself). If treatment is effective, the greatest improvements were expected between Time 2 and Time 3. All interviews were conducted by business people from a range of businesses in the local area, with different (and unfamiliar) interviewers at each assessment point. The interviewers had varying degrees of experience with interviews and with SLCN and none received training prior to the assessment.

All mock interviews were video recorded and sent to research students for off-line coding of the *positive verbal, positive nonverbal, negative verbal* and *negative nonverbal* social communication behaviours outlined in Table 9.1.

Table 9.1 Examples of social communication behaviours evaluated in mock interview videos at each assessment time (for further details see Mathrick, Meagher, & Norbury, 2017).

Measures	Example behaviours
Positive nonverbal behaviours	Eye contact, nodding
Negative nonverbal behaviours	Slouching, fidgeting, inappropriate facial expression or intonation
Positive verbal behaviours	Responds to verbal comments and questions, requests clarification, uses concrete examples
Negative verbal behaviours	Use of slang/inappropriate language, irrelevant comments, interrupts, minimal verbal response
Pre-interview behaviours	Shakes hands, introduces self
End interview behaviours	Stands up when interviewer stands up, says thank you

Coders were blind to time of interview, participant diagnosis, and individual treatment goals. Due to variation in the length of the interviews, we adjusted raw counts by the number of speaking turns to give the proportion of behaviours per speaking turn.

The impact of the interview skills intervention programme

There was considerable within-group variation in social communication at all time points, but over the three time points, scores improved in the expected direction on all four outcome measures. As a group, our participants showed significant (p < .05) increases in *positive nonverbal* behaviours and significant decreases in *negative nonverbal* behaviours. The former gave the clearest evidence of a treatment effect, with no change between T1 and T2, but significant change between T2 and T3 ($p = .005$). The decrease in *negative nonverbal* behaviours was more gradual, with significant differences only evident between T1 and T3 ($p = .045$). Change in *positive and negative verbal* behaviours did not reach levels of statistical significance ($ps = .18$ and $.08$ respectively), though the difference in means between T1 and T3 were of moderate-to-large effect size (Cohen's *d* = .78 and 1.10). See Mathrick, Meagher, & Norbury (2017) for further details.

The personalized memory prompts developed by the students through the interview skills training have also been used in real college interviews. The students also valued this resource as they have taken their interview packs with them when they have left school, demonstrating the importance and value that they place on this module, and the resources produced within it.

These results are encouraging, although require replication in larger samples using more robust treatment designs – for example using random allocation to treatment and treat-as-usual groups. The wide variation in diagnoses, severity of language and cognitive impairments and the presence of ASD-symptoms may all contribute to the variation in behaviour observed at all time points. Our student population was too small to test these effects rigorously. This is a challenge for school-based research, but represents an ecologically valid approach as clinical populations are by nature heterogeneous. Variation in outcome may not solely be due to student characteristics, as we also noted that *interviewers* varied considerably in their skills at interviewing individuals with SLCN. One avenue for future research and practice might be training employers to accommodate SLCN in interviews, in order to elicit optimal responses.

Breaking into Society: Increasing understanding of non-literal language by discussing song lyrics

Rationale for interventions for non-literal language

A considerable body of research has identified processing language in context as a key deficit for children with ASD (Loukusa, Leinonen, Kuusikko, et al., 2006), although there is growing recognition that non-literal language poses significant challenges for older children and teenagers with a range of clinical conditions (Norbury, 2005). There is considerable debate about the source of non-literal language and context processing deficits (Bishop & Norbury, 2005; Martin & McDonald, 2004; Rajendran, Mitchell, & Rickards, 2005). Most theories arise from the study of ASD and include theory of mind (Baron-Cohen, Leslie, & Frith, 1985), weak central coherence (Frith, 1989), and executive functioning (Ozonoff, Pennington, & Rogers, 1991). The 'theory of mind' hypothesis posits that individuals must understand that the speaker intends a non-literal message in order to trigger such an interpretation (Happe, 1993). Weak central coherence proposes that individuals with ASD focus on local detail at the expense of holistic meaning (Happe, 1999). Such a style of processing would make using context more challenging. Executive function is an umbrella term for a number of skills implicated in cognitive control, including attention, working memory, inhibition, and flexible thinking. Executive function may impact on comprehension of figurative language because individuals struggle to inhibit the literal meaning, or to be flexible enough to hold multiple interpretations in their mind long enough to select the meaning most appropriate to a given situation.

However, numerous studies have shown that deficits in using context to resolve ambiguous language (e.g., words like 'bank' or phrases such as 'pull your socks up') is not specific to ASD, and even within the ASD population these deficits are more evident in individuals who have impaired structural language skills (Gernsbacher & Pripas-Kapit, 2012). Indeed, deficits in understanding figurative language can be just as pronounced in adolescents with SLI as it is in those with ASD (Norbury, 2005). This work highlights the need to address core aspects of language, vocabulary, in-depth word knowledge, and grammar to support use of linguistic context, regardless of clinical diagnosis.

Rajendran et al. (2005) used dialogue-based tasks to explore comprehension of figurative expression in a more naturalistic way. Their study measured verbal ability, executive function and age, and asked which of these factors predicted success with understanding idioms, responding to inappropriate requests and sarcasm. They demonstrated that verbal ability, executive function, and diagnosis (ASD versus Tourette's syndrome) all predicted the ability to understand a figurative expression. Handling inappropriate requests was also predicted by age, as well as verbal ability, executive ability, and diagnosis.

Individuals with SLCN find figurative language challenging, but there is a paucity of research to inform interventions, particularly during adolescence. Given the frequency with which figurative and non-literal language is used, starting in the classroom (Colston & Kuiper, 2002; Lazar, War-Leaper, Nicholson, & Johnson, 1989) and beyond into society (Nicoll, 2016), there is a need for intervention programmes that target these skills. At St Catherine's we have developed a programme which focuses on making use of context to figure out non-literal language, and we use comprehension of song lyrics to motivate our students.

1. Listening to the intervention song

2. Following the words whilst listening

3. Thinking about it a verse at a time

4. Working out the context – what is happening

5. Using colours to highlight and answer *wh*- questions (when, where, who and what)

6. Picking out words or phrases not understood

7. Finding pictures from an internet search or drawing a picture to go with the word or phrase

8. Using the picture to think about the meaning (usually literal meaning)

9. If the literal meaning does not make sense, using the context (when, where, who and what was said before and after) to think what the slang and sayings could mean

10. Discussing the meaning outside of the song; who might use the words, and the ideas around register, i.e., with whom it is appropriate for students and with whom it is not

Figure 9.1 The intervention sessions context strategy.

Intervention description for increasing understanding of non-literal language using song lyrics

St Catherine's 'Language through Lyrics' module focuses on using a context strategy to understand song lyrics, highlighting slang and non-literal language. Song lyrics were used as it was motivational for the young people. Due to small class sizes the pilot study was carried out over three years and was comprised of 34 young people in groups of 1–12 participants aged 17–18 years old. The participants receiving the 'Language through Lyrics' therapy module all have persistent SLCN. They all received 12 group therapy sessions of 45 minutes each as part of their timetabled lessons. The song used in therapy was 'Fit But You Know It' by The Streets (Skinner, 2004). This song was used every week, breaking it down a verse at a time.

Figure 9.1 shows the steps the intervention sessions use to help the students break down the meaning of the non-literal language.

The students produced a 'context page' with steps from Figure 9.1 and pictures answering some of the *wh-* questions (see Figure 9.2).

For each verse the students highlighted the 'when', 'where', 'who', 'what'

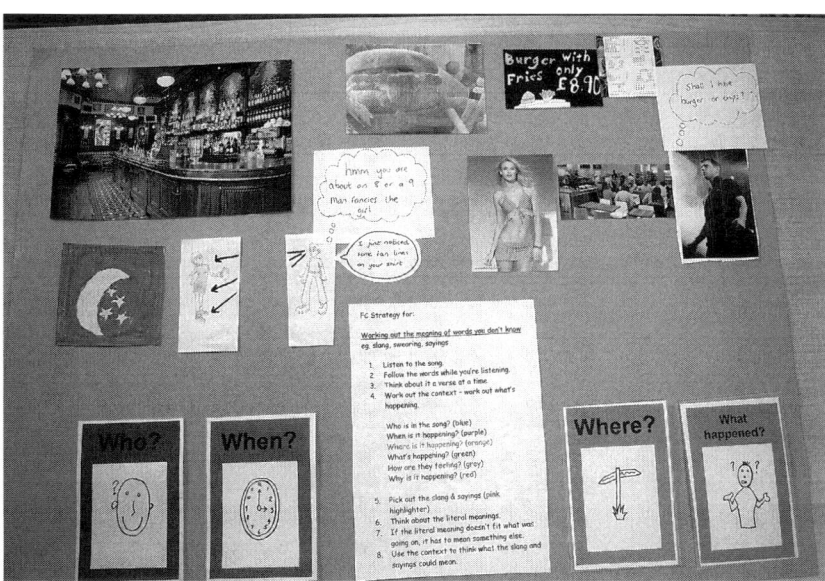

Figure 9.2 An example of the students' work on 'the context page'.

information and put the pictures from their internet search or what they had drawn around the verse. If the picture was literal (which it usually was), they put a cross by it and thought of what the non-literal meaning could be, by using the strategy (see step 9 of Figure 9.1), thinking about the context (the answers to the *wh*- questions) and what was sung before and after to work out the meaning (see Figure 9.3 for their work on verse 1).

As the example verse shows, the song was chosen as it contains a lot of non-literal language and slang to analyze. For example, the singer described a girl as 'fit', an expression that has a literal interpretation that would be different to the intended meaning of 'physically attractive'. Students used contextual cues such as rejecting the literal picture, then thinking about 'when', 'who', 'where', and 'what' information and looking at what was sung before and after (steps 7–9 of Figure 9.1) to arrive at the intended, non-literal meaning. This song was also chosen as it is a narrative about a man on holiday who sees a fit girl, what he does about this, and then, when she rejects him, comes to the conclusion that it doesn't matter as he has a girlfriend at home anyway. Songs with a narrative work better for the context strategy (the 'when', 'who', 'where', 'what'), as well as providing imagery to more easily facilitate locating

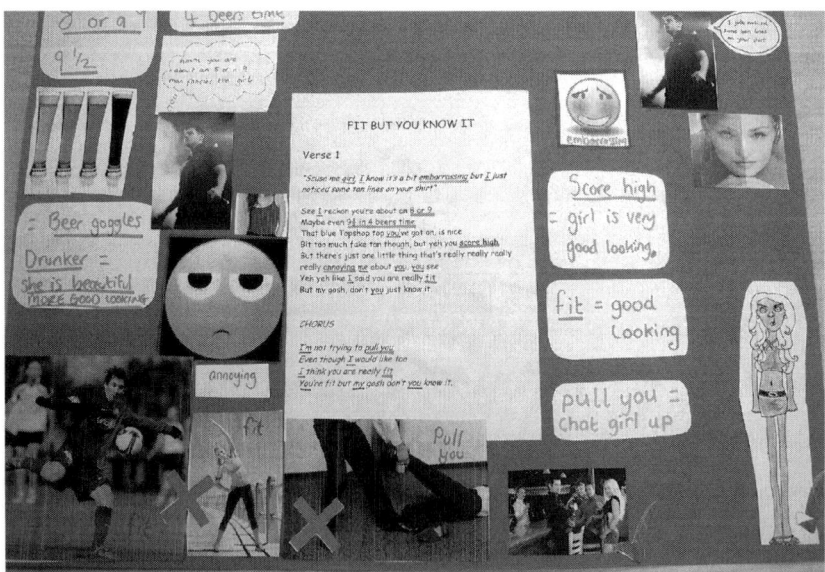

Figure 9.3 An example of verse 1 produced by the students as part of the therapy.

the pictures on the internet. Although old, the song still seemed to appeal to the students, as the themes remain adolescent – the man is out 'on the pull', there is some swearing, it involves alcohol, and so on. As part of the sessions, students are also encouraged to bring in any song lyrics of music they listen to, as this helps them understand the meaning. They can be quite shocked about the meaning of the songs they happily sing along to, and have a greater understanding of why it is not appropriate to sing them loudly when walking through town or on the bus.

Throughout therapy students also practise appropriate responses to hearing slang and swearing in the song. At the beginning of therapy some students respond by giggling loudly, shouting that they heard a swear word, covering their ears, or leaving the room. All of these are not appropriate for their age, and would not be acceptable in the community (for example, in town or in the pub). Although not quantifiably measured, therapists felt through clinical observation that the students' reactions to the language became more appropriate over the course of therapy.

Outcome measure for non-literal language

The outcome measure was based on a different song to the song used in intervention, as the students had worked on the intervention song for so many weeks and we wanted the outcome measure to be a test of applying the strategy (see Figure 9.1) – not a test of remembering what they had done in therapy. The song 'Sk8er Boi' (Avril Lavigne) was chosen as it also contains an abundance of non-literal language and slang; it also has a narrative, a girl who declines to 'go out' with a boy she likes because of her friends' opinions and then later regrets this. Students were given lyrics to the song pre- and post-therapy, and were asked to highlight non-literal phrases and any words or phrases they did not understand. Alongside the song lyrics they answered 10 open-ended questions regarding lyric meaning, but could move on to 10 multiple-choice options if necessary. The open-ended and multiple-choice questions asked about the meanings of the same 10 phrases. The students had a copy of the lyrics so that they could use the context to work out the meaning if they applied the strategy. The open-ended questions just asked what a phrase in the song meant, e.g.,

Look at the phrase below and say what it means in the song

Stuck up their nose

None of our students were able to express the meaning of all non-literal phrases in open-ended questions, so the open-ended question sheets were taken away when they were asked to complete the multiple-choice questions. Each multiple-choice question contained a literal answer, an associated answer, and the correct non-literal answer. The order of the type of answers was mixed up so it was not the same for each question. An example is:

What does the saying mean:

"Stuck up their nose"

(a) They had something in their nose

(b) They think they are better than the skater boy

(c) Skater boy is tall so they had to look up to him

In the example above the literal answer is (a), the non-literal answer is (b), and the associated answer is (c).

The student's persistent SLCN often means they have severe difficulties with expressive language. We did not feel that the open-ended questions alone allowed them to demonstrate all that they understood about the non-literal language – they simply don't have the words to express it, and are often frustrated that they cannot demonstrate their knowledge or post-therapy progression. Because of this, the multiple-choice questions are used as well, as they scaffold some of the language needed to help the students demonstrate their understanding. As multiple-choice inevitably contains some element of chance, using both open-ended and multiple-choice questioning seemed to be the most robust way of demonstrating knowledge beyond pure chance.

Evaluation results

The results indicate the students improved in their ability to identify non-literal phrases in the song lyrics. They also achieved higher accuracy scores for open-ended and multiple-choice questions, demonstrating an increased understanding of non-literal language. Where multiple-choice scores had gone down, the corresponding open-ended score had always gone up. Table 9.2 shows each student's pre- and post-measure score. Results are promising, though they should be interpreted with caution due to limitations in the evaluation design (for example, a lack of a repeated baseline means we cannot rule out practice effects).

Table 9.2 34 individual students' pre- and post- scores on assessment measuring understanding of non-literal language using the song by Avril Lavigne, 'Sk8ter Boi', for both open-ended and multiple-choice questions. Note: a score of 10 represents a ceiling score.

Student	Question Sheet 1 (Open ended ?s) TIME 1	Question Sheet 1 (Open ended ?s) TIME 2	Question Sheet 2 (Multiple choice ?s) TIME 1	Question Sheet 2 (Multiple choice ?s) TIME 2
1.	4	8 ↑	9	10 ↑
2.	0	2 ↑	3	4 ↑
3.	0	1 ↑	5	6 ↑
4.	0	1 ↑	2	4 ↑
5.	3	6 ↑	7	9 ↑
6.	0	0 ↔	3	3 ↔
7.	1	3 ↑	6	8 ↑
8.	1	2 ↑	6	8 ↑
9.	2	3 ↑	7	9 ↑
10.	0	3 ↑	4	8 ↑
11.	2	6 ↑	8	6 ↓
12.	0	4 ↑	6	9 ↑
13.	0	2 ↑	5	5 ↔
14.	5	8 ↑	9	10 ↑
15.	2	3 ↑	7	10 ↑
16.	4	5 ↑	9	10 ↑
17.	1	3 ↑	9	6 ↓
18.	0	3 ↑	6	8 ↑
19.	0	8 ↑	8	9 ↑
20.	0	4 ↑	5	7 ↑
21.	2	6 ↑	9	7 ↓
22.	0	0 ↔	2	2 ↔
23.	0	6 ↑	8	9 ↑
24.	0	2 ↑	2	1 ↓
25.	0	2 ↑	3	9 ↑
26.	2	4 ↑	7	5 ↓
27.	1	3 ↑	3	7 ↑
28.	1	8 ↑	0	10 ↑
29.	1	5 ↑	7	8 ↑
30.	1	5 ↑	8	8 ↔
31.	0	2 ↑	2	5 ↑
32.	4	10 ↑	9	10 ↑
33.	4	7 ↑	10	9 ↓
34.	0	3 ↑	5	6 ↑
TOTAL	41	138 ↑	199	245 ↑

Mean raw scores on assessment of figurative language comprehension pre- and post-therapy

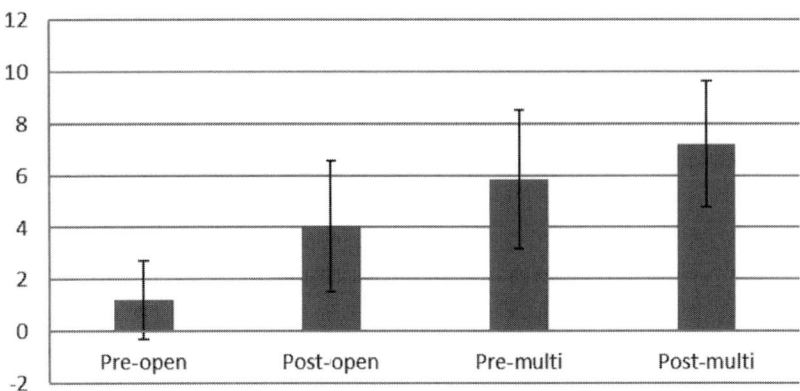

Figure 9.4 Results of pre- and post-assessment for open-ended questions (two bars on the left) and multiple-choice questions (two bars on the right) for 34 students. Raw scores are shown on the y-axis. The error bars represent the standard deviation and show considerable variation in performance (data from Mathrick, Meagher, Morey, & Masterson, 2014).

To look at the scores on assessment pre- and post-therapy for both open-ended questions and multiple-choice questions as a group, rather than individually, see Figure 9.4.

For students with floor scores (scaled scores of 3) on the CELF (Semel, Wiig, & Secord, 1995), progress was more difficult to demonstrate using open-ended questions. Six students with floor scores made an average gain of 2.83 points on the open-ended questions, but an average gain of 5.00 points on the multiple-choice questions. Thus, it is important to take into account response demands when measuring outcome.

There were only two of 34 students (students 6 and 22 in Table 9.2) who did not show evidence of improvement in either measure; both of these students had the most severe expressive language difficulties and found it hard to explain their answers in the open-ended questions. However, analysis of error responses on the multiple-choice questions showed that, while prior to intervention they had chosen literal interpretations, after intervention they were more likely to select an associated, but not literal, response. It therefore appeared that they recognized the literal meaning was incorrect but could not retain all the information necessary to work out the non-literal meaning.

For the majority of students, there was a decrease in the number of lyrics they highlighted as not understanding between 'Time 1' (pre-) and Time 2' (post-therapy) assessment. Interestingly, the same two students mentioned above (students 6 and 22 in Table 2) showed an increase in the number of song lyrics they highlighted as not understanding between these assessment points – suggesting that after therapy they had an increased awareness that slang and non-literal language exist but still found it hard to process the language to establish the meaning.

The impact of the language through lyrics module

To summarize, if students have awareness that non-literal language exists, they are able to identify it and work out the intended meaning. Avoiding overly-literal interpretations of non-literal language can also avoid exaggerated behaviour in the face of figurative language (for example, in a café, overhearing the phrase "he shot himself in the foot", then ducking under the table and asking "Where's the gun?"). Therefore, intervention that targets the understanding of non-literal language has functional relevance. We hope that the programme would not only impact on understanding the lyrics of popular music, but that skills would generalize to conversations with peers, family, friends and colleagues, and to maintain appropriate social interactions in a society where non-literal language and slang occur frequently.

Conclusions

Preparing a young person with SLCN for a successful transition to adulthood is important in order to prevent adverse effects on self-esteem, independence, and economic success (Conti-Ramsden & Durkin, 2012; Howlin, Mawhood, & Rutter, 2000). In addition, the introduction of Education, Health and Care Plans (EHCP) in England and Wales (Spivack, Craston, Thom, & Carr, 2014) provides a legal document outlining the need and support for young people through to age 25 years, and creates a new impetus for clinical and educational practitioners to focus on the transition from childhood to adulthood, and from education to employment.

The programmes outlined in this chapter demonstrate how intervention for adolescents' social communication skills can be functional, relevant and effective. As frontline practitioners, we need to ensure speech and language therapy is mandated in EHCPs for older students, to ensure that transition to adulthood is effectively supported. Focusing on areas such as social communication and developing interview skills are all key to empowering young people to take steps towards social and financial independence.

Reflective questions

1. What skills do young people need to successfully transition to adulthood?

2. How would you convince a manager, headteacher, parent, or teacher that working on social communication and interaction skills are as important as working towards qualifications?

3. Choose a song you like, look up the lyrics on the internet, and reflect on the content. Is there any non-literal language and figurative language within the lyrics? Could you use this song as a motivating framework for working with young people with SLCN on non-literal language?

4. Think of a young person who is about to transition to sixth form or leave college. What are the priorities for them in relation to adulthood?

References

Baron-Cohen, S., Leslie, A.M., & Frith, U. (1985). Does the autistic child have a theory of mind? *Cognition, 21*(1), 37–46.

Bishop, D.V.M. (2017). Why is it so hard to reach agreement on terminology? The case of developmental language disorder (DLD). *International Journal of Language and Communication Disorders, 52*(6), 671–680.

Bishop, D.V.M. & Norbury, C.F. (2005). Executive functions in children with communication impairments, in relation to autistic symptomatology: 2: Response inhibition. *Autism, 9*, 29–43.

Buzan, T. (1974). *Use Your Head*. London: BBC Books.

Caroll, C. & Dockrell, J. (2010). Leaving special school: Post-16 outcomes for young adults with specific language impairment. *European Journal of Special Needs Education, 25*(2), 131–147.

Clegg, J., Hollis, C., Mawhood, L., & Rutter, M. (2005). Developmental language disorders – a follow up in later adult life. Cognitive, language and psychosocial outcomes. *Journal of Child Psychology and Psychiatry, 46*(2), 128–149.

Colston, H.L. & Kuiper, M.S. (2002). Figurative language development research and popular children's literature: Why we should know "Where the Wild Things Are". *Metaphor and Symbol, 17*(1), 27-43.

Conti-Ramsden, G. & Durkin, K. (2012). Post-school educational and employment experiences of young people with Specific Language Impairment. *Language, Speech, and Hearing Services in Schools, 43*, 507-520.

Conti-Ramsden, G., Botting, N., & Durkin, K. (2008). Parental perspectives during the transition to adulthood for adolescents with a history of specific language impairment. *Journal of Speech, Language and Hearing Research, 51*, 84-96.

Ebbels, S. (2014). Effectiveness of intervention of grammar in school-aged children with primary language impairments: A review of the evidence. *Child Language Teaching and Therapy, 30*(1), 7-40.

Frith, U. (1989). *Autism: Explaining the Enigma.* Malden: Blackwell Publishing.

Gernsbacher, M.A. & Pripas-Kapit, S.R. (2012). Who's missing the point? A commentary on claims that autistic persons have a specific deficit in figurative language comprehension. *Metaphor and Symbol, Special Issue: Autism and Non-literal Language, 27*(1), 93-105.

Grinnell, R.M. & Lieberman, A. (1977). Teaching the mentally retarded job interview skills. *Journal of Counseling Psychology, 24*(4), 332-337.

Hall, C., Sheldon-Wildgen, J., & Sherman, J.A. (1980). Teaching job interview skills to retarded clients. *Journal of Applied Behavior Analysis, 13*(3), 433-442.

Happe, F.G.E. (1993). Communicative competence and theory of mind in autism: A test of relevance theory. *Cognition, 48*(2), 101–119.

Happe, F.G.E. (1999). Review autism: Cognitive deficit or cognitive style? *Trends in Cognitive Sciences, 3*(6), 216–222.

Howlin, P., Mawhood, L., & Rutter, M. (2000). Autism and developmental receptive language disorder: A follow-up comparison in early adult life. II: Social, behavioural, and psychiatric outcomes. *Journal of Child Psychology Psychiatry, 41*(5), 561-578.

Kelly, J.A., Wildman, B.G., & Berler, E.S. (1980). Small group behavioral training to improve the job interview skills repertoire of mildly retarded adolescents. *Journal of Applied Behavior Analysis, 13*(3), 461-471.

Lavigne, A., Spock, S., Christy, L., & Edwards, G. (2002). 'Sk8er Boi' from the album 'Let go', performed by Avril Lavigne, produced by The Matrix.

Lazar, R.T., War-Leeper, G.A. Nicholson, C.B., & Johnson, S. (1989). Elementary school teachers' use of multiple meaning expressions. *Language, Speech, and Hearing Services in Schools, 20*, 420-430. Doi:10.1044/0161-1461.2004.420

Loukusa, S., Leinonen, E., Kuusikko, S., Jussila., K., Mattila, M.-L., Ryder, N., Ebeling, H., & Moilanen, I. (2007). Use of context in pragmatic language comprehension by children with Asberger Sydrome or high-functioning autism. *Journal of Autism and Developmental Disorders, 37*(6), 1049-1059.

Martin, I. & McDonald, S. (2004). An exploration of causes of non-literal language problems in individuals with Asperger Syndrome. *Journal of Autism and Developmental Disorders, 4*(3), 311-328.

Mathrick, R. & Meagher, T. (2012). *Interview Skills Training for Young People with SLCN.* St Mabyn: Stass Publications.

Mathrick, R., Meagher, T., Morey, K., & Masterson, N. (2014). Language through lyrics. St Catherine's School and Sixth Form. Poster presented at RCSLT Conference 2014, Leeds, UK.

Mathrick, R., Meagher, T., & Norbury, C. (2017). Evaluation of an interview skills training package for adolescents with speech, language and communication needs. *International Journal of Language and Communication Disorders, 52*(6), 786-799.

Mok, P.L.H., Pickles, A., Durkin, K., & Conti-Ramsden, G. (2014). Longitudinal trajectories of peer relations in children with SLI. *Journal of Child Psychology and Psychiatry, 55*(5), 516-527.

Nicoll, L. (2016). All singing all dancing: Methods to evaluate and develop idiom skills in 9 to 17 year olds with DLD. Royal College of Speech and Language Therapists Research Champion Workshop 2016, London, UK.

Norbury, C.F. (2005). Barking up the wrong tree? Lexical ambiguity resolution in children with language impairments and autistic spectrum disorders. *Journal of Experimental Child Psychology, 90*(2), 142–171.

Norbury, C.F. (2014). Practitioner review: Social (pragmatic) communication disorder, conceptualization, evidence and clinical implications. *Journal of Child Psychology and Psychiatry, 55*(3), 204–216.

Ozonoff, S., Pennington, B.F., & Rogers S.J. (1991). Executive function deficits in high-functioning autistic individuals: Relationship to theory of mind. *Journal of Child Psychology and Psychiatry, 32*(7), 1081–1105.

Rajendran, G., Mitchell, P., & Rickards, H. (2005). How do individuals with Aspergers Syndrome respond to non-literal language and inappropriate requests in computer-mediated communication? *Journal of Autism and Developmental Disorders, 35*, 429-443.

Rao, P.A., Beidel, D.C., & Murray, M.J. (2007). Social skills interventions for children with Asperger's Syndrome or high-functioning autism: A review and recommendations. *Journal of Autism and Developmental Disorders, 38*, 353-361.

Semel, E., Wigg, E.H., & Secord, W.A. (1995). *CELF: Clinical Evaluation of Language Fundamentals, 3rd ed.* London: The Psychological Cooperation.

Shattuck, P.T., Narendorf, S.C., Cooper, B., Sterzing, P.R., Wagner, M., & Taylor, J.L. (2012). Postsecondary education and employment among youth with an autism spectrum disorder. *Paediatrics, 129*(6), 1042-1049.

Skinner, M. (2004) 'Fit but You Know It' from the album 'A Grand Don't Come For Free', performed by 'The Streets', produced by Mike Skinner.

Spivack, R., Craston, M., Thom, G., & Carr, C. (2014). *Special Educational Needs and Disability Pathfinder Programme Evaluation Thematic Report: The Education, Health and Care (EHC) Planning Pathway for Families that are New to the SEN System.* Research Report January 2014. London: Department for Education.

Strickland, D.C., Coles, C.D., & Southern, L.R. (2013). JobTIPS: A transition to employment program for individuals with autism spectrum disorders. *Journal of Autism Developmental Disorders, 43,* 2472–2483.

Whitehouse, A.J.O., Watt, H.J., Line, E.A., & Bishop, D.V.M. (2009). Adult psychosocial outcomes of children with specific language impairment, pragmatic language impairment and autism. *International Journal of Language and Communication Disorders, 44,* 511-528.

Yew, S.G.K. & O'Kearney, R. (2013). Emotional and behavioural outcomes later in childhood and adolescence for children with SLI: Meta-analyses of controlled prospective studies. *Journal of Child Psychology and Psychiatry, 54*(5), 516–524.

Acknowledgements

This chapter would not have been possible without the hard work and dedication of the St Catherine's School and Sixth Form Isle of Wight students and Speech and Language Therapy Department. Many thanks to:

Tina Meagher: Head of Therapy who has whole-heartedly supported both projects, jointly carried out the initial interview skills pilot, and has supported the interview skills and language through lyrics therapy for the research in this chapter.

Nicola Masterson, and Kayleigh Sparkes: For delivering interview skills training, and language through lyrics therapy for the research in this chapter.

Rachael Parsloe: For supporting the delivery of language through lyrics therapy which is outlined in this chapter.

Also many thanks to the university students at Royal Holloway, London University for their hard work coding the interview skills videos: Agnes Banyai, Monisha Nahar and Sara Schamborg.

10 Adolescence and augmentative and alternative communication

Martine Smith

Learning outcomes

The chapter will enable readers to:

- Describe the multimodal nature of AAC systems

- Consider the needs of adolescents who use AAC

- Identify the potential of AAC in supporting access to participation in learning, social, leisure and vocational opportunities

- Identify four key areas to consider when devising interventions to support adolescents who use AAC

- Recognize the key challenges that this stage of development poses for interventions focused on increasing access to and use of AAC

Introduction

The speech, language and communication needs and challenges of adolescents have been well articulated across all the chapters in this volume. This chapter focuses on a specific group of young people, those who must navigate this developmental transition using augmentative and alternative communication (AAC). Their ways of communicating may not be easily recognized or interpreted by potential communication partners and their access to satisfying and fulfilling interaction experiences may be challenged by barriers outside their control, including technological barriers, the attitudes of those with whom they come into contact, as well as their own language and communication abilities. Before delving further into the unique and universal challenges these young people face, consider the following scenarios.

Gary is a 14-year-old student who has severe cerebral palsy that compromises his ability to control most of his body apart from eye movements. Although he has no difficulty in understanding spoken language, Gary can only produce some vocal sounds, but no words that can be understood. He can communicate a surprising amount by using his eyes and facial expression with people who know him well, but these modes largely limit him to communicating about things in the here-and-now so he uses a Speech Generating Device (SGD) or Voice Output Communication Aid (VOCA) for much of his communication. His SGD is a tablet computer with dedicated software for communication purposes and he can select messages or spell out words using an eye-tracking interface. Using this mode of communication is slow and physically tiring and it can also be difficult to manage conversation flow, given that he needs to look directly at his SGD rather than at his communication partner, and the voice output lacks prosody and is often difficult to understand in noisy group settings. However, for Gary's team the SGD is seen as essential in supporting his integration and academic progress in his mainstream secondary school.

Megan is aged 16 and attends a special school. Like Gary, she has very little intelligible speech. She walks with an unsteady gait and has sufficient hand control to grip a thick pen. Megan has significant learning difficulties and does not easily understand the spoken language of her environment. She understands many manual signs, but her somewhat limited hand control means that her own attempts at signing are not easily understood. She relates well to picture symbols and has a large folder containing pages of symbols categorized by topic and activity. Megan can find most of the symbols in her folder, but rarely uses the symbols spontaneously for communication. Several different types of SGDs have been trialled with Megan, but the physical force she sometimes uses to select a symbol on a screen has raised concerns about the potential risks and benefits of purchasing a device. For the moment, the main emphasis is on increasing the presence and visibility of picture symbols in her environment to support her understanding of her world and reduce some of the challenging behaviours that are disruptive in the classroom and the home setting.

Introduction

In both the above scenarios access to spoken language is restricted and alternative modes of communication are recruited to support or enhance language and communication. The term augmentative and alternative communication (AAC) is used to refer to the use of multiple modes of communication to compensate for an impairment in the ability to understand spoken language or to produce speech that is sufficiently intelligible to enable participation in communication interactions. For some people, AAC serves primarily as an expressive mode of communication, to bypass speech production difficulties or to supplement speech intelligibility. For others, AAC modes are an important support for language as well as speech, scaffolding understanding as well as supporting expressive communication.

An AAC system is a complex integration of all the modes of communication available to an individual. Some modes (such as facial expression, eye gaze and gesture) are used by all communicators, although these modes may assume a role and prominence that is different for an individual who has very limited speech. Other modes may be more exceptional, including the use of a manual signing system, picture symbols or speech-generating devices such as an iPad. In this context, *unaided communication* refers to the use of communication modes that draw on the physical resources of the communicator, such as gesture, facial expression or eye gaze. By contrast, *aided communication* involves the recruitment of additional physical resources, ranging from high-tech devices including tablet computers with speech output, to low-tech or no-tech devices that allow only a single message to be stored and retrieved, or communication boards or folders of pictures symbols. All communicators who use aided communication also use unaided modes; in fact, evidence to date suggests that unaided modes are relied on to a far greater extent than aided modes, even if the latter are powerful computer-based devices (e.g., Clarke & Wilkinson, 2007; Simpson, Beukelman, & Sharpe, 2000).

Despite the potential of AAC to enhance communication and participation, integrating aided communication into everyday life and interaction experiences can be very difficult. Many survey studies have pointed towards a rejection of aided communication, both high- and low-tech, by potential users and their families, with estimates of abandonment of 30% not uncommon (Allaire, Gressard, Blackman, & Hostler, 1991; Johnson, Ingelbret, Jones, & Ray, 2006). Rejection can occur at any developmental stage, and may indeed reflect developmental progress, growing out of the capacity of a device to support communication (Scherer, 2005). However, there are features unique to the adolescent period that suggest this may be a particularly critical stage when young people assert their autonomy and desire to communicate in a way that fits with their own sense of self.

Defining the population: Who are we talking about?

Although the terms 'people who use AAC' or 'AAC users' are widely used, as the two vignettes at the start of this chapter illustrate, these umbrella terms cover a very wide range of individuals who have very different abilities, needs and aetiological conditions associated with AAC use. One attempt at establishing the prevalence of need for use of AAC in the UK (Enderby, Judge, Creer, & John, 2013), estimated that 0.5% of the population may require AAC, equating to 529 people per population of 100,000. While adults with acquired disabilities are likely to account for more than half this group, four groups of conditions were identified as often leading to a need for young people to use AAC: (1) congenital conditions, such as cerebral palsy or profound and multiple learning difficulties; (2) developmental disorders including learning disabilities and autism spectrum disorders; (3) acquired neurological conditions, such as brain injury; and (4) progressive neuromuscular conditions (e.g., muscular dystrophy or Friedrich's Ataxia).

Within each of these groups, the proportion of young people needing access to AAC may also vary considerably. Those with overt speech difficulties, often related to a physical disability such as cerebral palsy, are most likely to be identified. In the SH&PE population study (Cockerill, Elbourne, Allen, et al., 2013), Cockerill and colleagues assessed the speech of 224 young people with cerebral palsy aged between 16 and 18. The majority (62%) presented with impaired speech intelligibility and 32% (n=72) had been provided with AAC. Remarkably similar figures were reported from a population study of younger children with cerebral palsy in western Sweden (Himmelmann, Lindh, & Cooley Hidecker, 2013). It is far more difficult to capture data on use of AAC by young people with learning disabilities or autism spectrum disorders. In part, this may be because the potential language benefits of AAC are not always recognized as easily (Enderby et al., 2014); in part, it may reflect the fact that the need to use AAC may be a very fluid picture in young people with learning disabilities or autism, as speech production abilities may change over time and become more functional as a mode of communication. However, even without clear population data, it is evident that a significant number of young people enter adolescence with speech, language and communication needs that could benefit from AAC systems and strategies.

Creating a communicatively accessible environment for AAC use

In order for the potential benefits of AAC to be fulfilled, the environment must accommodate to the unique demands and opportunities AAC offers; it must become communicatively accessible (von Tetzchner & Stadskleiv, 2016). An environment that is communicatively accessible for an adolescent who uses AAC is one where AAC options are available, accessible, accepted and supported.

Availability of AAC

A fundamental requirement for effective use of AAC, particularly aided communication, is that the aided mode is present and available within the environment. There is reliable evidence to suggest that not all young people who could use AAC are provided with appropriate and relevant AAC supports (Enderby et al., 2013). This problem is not unique to adolescents, and often reflects funding constraints that limit choices of aided communication options, or uncertainty on the part of support teams as to the most appropriate and effective AAC system to recommend (Baxter, Enderby, Evans, & Judge, 2012). Even if a system has been provided, it may not be available across environments. For example, Cockerill et al. (2013) found that only 12 of the 52 adolescents for whom AAC systems had been provided had these systems available to them across home and school environments; 21 of the 34 participants who used high-tech voice output devices only had access to these devices in school. Wickenden (2011a, 2011b) conducted an 18-month anthropological study of nine adolescents aged 10 to 15 years, all of whom had cerebral palsy. She describes pushing Terry, aged 14, on a school fieldtrip, trying to have a conversation, and reflecting later in her journal that she was "very aware of how difficult it is for him to make active conversation in this setting, as he didn't have his VOCA so he really has very little means of initiating any predictable conversation" (Wickenden, 2011a, p.20).

Accessibility of AAC

Even if an aided communication option is available in the environment, it may not be independently accessible to the adolescent who is expected to use it. Communication boards may sit in schoolbags or on a table at a distance from the student, who may rely on others to position it appropriately. Similarly, even if a device is physically within reach, a student may not be able to independently set it up for use, connect switches, turn it on or change the volume settings. Devices accessed through eye-tracking technology may easily become inaccessible due to physical movement that interferes with the calibration of the eye gaze. These challenges of ensuring a device is accessible are not unique to adolescents, but at a life stage when autonomy and independence assume a new relevance, reliance on others to ensure that a key communication mode is accessible may be a significant barrier to using AAC.

Acceptance of AAC as a valid and valued mode of communication

Von Tetzchner and Stadskleiv (2016) highlight the responsibility of all communication partners to acknowledge and value communication expressed through aided means as part of creating a communicatively accessible environment. Adolescents may be particularly sensitive to the attitudes of others towards their modes of communication. Even adolescents who see their SGD as critical to their participation in life often encounter limited awareness, negative attitudes and barriers as they negotiate their daily routines. Over the course of the study by Wickenden (2011a, 2011b), the participants and their parents discussed the challenges they experienced when people unfamiliar with their communication systems regarded them as objects of curiosity, or when they were ignored or patronized. The teenagers attributed many of these negative experiences to the fact that they used aided communication, were unable to speak and so were often assumed to be unable to understand. As one adult consultant to the research project, Katie, who used AAC, expressed it, "it is tempting to think that less talk means fewer ideas" (Wickenden, 2011a, p.14). Although it is just as likely that their physical impairments impacted on attitudes of unfamiliar people in their environment, being unable to speak and address these reactions directly likely creates an additional barrier.

There is some evidence that, overall, children (Beck, Fritz, Keller, & Dennis, 2000), adolescents (Beck, Thompson, Kosuwan, & Prochnow, 2010) and adults

(McCarthy & Light, 2005; Soto, 1997) have more positive attitudes to high-tech communication devices than to low-tech options. As the use of technology generally becomes more pervasive, it seems likely that the 'fear factor' reported in early studies of aided communication technology will quickly become a thing of the past, particularly among younger people, including adolescents. Nonetheless, the importance of peer acceptance and image may lead some young people to reject aided communication in order to minimize difference from peers. Acceptance of AAC on the part of the environment is important, but not sufficient. While young children who use AAC have expressed positive attitudes towards their AAC devices as 'cool' (Clarke, McConachie, Price, & Wood, 2001), individual adolescents who use AAC may struggle to decide whether the potential gain from using AAC compensates for the attention that aided modes may attract. For example, Stevenson (2001) describes Laura, who at the age of 16 began to refuse to have her voice output device mounted on her chair, even though her rehabilitation team reduced the size of her head switches to her specifications and her mother provided leopardskin covers for the switches to make them more cosmetically acceptable. In a similar vein, five young adolescent aided communicators who were interviewed in their residential setting (Smith & Kenny, cited in Smith, 2005a) expressed reservations about using aided communication in public. Two participants referred to the fear that it would make them "even more different" and one expressed concern that "people think it is a toy for me, not for communication" (p.75). At a life stage when image and identity assume particular importance, fitting in may mean pushing AAC out.

Support afforded for use of AAC

The final characteristic of a communicatively accessible environment is that it is one where there are sufficient supports in place to scaffold effective use of AAC, both practically in terms of technical support and training, as well as intervention supports. Poor reliability of devices and lack of technical support are frequently cited as frustrating barriers to effective use of aided communication (e.g., Baxter et al., 2012; Judge & Townend, 2013; Smith & Connolly, 2008; Wickenden, 2011a, 2011b). The teenagers who participated in Wickenden's study (2011a) expressed their wishes for access to appropriate and reliable technology, described as key elements in facilitating their independence and autonomy.

Secondary school differs in many fundamental ways from the relatively stable and controlled environment of primary school. Students entering their adolescent years may find themselves navigating multiple different classrooms, class groupings and teachers, as well as complex peer group interactions. Having access to a reliable source of support and contact to ease these transitions may be critical, not only to effective use of AAC but to effective participation in all aspects of school life (e.g., Stoner, Angell, & Bailey, 2010). At the same time, navigating these transitions through the assistance of another person may present its own difficulties, creating tensions between emerging desires for autonomy and independence.

Defining a role for AAC in adolescence

While AAC has the potential to greatly enhance communication opportunities, its ultimate purpose is not to enhance communication but rather to enable access to the range of activities that communication normally affords: participation in society, in academic, social, leisure and vocational opportunities, as well as the development of autonomy and self-determination. Within each of these domains, AAC may play a unique role but may also pose particular intervention challenges.

The role of AAC in supporting participation for learning

Adolescence sees the increasing emergence of meta-cognitive skills, such as paying attention to and monitoring one's own learning (Lee & Freire, 2003; Paul & Norbury, 2012). However, language remains the primary vehicle through which the academic curriculum is accessed, while the academic curriculum itself becomes increasingly important as a source of language learning for young people (Nippold, 1998, 2000). Many adolescents who use AAC encounter significant barriers to academic progress over these years, including difficulties in acquiring effective literacy skills (Bryen, Potts, & Carey, 2007; Smith, 2005b; Smith, Dahlgren Sandberg, & Larsson, 2009). Unless they achieve effective literacy skills, they may encounter unique language-learning difficulties related to mismatches between the external vocabulary available to them in their aided AAC component and their internal lexical development. They are dependent on others to ensure that the vocabulary they need is stored in their aided system; having the relevant and appropriate vocabulary has been found to be one of the most important factors determining whether or not aided communication is useful and used (Judge & Townend, 2013; Murphy, Maraková, Collins, &

Moodie, 1996; Senner, 2011). For support staff, keeping pace with vocabulary needs and finding time to program or provide requisite vocabulary may place significant organizational demands. Furthermore, adolescents who use AAC must not only master the conceptual, semantic and lexical properties of a wide range of new terms in order to engage with the curriculum, they must also learn where these items are stored and how to access them.

The role of AAC in supporting participation in social opportunities

Adolescence has been characterized as a group experience (Turkstra, 2000), where the rate, quantity and pace of language use increase as group interactions with peers assume new importance (Bergevin, Bukowski, & Miners, 2003; Larson & McKinley, 1998; Turkstra, Ciccia, & Seaton, et al., 2003). Language style and code switching are important for in-group identification (Nippold, 1998; Turkstra, 2000), as is humour, often expressed through language (Henry, Reed, & McAllister, 1995). For any adolescent, these fast-paced interactions, with layered levels of meaning within group contexts, involve new learning. For adolescents using aided communication, the challenges are even greater – for both the adolescents and those involved in supporting them. Many young people who use AAC may enter adolescence with fragile interaction skills. Senner (2011) asked 21 parents of adolescents and young adults who used SGDs (aged 16 to 21 years) to rate the interaction skills of these young people, using an online version of the Pragmatic Profile of the *Clinical Evaluation of Language Fundamentals* (CELF-4; Semel, Wiig, & Secord, 2004). While the ability to use greetings effectively was identified as a clear strength for this group, extending conversations, asking questions and using peer-appropriate language were all areas where parents identified significant learning needs. Even where peer-appropriate language is available, the sheer pace of group talk may make it difficult for an adolescent using aided communication to contribute in synchrony with the group, while the nuances of layered meaning may be particularly difficult to convey through graphic symbol-based communication systems or voice output systems that have limited capacity for expressing prosody or intonation.

In addition to these challenges, effective social participation now involves not only face-to-face interaction, but also distance communication in various social media platforms and text-based messaging systems. These emerging social networks offer new opportunities for adolescents who use AAC: they largely remove the time pressure that makes equal participation in face-to-face interaction so difficult. Although many media platforms require both traditional and digital literacy skills, they also offer opportunities to connect with peers using photographs, visual images, symbols and videos, thereby creating new opportunities for equalizing communication interactions. Research in this area is only now emerging, but it is clear that many young people who use AAC are keenly motivated to engage with social media (Hynan, Goldbart, & Murray, 2015) and recognize the benefits it offers in terms of building social networks, promoting independence and supporting reciprocity in communication (Caron & Light, 2016). Despite these advantages, access to the internet is not always easy for young people who use AAC; literacy difficulties, technology problems and lack of supports often combine to reduce the extent to which adolescents manage to engage (e.g., Raghavendra, Wood, Newman, & Lawry, 2012b).

Stable and robust social networks are important for many reasons, not least of which is the support they offer to the development of self-confidence and a positive sense of self. They are important in the long term as a protection against loneliness and in supporting physical and mental health (Cacioppo, Fowler, & Christakis, 2009; Cacioppo, Hawkley, & Thisted, 2010). They have also been identified as valuable in leveraging employment opportunities for young people with disabilities (Bryen, 2006). An important role for AAC is to enable adolescents to develop, sustain and expand their social networks.

The role of AAC in supporting participation in leisure opportunities

Leisure activities represent an important context for developing social networks that differ from the networks present in structured activities. Leisure activities bring together people who share common interests and motivations; they have a voluntary dimension that implies choice and control. This aspect of leisure activities was highlighted by the 12 young people interviewed by King, Gibson, Mistry, et al. (2014), seven of whom used AAC. For these participants, control over choices about activities and levels of participation were linked to a sense of independence. For the seven participants who used AAC, additional factors impacted on their choice of leisure activities, including the organizational and physical demands an activity implied for themselves and for their families. As noted by these authors, leisure activities for the participants who used AAC required significant "planning, support and structure in advance and throughout" (p.1632) (see also Hajjar, McCarthy, Beningno, & Chabot, 2016).

Deciding whether or not to participate in a leisure activity is in part influenced by comparing the potential benefit to the implied costs. Key benefits reported by the adolescents in the study by King et al. were (not surprisingly) fun and a sense of belonging. These simple but powerful motivators may be easily overlooked in what these authors describe as a risk of "over-therapizing" (King et al., 2014, p.1626) young people with disabilities.

The sense of belonging, of control and of choice that leisure activities afford may depend to a large extent on having access to a mode of communication that allows connections to be made with peers in such activities. Appropriate modes of communication offer a means of expressing choice and exerting control, but must also be available, interpretable and accepted within those activities. In their study of participation of young people with complex communication needs in active recreation activities, Hajjar et al. (2016) found that often aided communication systems were left at home, to avoid any risk of damage or loss or because they were difficult to integrate into the environment of the leisure activity. While it is likely to always be the case that a swimming pool is out of bounds for an iPad as a communication aid, alternative solutions are needed. Adolescents who use AAC should not have to choose between swimming and communicating, but instead should have the opportunity to choose whether or not to communicate while swimming.

The role of AAC in supporting participation in vocational opportunities

Mid- to late-adolescence is often a time when future life choices start to crystallize, with attention turning to vocational options and the potential for independent living. The stark reality of finding employment in a competitive work environment can be daunting. Successful transitions to further education or employment are most often underpinned by strong communication and literacy skills and rich social networks, as well as supportive families who are often the unsung advocates and enablers of these positive outcomes (Bryen, 2006; Lund & Light, 2007b; McNaughton & Arnold, 2010). In order to demonstrate their communication skills and to build their literacy abilities, adolescents need support to maintain and develop their competence in using the full range of communication modes available to them, including aided communication. Often at this stage, they may both physically and linguistically outgrow existing communication devices and face the challenge of developing a range of new operational skills, precisely at a stage when they may also wish to assert their independence and autonomy in choosing not to use a mode that identifies them as different to their peers (e.g., Lund & Light, 2007a).

The role of AAC in supporting transitions

The transition across adolescence towards independence and autonomy as an adult is an exciting but anxiety-inducing stage for adolescents and families alike. Over this period, communication is crucial in supporting successful negotiation of conflict, of distancing, of reassurance and for establishing new relationships. While all parents view approaching adulthood for their children with a degree of trepidation, for parents of children with disabilities the fears and anxieties are greatly increased. Balancing the needs of a young person to develop independence against the risks when that young person cannot use speech to communicate is difficult for all concerned. Many of the young people interviewed by Wickenden (2011a) wished for more opportunities to independently go out to cafés, pubs, clubs and bowling and all the other places where young people socialize. They wished for more same-age peers without disabilities, so that any help they needed could be provided by peers rather than adults, and so that, as one participant expressed it, parents could 'butt out' (p.19). Many parents struggle with stepping back and establishing boundaries as their children move through adolescence. However, if a parent feels that an adolescent is unable to communicate effectively without their being physically present, it may not be possible for them to simply step back and 'butt out'.

Building interventions to support adolescents who use AAC

Expectations that young people with disabilities, including those who use AAC, should participate fully in all aspects of life have changed dramatically over the past decades, even if the reality of meeting those expectations has lagged somewhat behind (McNaughton & Bryen, 2007; McNaughton, Light, & Gulla, 2004). Some of the themes explored in this chapter point to important considerations for harnessing the potential of AAC to maximize the benefits to adolescents as they move towards the next stage in life. Four points for consideration are outlined here.

Vocabulary, vocabulary, vocabulary

People who use aided communication have a unique reliance on others to ensure that they have the words they need to navigate their lives. There are four domains of vocabulary that merit consideration when planning for adolescents using AAC.

1. One domain is academic, building a system which ensures that vocabulary needs are identified and there are mechanisms in place to ensure that these needs can be met.

2. A second is social – ensuring access to the kind of language that enables a young person to fit in with a peer group, to joke, to curse, to tease and to connect.

3. A third emerges in later adolescence: the need for vocabulary that is appropriate and specific to the workplace or to future educational or vocational opportunities.

4. Adolescents also need to be able to protect themselves, to report crime and abuse and to manage often complex healthcare issues.

Based on her work with adults who use AAC, Bryen (2008) developed vocabulary lists as a resource for those working with adolescents and adults facing important life transitions. These lists provide vocabulary related to: (a) college life; (b) emergency preparedness; (c) employment; (d) sexuality, intimacy and sex; (e) reporting crime and abuse; (f) managing personal and assistance services; (g) managing healthcare; and (h) using transportation.

In addition to planning for vocabulary programming and updating, adolescents need to be supported to develop strategies to monitor their own vocabulary needs, to take responsibility for requesting vocabulary or programming themselves, and to develop a system that ensures that vocabulary maintenance is an embedded dynamic process, constantly evolving.

Building social networks

Communication skills offer a passport to participation in society, but they are simply a tool to be used in interaction. The activity of communicating needs to be embedded in sustainable social networks. Research suggests that the social networks of young people who use AAC are restricted relative to peers, and disproportionately rely on adults or on individuals paid to be present in their lives (e.g., Raghavendra, Olsson, Sampson, et al., 2012a). From the point of view of young people themselves (Wickenden, 2011a) and of their families, encouraging friendships and social connections are key priorities (Angelo, Kokoska, & Jones, 1996; Marshall & Goldbart, 2008, Tavares & Peixoto, 2003), with parents sometimes trying to engineer opportunities for friendships to evolve even if their adolescent children are uncomfortable with this perceived interference (Wickenden, 2011a). Identifying and using adolescents' social networks as the starting point in planning intervention, using tools such as the Social Network Inventory (Blackstone & Hunt-Berg, 2012) creates the potential for supporting sustainable social interaction opportunities – without which effective communication skills may have little functional value.

One intervention strategy with an emerging evidence base involves harnessing peers as intervention partners, both to guide intervention decisions and to implement intervention goals. For example, Lilienfeld and Alant (2005) described an intervention with Simon, a 15-year-old student who used AAC. In this study, Simon identified barriers limiting his own communication with peers (e.g., the need to give him time to formulate messages; the importance of highlighting when a message was not understood; identifying behaviours that blocked effective communication). Using this information, eight adolescent peers participated in a series of workshops, each focused on a specific difficulty Simon had identified. Peers worked together with Simon to identify solutions to the problems, and identified an action leader to implement the solution, promoting their active engagement with both the problem and the solution. Follow-up evaluation indicated that Simon communicated more frequently (more interactions per hour of observation), for longer (the duration of interactions increased, with more and longer contributions from Simon), for a wider range of purposes (including teasing, humour and sarcasm), and more successfully (fewer interruptions or ignoring of Simon's contributions). Enabling peers to actively support use of AAC may take careful planning and requires sensitivity to the group dynamic and the potential risk of assigning a role of 'problem' or 'neediness' to the adolescent who uses AAC. However, even without direct involvement in intervention, three strategies have been proposed to promote success peer interactions (Hunt, Doering, Maier, & Mintz, 2009). These are: (a) providing relevant and accessible information to peers; (b) identifying and making available a range of communication modes to support social interactions, rather than relying on a single mode; and (c) providing structured support for interaction opportunities.

Finally, social networks can also be fostered and supported in an online environment. Young people need to be aware of the risks involved in these media, and need guidance on how to stay safe. However, the opportunities they offer have potentially unique benefits for young people who use aided communication. Online social networks support interactions where participants can choose how they wish to present themselves, where they can connect with others who share similar experiences, even if geographically distant. These interactions generally involve some engagement with text, so may also have spinoff benefits for literacy skills that otherwise seem to present a particular challenge for young people who use AAC (Hynan et al., 2015). They may also offer opportunities for participating in mentoring programmes that not only support skill development but also create opportunities for building communities with a shared experience (Cohen & Light, 2000; Light, McNaughton, Krezman, et al., 2007).

Curriculum

Supporting adolescents who use AAC to navigate the complex range of classroom environments and subject domains of the secondary school environment requires setting in place a system where key personnel within the school setting are designated as responsible for problem-solving immediate communication difficulties and planning for curriculum needs (Soto, Muller, Hunt, & Goetz, 2001; Stoner et al., 2010). Without clear lines of responsibility and designated key personnel, adolescents may be left to overcome these difficulties on their own. The case study by Stoner et al. (2010) suggests that, even with the best of intentions on the part of all staff, lack of a clear line of responsibility for troubleshooting and planning can thwart the best efforts of those involved. Equally essential is that these key individuals are supported to acquire the knowledge and skills that will enable them to quickly and easily overcome difficulties such as minor technical problems, or to link with teachers to determine vocabulary needs for specific classes and ensure that the necessary programming is completed.

Adolescents need to be supported to negotiate and make choices about where, with whom and to what purpose they use their range of communication modes. Using aided communication for prolonged periods of time can be both physically and cognitively exhausting (Murray & Goldbart, 2009; Smith & Connolly, 2008) and may represent an additional load on what most adolescents already experience as a tiring school day. For this reason, changes in pace may need to be negotiated, with opportunities to review and reorganize schedules and activities. Finally, language and literacy skills are the key pillars of curriculum access. Both are domains of activity where learning may extend across the lifespan. Given the special role that literacy plays in the communication opportunities available to young people who use AAC, building language and literacy skills should be an ongoing curriculum focus across their school years and potentially beyond.

Supporting independence, autonomy and choice

Over the past decade, a growing body of research has emerged documenting the experiences of adults who use AAC as they reflect back on their earlier experiences and current situations (Dattilo, Estrella, Estrella et al., 2008; Hemsley, Balandin, & Togher, 2008; Lund & Light, 2006, 2007a, 2007b). It is clear that the transition across adolescence into adulthood is not always easy and that in many cases the outcomes for young adults are not as positive as they would have hoped (e.g., Hamm & Mirenda, 2006). Developing meaningful relationships, living independently, managing personal care and support staff and finding gainful employment are challenges for all young people, but are even greater for those whose communication is not easily understood by others and who may also be physically dependent. The right of adolescents to communicate how they wish, including the right not to use AAC, must be respected. The responsibility of those supporting them is to ensure that the choice is an informed one, that the opportunities to use AAC are available and are at least as accessible as other options, and that the door remains open to return to skill building, should the need arise. Part of this planning must address the need for young people to be able to independently set up their own communication systems, currently often an apparently insurmountable challenge (Hunt-Berg, 2005), but an area where future technological developments seem to be focusing welcome attention (Judge & Townend, 2013; McNaughton & Bryen, 2007).

One of the key gaps in supporting autonomy and independence identified by families and adults who use AAC is access to trained personnel across the later adolescent and early adult years, as service structures, responsibilities and resources shift in the reality of the post-school environment (Hamm & Mirenda, 2006). Planning for this transition is an important step in ensuring that the bridge from adolescence to adulthood is sufficiently strong to meet the demands likely to be faced both by adolescents who use AAC and their families. Negotiating these kinds of supports may involve breaking down traditional service boundaries to facilitate seamless transitions.

Summary and conclusions

Adolescents who use AAC face all the challenges of their peers as they negotiate this dynamic, exciting stage of development. Some of the battles they encounter are unique, navigating as they must the physical, attitudinal and technological barriers that are sometimes associated with the use of aided communication. However, in many more respects they are just like all other adolescents, striving to establish their own identity, autonomy and make friends with whom they can relax, share and compete. The young people interviewed by Wickenden (2011a) continuously emphasized their desire to be seen as typical teenagers, sociable, funny and interesting in their own right. They expressed a wish that they not be defined by their disability, that people talk to them as teenagers and young adults ("treat me as a person", Ted, aged 14; "don't be scared of me, talk to me as normal", Prakash, aged 14, both from Wickenden, 2011a, p.24). Effective use of AAC offers one tool to support young people expressing who they are and defining how they fit into a range of different social networks. The many challenges associated with achieving effective use of AAC that have been described in this chapter are simply a reminder of the complexity of interventions to support participation in society, when communication skills differ from those of the society in which participation is sought.

Reflective questions

1. What are the potential challenges that use of aided communication poses for adolescents' self-esteem and identity? How might these challenges be addressed in interventions?

2. What are the risks associated with harnessing the input of peers as intervention agents and how could those risks be mitigated?

3. How could the potential of social media be exploited to support the development of language and literacy skills for adolescents who use AAC?

4. When might it be appropriate to require an adolescent to use aided communication, even if she/he has indicated a desire to use unaided modes of communication only?

5. What are the structural barriers to identifying key personnel with designated responsibility for supporting the technical needs of an adolescent who uses aided communication? How might those barriers be addressed?

References

Allaire, J., Gressard, R., Blackman, J., & Hostler, S. (1991). Children with severe speech impairments: Caregiver survey of AAC use. *Augmentative and Alternative Communication, 7*, 248-255.

Angelo, D., Kokoska, S., & Jones, S. (1996). Family perspective on Augmentative and Alternative Communication: Families of adolescents and young adults. *Augmentative and Alternative Communication, 12*, 13-20.

Baxter, S., Enderby, P., Evans, J., & Judge, S. (2012). Barriers and facilitators to the use of high-technology augmentative and alternative communication devices: A systematic review and qualitative synthesis. *International Journal of Language and Communication Disorders, 47*, 115-129.

Beck, A., Fritz, H., Keller, A., & Dennis, M.L. (2000). Attitudes of school-aged children toward their peers who use augmentative and alternative communication. *Augmentative and Alternative Communication, 16*, 13-26.

Beck, A., Thompson, J.R., Kosuwan, K., & Prochnow, J.M. (2010). The development and utilization of a scale to measure adolescents' attitudes towards peers who use augmentative and alternative communication. *Journal of Speech, Language & Hearing Research, 53*, 572-587.

Bergevin, T., Bukowski, W., & Miners, R. (2003). Social development. In: A. Slater & G. Bremner (Eds), *An Introduction to Developmental Psychology.* Oxford: Blackwell Publishing.

Blackstone, S. & Hunt-Berg, M. (2012). *Social Networks: A Communication Inventory for Individuals with Complex Communication Needs and their Communication Partners (Revised).* CA: Attainment Company.

Bryen, D. (2006). Job-related social networks and communication technology. *Augmentative and Alternative Communication, 22*, 1-9.

Bryen, D. (2008). Vocabulary for socially-valued adult roles. *Augmentative and Alternative Communication, 24*, 294-301.

Bryen, D., Potts, B., & Carey, A. (2007). So you want to work? What employers say about job skills, recruitment and hiring employees who rely on AAC. *Augmentative and Alternative Communication, 23*, 126-139.

Cacioppo, J., Fowler, J., & Christakis, N. (2009). Alone in the crowd: The structure and spread of loneliness in a large social network. *Journal of Personality and Social Psychology, 97*, 977-991.

Cacioppo, J., Hawkley, L., & Thisted, R. (2010). Perceived social isolation makes me sad: 5-year cross-lagged analyses of loneliness and depressive symptomatology in the Chicago health, aging and social relations study. *Psychology and Aging, 25*, 453-463.

Caron, J. & Light, J. (2016). Social media experiences of adolescents and young adults with cerebral palsy who use augmentative and alternative communication. *International Journal of Speech-Language Pathology, 19*, 30-42.

Clarke, M. & Wilkinson, R. (2007). Interaction between children with cerebral palsy and their peers 1: Organizing and understanding VOCA use. *Augmentative and Alternative Communication, 23*, 336-348.

Clarke, M., McConachie, H., Price, K., & Wood, P. (2001). Views of young people using augmentative and alternative communication systems. *International Journal of Language and Communication Disorders, 36*, 107-115.

Cockerill, H., Elbourne, D., Allen, E., Scrutten, D., Will, E., McNee, A., Fairhurst, C., & Baird, G. (2013). Speech, communication and use of augmentative communication in young people with cerebral palsy: The SH&PE population study. *Child: Care, Health and Development, 40*, 149-157.

Cohen, K. & Light, J. (2000). Use of electronic communication to develop mentor-protégé relationships between adolescent and adult AAC users: Pilot study. *Augmentative and Alternative Communication, 16*, 227-238.

Dattilo, J., Estrella, G., Estrella, L.J., Light, J., McNaughton, D., & Seabury, M. (2008). "I have chosen to live life abundantly": Perceptions of leisure by adults who use augmentative and alternative communication. *Augmentative and Alternative Communication, 24*, 16-28.

Enderby, P., Judge, S., Creer, S., & John, A. (2013). Examining the need for provision of AAC methods in the UK. *Advances in Clinical Neuroscience and Rehabilitation, 13*, 20-23.

Hajjar, D., McCarthy, J., Beningno, J., & Chabot, J. (2016). "You get more than you give": Experiences of community partners in facilitating active recreation with individuals who have complex communication needs. *Augmentative and Alternative Communication, 32*, 131-142.

Hamm, B. & Mirenda, P. (2006). Post-school quality of life for individuals with developmental disabilities who use AAC. *Augmentative and Alternative Communication, 22*, 134-147.

Hemsley, B., Balandin, S., & Togher, L. (2008). "I've got something to say": Interaction in a focus group of adults with cerebral palsy and complex communication needs. *Augmentative and Alternative Communication, 24*, 110-122.

Henry, F.M., Reed, V., & McAllister, L. (1995). Adolescents' perceptions of the relative importance of selected communication skills in their positive peer relationships. *Language Speech & Hearing Services in Schools, 26*, 263-272.

Himmelmann, K., Lindh, K., & Cooley Hidecker, M.J. (2013). Communication ability in cerebral palsy: A study from the CP register of western Sweden. *European Journal of Paediatric Neurology, 17*, 568-574.

Hunt, P., Doering, K., Maier, J., & Mintz, E. (2009). Strategies to support the development of positive social relationships and friendships for students who use AAC. In: G. Soto & C. Zangari (Eds), *Practically Speaking: Language, Literacy and Academic Development for Students with AAC Needs*. Baltimore, MD: Paul H Brookes.

Hunt-Berg, M. (2005). The Bridge School: Educational inclusion outcomes over 15 years. *Augmentative and Alternative Communication, 21*, 116-131.

Hynan, A., Goldbart, J., & Murray, J. (2015). A grounded theory of Internet and social media use by young people who use augmentative and alternative communication (AAC). *Disability and Rehabilitation, 37*, 1559-1575.

Johnson, J.M., Inglebret, E., Jones, C., & Ray, J. (2006). Perspectives of speech language pathologists regarding success versus abandonment of AAC. *Augmentative and Alternative Communication, 22*, 85-99.

Judge, S. & Townend, G. (2013). Perceptions of the design of voice output communication aids. *International Journal of Language and Communication Disorders, 48*, 366-381.

King, G., Gibson, B., Mistry, B., Pinto, M., Goh, F., Teachman, G., & Thompson, L. (2014). An integrated methods study of the experiences of youth with severe disabilities in leisure activity settings: The importance of belonging, fun and control and choice. *Disability and Rehabilitation, 36*, 1626-1635.

Larson, V.L. & McKinley, N.L. (1998). Characteristics of adolescents' conversations: A longitudinal study. *Clinical Linguistics and Phonetics, 12*, 183-203.

Lee, K. & Freire, A. (2003). Cognitive development. In: A. Slater & G. Bremner (Eds), *An Introduction to Developmental Psychology.* Oxford: Blackwell Publishing.

Light, J., McNaughton, D., Krezman, C., Williams, M.B., Gulens, M., Galskoy, A., & Umpleby, M. (2007). The AAC Mentor Project: Web-based instruction in sociorelational skills and collaborative problem solving for adults who use augmentative and alternative communication. *Augmentative and Alternative Communication, 23*, 56-75.

Lilienfeld, M. & Alant, E. (2005). The social interaction of an adolescent who uses AAC: The evaluation of a peer-training program. *Augmentative and Alternative Communication, 21*, 278-294.

Lund, S. & Light, J. (2006). Long-term outcomes for individuals who use augmentative and alternative communication: Part I - What is a "good" outcome? *Augmentative and Alternative Communication, 22*, 284-299.

Lund, S. & Light, J. (2007a). Long-term outcomes for individuals who use augmentative and alternative communication: Part II - Communication interaction. *Augmentative and Alternative Communication, 23*, 1-15.

Lund, S. & Light, J. (2007b). Long-term outcomes for individuals who use augmentative and alternative communication: Part III - Contributing factors. *Augmentative and Alternative Communication, 23*, 323-335.

Marshall, J. & Goldbart, J. (2008). "Communication is everything I think." Parenting a child who needs Augmentative and Alternative Communication (AAC). *International Journal of Language and Communication Disorders, 43*, 77-98.

McCarthy, J. & Light, J. (2005). Attitudes toward individuals who use Augmentative and Alternative Communication: Research review. *Augmentative and Alternative Communication, 21*, 41-55.

McNaughton, D. & Arnold, A. (2010). Supporting positive employment outcomes for individuals who use AAC. *Perspectives on Augmentative and Alternative Communication, 19*, 51-59.

McNaughton, D. & Bryen, D. (2007). AAC technologies to enhance participation and access to meaningful societal roles for adolescents and adults with developmental disabilities who require AAC. *Augmentative and Alternative Communication, 23*, 217-229.

McNaughton, D., Light, J., & Gulla, S. (2004). Opening up a 'Whole New World': Employer and co-worker perspectives on working with individuals who use Augmentative and Alternative Communication. *Augmentative and Alternative Communication, 19*, 235-253.

Murphy, J., Marková, I., Collins, S., & Moodie, E. (1996). AAC systems: Obstacles to effective use. *European Journal of Disorders of Communication, 31*, 31-44.

Murray, J. & Goldbart, J. (2009). Cognitive and language acquisition in typical and aided language learning: A review of recent evidence from an aided communication perspective. *Child Language Teaching and Therapy, 25*, 7-34.

Nippold, M. (1998). *Later Language Development: The School-age and Adolescent Years.* Austin, TX: Pro-Ed.

Nippold, M. (2000). Language development during the adolescent years: Aspects of pragmatics, syntax, and semantics. *Topics in Language Disorders, 20*, 15-28.

Paul, R. & Norbury, C. (2012). *Language Disorders from Infancy Through Adolescence: Listening, Speaking, Reading, Writing and Communicating, 4th ed.* St Louis, MI: Elsevier Mosby.

Raghavendra, P., Olsson, C., Sampson, J., McInerney, R., & Connell, T. (2012a). School participation and social networks of children with complex communication needs, physical disabilities and typically developing peers. *Augmentative and Alternative Communication, 28*, 33-43.

Raghavendra, P., Wood, D., Newman, L., & Lawry, J. (2012b). Why aren't you on Facebook? Patterns and experiences of using the Internet among young people with physical disabilities. *Technology and Disability, 24*, 149-162.

Scherer, M. (2005). *Living in the State of Stuck: How Assistive Technology Impacts the Lives of People with Disabilities.* Cambridge, MA: Brookline Books.

Semel, E., Wiig, E.H., & Secord, W. (2004). *Clinical Evaluation of Language Fundamentals, 4th ed.* Boston, MA: Pearson.

Senner, J.E. 2011. Parent perceptions of pragmatic skills in teens and young adults using AAC. *Communication Disorders Quarterly, 32*, 103-108.

Simpson, K.O., Beukelman, D.R., & Sharpe, T. (2000). An elementary student with severe expressive communication impairment in a general education classroom: Sequential analysis of interactions. *Augmentative and Alternative Communication, 16*, 107-121.

Smith, M. (2005a). The dual challenges of aided communication and adolescence. *Augmentative and Alternative Communication, 21*, 67-79.

Smith, M. (2005b). *Literacy and Augmentative and Alternative Communication.* London: Elsevier Academic Press.

Smith, M. & Connolly, I. (2008). Roles of aided communication: Perspectives of adults who use AAC. *Disability and Rehabilitation: Assistive Technology, 3*, 260-273.

Smith, M., Dahlgren Sandberg, A., & Larsson, M. (2009). Reading and spelling in children with severe speech and physical impairments: A comparative study. *International Journal of Language and Communication Disorders, 44*, 864-882.

Soto, G. (1997). Special education teacher attitudes toward AAC: Preliminary survey. *Augmentative and Alternative Communication, 13*, 186-197.

Soto, G., Muller, E., Hunt, P., & Goetz, L. (2001). Critical issues in the inclusion of students who use augmentative and alternative communication: An educational team perspective. *Augmentative and Alternative Communication, 17*, 62-72.

Stevenson, P. (2001). The impact of adolescence on the use of voice output communication aids. In: H. Cockerill & L. Carroll-Few (Eds), *Communicating Without Speech: Practical Augmentative and Alternative Communication.* Cambridge: MacKeith Press, Cambridge University Press.

Stoner, J., Angell, M., & Bailey, R. (2010). Implementing Augmentative and Alternative Communication in inclusive educational settings: A case study. *Augmentative and Alternative Communication, 26*, 122-135.

Tavares, L. & Peixoto, A. (2003). Late development of independent conversation skills with manual and graphic signs through joint activities. In: S. von Tetzchner & N. Grove (Eds), *Augmentative and Alternative Communication: Developmental issues.* London: Whurr.

Turkstra, L.S. (2000). Should my shirt be tucked in or left out? The communication context of adolescence. *Aphasiology, 14*, 349-364.

Turkstra, L.S., Ciccia, A., & Seaton, C. (2003). Interactive behaviors in adolescent conversation dyads. *Language Speech & Hearing Services in Schools, 34*, 117-127.

von Tetzchner, S. & Stadskleiv, K. (2016). Constructing a language in alternative forms. In: M. Smith & J. Murray (Eds), *The Silent Partner? Language, Interaction and Aided Communication.* Guildford: J&R Press.

Wickenden, M. (2011a). 'Talk to me as a teenager': Experiences of friendship for disabled teenagers who have little or no speech. *Childhoods Today, 5*.

Wickenden, M. (2011b). Talking to teenagers: Using anthropological methods to explore identity and the lifeworlds of young people who use AAC. *Communication Disorders Quarterly, 32*, 151-163.

Part III

School-level support for adolescents with language disorders

11 Creating language-accessible secondary classrooms

A professionally collaborative approach to supporting adolescents with language difficulty

Julia Starling

Learning outcomes

This chapter will enable readers to:

- Present the rationale underlying an evidence-based, professionally collaborative model of service delivery

- Discuss the impact of the secondary school learning environment on the academic progress of students with language difficulty

- Describe how speech and language therapists can work with teachers to create language-accessible secondary classrooms, to provide sustainable, inclusive support for students with language difficulty

- Describe adjustments that can be made to teachers' oral and written instructional language

---

Introduction

This chapter presents an evidence-based approach to supporting students with language difficulty through changes made to teachers' instructional language (Starling, Munro, Togher, & Arciuli, 2012). There are a great many challenges undermining the provision of effective support for adolescents with language-based learning difficulties (e.g., Prelock, 2000; Starling, Munro, Togher, & Arciuli, 2011). A professionally collaborative programme, such as that outlined below, has been shown to provide an alternative approach to intervention that is effective in both the short and long term. The programme, which was evaluated by a randomized controlled trial (RCT) at the University of Sydney (Starling et al., 2012), involves an intervention that targets in-class, inclusive support of students with language difficulty. Mainstream secondary teachers are trained by a speech-language therapist (SLT) in ways to modify their oral and written instructional language. For the RCT, an interactive training programme was implemented through regular face-to-face meetings over the course of a school term (10 weeks).

In summary, results demonstrated significantly increased use of the instructional language modification techniques by the trained teachers when compared to the control group of untrained teachers, with this use maintained over at least one further school term. A group of Year 8 (13-14-year-old) students with language difficulty in both experimental and control (wait condition) schools was identified through a screening process. Results from the pre- and post-testing of the students in the trained teachers' classes were indicative of a significant improvement in the students' written expression and listening comprehension relative to the students in the untrained teachers' classes (Starling et al., 2012).

The intervention as presented here can be used as a sole language intervention approach or as part of a more diverse approach that also includes direct client support. In the Response to Intervention model (Bradley, Danielson, & Doolittle, 2005), this intervention fits well with a Tier 2 targeted approach, allowing SLTs to provide sustainable support for whole populations of secondary students with language difficulty. SLTs are then more able to focus valuable time and resources at the Tier 3 specialized level of support for students with more complex needs. Naturally, these decisions are dependent on many management factors including time and resource availability.

Barriers to learning in the secondary school classroom

The teaching of curriculum content, across subjects and grades, involves secondary teachers presenting their students with often highly complex oral and written instructional language (Whitmire, 2000). As a result, students with language difficulty may find themselves in a disadvantageous environment, unable to fully access much of the academic curriculum. SLTs are well aware of the disparity between the language abilities of students with language difficulty and the increasingly complex language-based learning demands of mainstream secondary classrooms (Starling et al., 2011). This is often an area of particular concern and focus when SLTs are planning an approach to intervention for their adolescent caseloads (Ehren, 2002).

As part of their regular teaching practices, secondary teachers across all subject disciplines use both oral and written language to interact with students. Using oral language, essential to students' learning (Alexander, 2012), teachers instruct, present information, review, summarize, question their students' knowledge and outline projects, assignments and assessment tasks. Using written language teachers present texts, worksheets, glossaries, board work and classroom and homework instructions. Students are required to attend to and process teachers' instructional language and, using their innate language abilities, comprehend, analyze, retain and demonstrate understanding and knowledge through using their own oral and written language (Nippold, 2007). Ultimately this understanding and retention of the curriculum is evaluated largely by means of written assignments, tests and exams.

Students with oral and written language difficulty, regardless of the type or severity of impairment, are at significant risk of academic failure (Law, Rush, Schoon, & Parsons, 2009; Snowling, Adams, Bishop, & Stothard, 2001), largely as they may not have the receptive and expressive language skills needed for proficient understanding and learning of the secondary academic curriculum. They may find new vocabulary and terminology overly complex (Nash & Donaldson, 2005), and the rate of delivery and amount of information presented at any one time too demanding (Hughes, Turkstra, & Wulfeck, 2009). They may be challenged with processing and retaining information (Archibald & Gathercole, 2006), also with demonstrating their knowledge through oral (Nippold, Mansfield, Billow, & Tomblin, 2009) and written expression (Dockrell, Lindsay, & Connelly, 2009).

Support for the collaborative approach

Addressing these issues through an inclusive, systems-based intervention has wide support (e.g., Lindsay & Dockrell 2008; Paul, 2007). Both Ehren (2002) and Larson and McKinley (2003) recommend modifying curriculum content as a particularly useful collaborative approach, having the potential to assist students with language difficulty with their academic progress and the development of curricular knowledge. In an editorial on the continuing need for SLTs to be more proactive in providing an intervention evidence base and more support for adolescents with language difficulty, Nippold (2010) also recommended that SLTs collaborate with secondary classroom teachers on making topic knowledge more accessible. Studies have highlighted the particular benefits of school-based collaborative interventions involving vocabulary enrichment to support secondary students with specific language impairment (Joffe, 2006; Murphy et al., 2017; Wilson, Nash, & Earl, 2010). A major goal of the collaborative process in the secondary school environment could therefore be to create 'language-accessible' learning environments that ensure increased accessibility to information and improved opportunities for learning for students with language difficulty.

Professional development as part of the collaborative process

Teachers' professional development (PD) on communication disorders, in particular language-based learning difficulties, is a regular part of many SLTs' caseload management programmes. Teachers identify PD on speech and language difficulties as high priority so that they can address inclusive teaching practices adequately (Dockrell & Lindsay, 2001). Literature in the field of education gives some specific guidance for ensuring the effectiveness of providing PD to teaching staff. In a synthesis of evidence-based research on all types of PD for teachers, it is reported that conditions common to successful training programmes, using student progress as a criterion, were those that were presented in a sustained and interactive manner, were site-based and presented by experts in the relevant field (Guskey & Yoon, 2008).

In the secondary school scenario, sustainability of teacher training could be ensured by embedding key ideas and strategies in on-site training that is implemented over a period of time. The goal of this sustained interaction between the trainer (SLT) and the trainees (teachers) would be to empower teachers to make conceptual and practical changes to their teaching practices, thereby optimizing opportunities for the generalization of skills and knowledge, and continued use of the learned techniques in the long term.

Objectives of the collaborative programme

Building on the guidance thus outlined, the overarching objective of the intervention presented in this chapter is for SLTs and teachers to work together over a period of time to create more language-accessible secondary classrooms. When this occurs there are many potential benefits for students with language difficulty, and the following are quite realistic expectations:

- The students are better able to access the language of the curriculum through information presented both orally and in print

- They are better able attend to, process, analyze, retain and use presented information in a wide range of learning situations

- They are better able to become more proactively engaged in learning through increased participation in class activities

- They are able to demonstrate an improved understanding of curriculum content in assignments, projects, tests and exams

- They are better able to develop and use a broader and more robust vocabulary, a cornerstone of well-developed language and literacy.

All of these empowering factors, in combination with improved receptive and expressive language skills, can positively impact aspects of the students' personal development and feelings of wellbeing as they come to view themselves as more able learners.

In such a professional collaboration, teachers bring curriculum content knowledge and teaching expertise and experience to the partnership; they can ensure that any intervention has immediate academic relevance and impact, and provide opportunities for skill practice and generalization. SLTs bring knowledge and experience of the nature and impact of language difficulty, and insight into the barriers to learning experienced by populations of students with language-based learning difficulties.

Modifying teachers' instructional language

1 Oral instructional language

Secondary teachers present much curriculum content and instruction through their oral language. For example, they explain, instruct, discuss, question, recap, summarize, explore, illustrate, and elaborate (Cazden & Beck, 2008). As a result, students spend a great deal of time listening to and processing teachers' oral presentations. The oral language of secondary classrooms can range from everyday, conversational interactions to highly complex technical and subject-specific content presentation.

SLTs and secondary teachers working collaboratively need to address the many oral language issues faced by students with language difficulty. As outlined previously, these may include: an underlying auditory processing difficulty affecting the ability to process and retain information and follow instructions; attention inhibition problems so that students may become easily distracted by sounds in the classroom other than the teacher's voice; and a slow rate of processing, so that extra time is needed to process information and organize their thoughts to produce a response (Hoffman & Gillam, 2004). Students with auditory processing and working memory difficulties are challenged when having to apply more cognitive resources than other students to listen and concentrate in class (Archibald & Gathercole, 2006). Students with overlapping language and attention deficits may have difficulties with regulating their attention to be alert for sustained periods in the classroom (Cohen, Vallance, Barwick, et al., 2000).

Targets of the collaborative interaction could therefore focus on the following aspects of teachers' classroom communication:

- The balance between teachers' oral communication and other forms of communication, for example visual aids, demonstrations, increased use of gesture, multisensory experiences (see Table 11.1a for specific strategy ideas)

- Oral questioning: adopting strategies aimed at increasing opportunities for students with language difficulties to participate in Q&A and group discussion activities (see Table 11.1b)

- The organization and sequencing of information to increase clarity of plans and purpose of learning curriculum content, and to clarify links between current and prior learning (see Table 11.1c)

- Ensuring that students can more readily comprehend the presented content, for example by reducing the complexity of vocabulary and length of sentences, by stressing key information, and by using explicit rather than implied information (see Table 11.1d)

- The oral presentation style of individual teachers, such as rate, volume, intonation and general intelligibility factors (see Table 11.1e).

An example of these target areas is as follows. Students with language difficulty often struggle to make links between new and previously-learned information,

Table 11.1 Increasing students' access to teachers' oral language (adapted from Starling, 2014).

Specific target	Strategy examples
(a) Assisting students with auditory processing and working memory difficulty	- Balance oral language delivery with visual aids and demonstrations. Visual aids can include posters, tables, mind maps, time lines and graphs - Supplement talking with gestures - Provide verbal and bullet point summaries of segments of information - Start each lesson with a step-by-step visual planner of the lesson content - Provide a visual 'homework alert', with the main objective and due-time information on a calendar, days and weeks clearly marked
(b) Addressing students' slow rate of processing and thought organization	- Allow more time for processing questions and forming responses. Allow 3–5 seconds processing/response time. The average time that teachers pause before moving on is less than 1 second (Rowe, 1986) - Scaffold oral questions, e.g., expect a single word answer, give a choice of two answers, start a sentence and expect a completion - Alert students to the content of likely questions when presenting new information, i.e., what they should listen out for
(c) Addressing students' gaps in having or recalling prior learning	- Overview the new topic, with oral explanation of the purpose for learning about it, and the links with previously-learned material - Oral and/or written summary of segments of presented information - Check for understanding and recall before moving on - Visual aids, e.g., a mind map, to demonstrate links between prior and current learning. Keep as a working document, add new information as presented
(d) Reducing the complexity of teachers' oral language	- Be direct, not indirect, with requests and instructions - Avoid sarcasm, innuendo and ambiguity - Repeat important instructions, emphasize key points - Check for complexity of vocabulary, sentence length
(e) Modifying aspects of teachers' speech, rate, volume and/or pitch to improve oral delivery	- Adjust the rate of delivery, the volume of speech and the use of pitch (intonation) to provide extra meaning - Talk facing the class, not the board - Be aware of using good eye contact, and ways to get the attention of students with attention difficulties - Use gesture, eyes and general body language to convey interest to the students

and indeed may not have truly 'learned' previously-taught information or concepts the first time around. In comparison, the more language-able students are often better able to build on prior knowledge. Teachers can support students with language difficulty by revisiting past topics and talking about how the information relates to the new topic content. Teachers can also verbally overview what is to be presented, the most important information to listen out for, and the overall purpose for learning the particular topic. They can also introduce some visual aids such as mind maps linking previous and new information, and/or videos encapsulating overviews of the topic content. Many students with language difficulty do not automatically understand at a 'big picture' macro level, as they are likely to be attempting to attend to and understand at a micro-detail level.

Further examples of specific oral language modification strategies are presented in Table 11.1.

2 Written instructional language

Secondary students are faced with a wealth of written language in all subject areas, with even the most practical, hands-on subjects such as Physical Education, Visual Arts, Drama, and Design and Technology incorporating a great deal of theory work. Teachers commonly instruct using textbooks, additional texts, worksheets, assignment and project instruction sheets, glossaries, and test and exam papers. Well-developed reading abilities (reading accuracy, comprehension and fluency) are essential attributes for independent learning in this environment.

The rationale behind a collaborative approach to facilitating modifications to teachers' written language used in the classroom is that students with language difficulty are likely to have as much of an issue (in some cases more) with written language as they are with their oral language abilities (e.g., Nippold, 2007). These problems become increasingly apparent as students move through the secondary grades, and are challenged with understanding, interpreting, retaining and responding to information presented in any form of written resource, in both print and electronic forms. Underlying these issues are any number of possible barriers: sentences or paragraphs that are long and grammatically complex; overuse of unfamiliar and complex vocabulary and terminology; overly dense text with few headings and graphic aids; important instructions that are 'buried' in a large amount of related text; and/or abstract, high order language that is difficult to analyze and interpret.

Modifications to the written language used by teachers can be at any level, from words and phrases, through sentences, to paragraphs and whole texts. Adjustments may be made to the presentation of instructions (assignments, assessments, tests and exams), and by developing ways to support students in producing their own written work. Similar to strategies applied to teachers' oral language, attention can be paid to preparing students ahead of time to the content of written resources (e.g., key vocabulary, purpose of the text, alerting them to overarching ideas and key details, and making links with previous learning); the use of visual aids to supplement written text; avoiding the use of long, complex sentences containing multiple ideas; and ensuring that key information is made explicit. See Table 11.2 for specific strategy ideas for increasing students' access to written language.

Supporting students to conduct research

Conducting research for academic work is a language-loaded activity at all levels, whether the internet or printed texts are involved. Students with language difficulty are likely to encounter problems at many levels, the first and probably most challenging being the appropriate use of key words when using search engines. This task requires flexibility of thinking and having a broad vocabulary. As an example, if students are researching biographic details on well-known people and the instruction includes a point such as 'What hurdles did (…) face in his life?', relevant information will only be found if synonyms for 'hurdles' are used such as 'difficulties, challenges, problems, or obstacles'. By inserting the person's name and the word 'hurdles' it is more likely that information will appear about an athletics career, which may not exist or be the most relevant information.

Having language and literacy difficulties will also significantly impact using alphabetized book indexes, reading large quantities of text from any resource (including the internet), extracting relevant details, synthesizing and linking different ideas and summarizing the gathered information. The SLT's role can be to raise teachers' awareness of these potential barriers and to demonstrate valuable strategies such as working with whole classes on synonym brainstorming before students commence independent research, assisting with accessible resource and website selection, and using strategies such as topic colour coding to assist with information selection and organization.

As an example, in a Science class the topic is the study of endangered species. First, the teacher invests time on some direct vocabulary instruction (see Section 3 below) and decides that the following 10 words are the most essential for the study of this topic: *endangered*, *extinct*, *vulnerable*, *environment*, *ecosystems*, *species*, *conservation*, *preservation*, *poachers* and *deforestation*. Included in the direct instruction is time spent on brainstorming synonyms, so that these words are available to the students for their research undertakings. The teacher and students then work together to decide on the different subtopics relevant to the study, and agree on five key areas: Endangered Species, Levels of Endangerment, Habitat, Threats, and Conservation. Each area is given a colour: Endangered Species (brown), Levels of Endangerment (orange), Habitat (green), Threats (red) and Conservation (blue). These colours are then used for identifying and organizing information at every point of the research process, be it in the students' own time, in small group work and in whole class work.

The use of these and other similar language-assistive strategies that increase the accessibility of information ensure that students disadvantaged in these highly language-oriented tasks have a greater opportunity to process information effectively, retain and subsequently demonstrate their ideas and knowledge.

Table 11.2 Increasing students' access to written language (adapted from Starling, 2014).

Specific target	Strategy examples
Reducing the complexity of teachers' written language	- Keep sentences short and to the point, one idea per sentence - Simplify the language, not the content - Keep language explicit and direct - Use sequenced step 'pointers' such as numbers or words (first, secondly, finally)
Using more accessible vocabulary	- Use words that are familiar to the students - Provide descriptions for unfamiliar or complex vocabulary - Pre-teach key vocabulary that will be encountered in forthcoming texts or learning situations - Explain the meanings of instructional words, e.g., evaluate, distinguish between, enumerate… - Check for ambiguity of language; ensure the meaning matches the context - Explain non-literal and figurative language in literal, explicit terms
Increasing the 'readability' of written resources	- Break up pages dense with text with the use of, for instance, boxes, tables, headings, and emboldened words - Use visual aids where relevant, such as icons for key terms that can be repeated whenever used - Break down densely written texts as a class activity involving all students, e.g., by analyzing the content of each paragraph, creating headings, creating mind maps for main ideas and associated details
Facilitating the understanding of assignment and test instructions	- Include the main instructions early in the text - Highlight the issue to be addressed in relation to the topic, so students know precisely what it is they are being asked to write about. State this at the start of written assignment sheets - Avoid using too many complex instructional terms and multipart instructions - Provide examples and models of expected answers on similar issues and topics

Further examples of specific written language modification strategies are presented in Table 11.2.

3 Increasing students' access to curricular vocabulary

The acquisition of a robust lexicon is fundamental to the development of language, literacy and academic skills in general (Biemiller, 2006; Perfetti & Strafura, 2014; see also Lowe & Joffe, this volume). Children who enter school with restricted vocabularies are likely to be at risk for being behind normal grade levels in their literacy and academic development (Hart & Risley, 2003), a situation that will continue throughout their school years unless these children receive direct and explicit vocabulary instruction. A common aspect of the profile of students with language difficulty is a restricted lexicon (Kan & Windsor, 2010; Steele & Mills, 2011). Poor ability with receptive and expressive language along with low reading levels and auditory processing difficulties lead to a reduced exposure to new vocabulary in texts, reduced ability to infer meanings from contexts, and reduced ability in extracting meaning and retaining unfamiliar vocabulary from teachers' oral presentations.

Exposure to new words

Secondary teachers across all subjects regularly introduce key vocabulary and terminology to their students, often at the start of each new topic. This curriculum-essential vocabulary may be unfamiliar, and introduced briefly or through glossary sheets handed out by the teacher or provided in textbooks. This may place students with language difficulty in a position of disadvantage, where they may feel overwhelmed with the number of new words to be learned, may not process them efficiently, and may not recognize them in print or know how to spell them.

There is often a list of words that a teacher can identify as being essential for the understanding and learning of a specific curricular topic. Teachers may want to be guided in their selection of these key words by asking themselves the following questions:

- Is the word essential for my students' in-depth understanding of the topic?

- Will the word be used repeatedly in my teaching?

- Will students have multiple opportunities to use the word in their oral discussions and written work?

- If the word is complex (e.g., multisyllabic, unusual spelling, not often encountered in everyday language), do I have some strategies for supporting the students' word learning?

Studies into typical word learning demonstrate that robust word knowledge will only occur if words are revisited on multiple occasions; a minimum of 12 repetitions in a range of contexts is suggested (Graves, 2006). For a word to be considered well established in a personal lexicon, there must be both depth and breadth of knowledge such as knowing its multiple meanings (e.g., *saw*: a saw/to saw, and *saw*, as in 'I saw'), and its etymology and metaphorical use (Ford-Connors & Paratore, 2015). The word can be understood and applied in a range of contexts (decontextualized). Most importantly (and this is particularly relevant for the introduction of new curricular vocabulary), students need to hear the word so they know its pronunciation, see it in print so they learn the correct spelling, understand its meaning (multiple meanings if relevant) and ultimately have opportunities to use the word in a range of situations, in both spoken and written language (Baumann, Kame'enui, & Ash, 2003).

Direct vocabulary instruction

Direct vocabulary instruction should underlie all SLT/teacher instructional language modification collaborations. Professionals can be guided by the seminal work of Isabel Beck and her colleagues (Beck, McKeown, & Kucan, 2013) in the formation of a three-tiered hierarchy of vocabulary. Beck et al.'s hierarchy, and models of intervention for vocabulary instruction, are outlined in detail in Lowe and Joffe's chapter on vocabulary enhancement in this publication.

Sharing ideas on the implementation of direct vocabulary instruction in the classroom is a practical and eminently achievable aspect of the collaborative process. The following outlines some general techniques and strategies that can be readily tailored to individual teacher's instructional needs. This hierarchical approach is based on Robert Marzano's (2009) six-step process for teaching academic vocabulary. In summary these steps involve:

1. Explain: Teachers provide a description, explanation or example of the new words.

2. Restate: Students are involved in creating descriptions in their own words, as whole class activities.

3. Show: Students are involved in creating visual representations of the word.

4. Discuss: Multiple opportunities are provided for students to hear, read, write and say the word in structured class activities.

5. Refine and reflect: Opportunities are created for the students to discuss and refine their word knowledge.

6. Apply in learning games: Teachers involve students in games allowing further word practice (Marzano, 2009).

During the collaboration, the SLT and teacher may discuss and agree on the selection of a core group of essential words prior to the introduction of a new topic, and together produce word descriptions in everyday, student-friendly language. Teachers then introduce these words to their students, linking words and meanings to previous knowledge and teaching. This essential step facilitates students' understanding of new and unfamiliar terms in the broader 'word and world knowledge' context. From the start, all students should be encouraged to be involved in interacting with the new word-learning process, such as contributing their own ideas about the meaning of the words (*sounds like…*, *looks like…, might mean…*). Where possible, teachers and students can work together to create visual icons of the key words, to facilitate understanding and recall through visual association for those students with relatively stronger visual, hands-on learning skills.

Teachers can also ensure that all students are directly involved in creating word descriptions and definitions that are relevant and which use familiar, student-friendly language. If this is not the case there is a danger that some students (especially those with language difficulty) will learn glossary definitions by rote, with little to no understanding of the actual meaning (Ford-Connors & Paratore, 2015). An example of difficult-to-access language in a definition is the following for the word 'improvise'. A standard dictionary definition is '*Compose or perform extempore*' (Moore, 2003). In contrast, a language-accessible description could be '*To produce something quickly by using whatever is available*'.

These, and additional, strategies for facilitating the access to, and knowledge and use of, secondary curricular vocabulary for students with language difficulty are outlined in Table 11.3.

Table 11.3 Teachers' use of robust vocabulary instruction techniques (adapted from Starling, 2014).

Specific target	Strategy examples
Prioritizing essential curricular vocabulary	- When starting on a new topic, select up to 10 words (maximum) that are essential for the basic understanding of the topic content - Present these words to students in clear, unambiguous definitions, where possible involving students in the creation of topic-relevant descriptions for the words - All new vocabulary should be presented in spoken and written forms, so students can hear and repeat the pronunciation (oral language) as well as be familiar with the spelling (written language) - Check that glossary definitions are in accessible language, and the meanings are relevant to the context of the topic
Maximizing opportunities to understand, recall and use new vocabulary	- Ensure multiple opportunities for the application of these words into students' learning - Expand the same strategies to the introduction of all other unfamiliar vocabulary - Ensure that students have many opportunities to use new vocabulary in their work - Demonstrate new vocabulary in a range of resources and situations
Demonstrate strategies for understanding unfamiliar vocabulary	- Show students how context can be used for working out what words mean - Provide direct instruction in morpheme analysis for complex words such as scientific terminology
Provide instruction in the use of relevant key words for researching information	- Discuss how key words work when using search engines - Brainstorm synonyms for topic research tasks

Conclusion

"If I had this knowledge when I first started teaching I think I would have been a better teacher from the start. It's taken me so many years to identify the fact that language is so important."

"The (program's) brought back the awareness that some kids, behaviour-wise, may play up simply because they can't do the work."

"This isn't rocket science, but it's an important wake-up call!"

These quotes are from teachers involved with the implementation of the collaborative programme that has been described in this chapter. Engaging students in the process of learning a broad curriculum can be a challenge for all secondary teachers, especially so when teachers have to address the additional learning needs of the students in their classes with language-based learning difficulties. A professionally collaborative approach to intervention has been shown, through rigorous research, to provide effective inclusive support for these students. A suite of suggested strategies and techniques has been presented, allowing each collaborative team the flexibility to create a tailor-made support programme.

Reflective questions

- For SLTs and other service providers: How does this model of service delivery fit with your current approach to providing supports and services to adolescents with language difficulty?

- For teachers: Has this information helped you to identify students in your classes who may have language difficulty? How will I recognize if there have been any benefits to their personal and academic progress as a result of the changes I have made to my teaching practices?

Case history

Mary is a History teacher at a large coeducational secondary school. She teaches a broad range of classes, from Years 7 to 12, and has everything from mixed ability to high-achieving student groups. Mary has been teaching for nine years, and loves her subject and the stimulation of her work. However, she often feels challenged by attempting to address the additional learning needs of many of her students, some of whom have diagnosed language-based learning difficulties. Because of her subject matter, Mary uses a high degree of both oral and written instructional language in her daily teaching practices. She is aware that many of these students have problems with processing information through their listening and reading, and have particular difficulties with retaining information and getting their ideas down in writing, an issue that is regularly highlighted in their poor test and exam performances.

Mary's biggest concern is that many of these students are disengaged in classroom activities; some of them are easily distracted or distract other students. Others are withdrawn, and rarely bring themselves to her attention. On the other hand, Mary is also aware of the amount of curriculum content she needs to cover in her lessons, and how unrealistic it would be to take time out of whole-class teaching to give these students individual help.

Mary decided to participate in a teacher training programme led by the school-based SLT, where she and some other teachers met with the SLT once a week for individual consultations. Over the course of a term Mary and the SLT worked together on oral and written instructional language modifications that she applied to her regular teaching practices.

Some examples of the modifications that she made to her classroom teaching involved the greater use of visual aids, such as mind maps and time lines; she ensured that all students understood the vocabulary of instruction such as 'evaluate, compare, consider and relate'; and she provided all students with, and discussed, printed content summary sheets at the end of each topic or sub-topic, using the information for competitive quizzes and games. The programme also involved learning the process of using direct instruction for key curriculum vocabulary, and Mary regularly identified 10 essential curricular words for extra instruction before the start of each new topic.

By the end of the term Mary was able to report that, based on pre- and post-vocabulary tests, and comparison with previous years' topic test results, students with additional learning needs such as language difficulties were showing a marked improvement in their knowledge and performance. Additionally, Mary reported anecdotal evidence of students' improved motivation and engagement in the learning process.

References

Alexander, R. (2012). Improving oracy and classroom talk in English schools: Achievements and challenges. Paper for DfE, http://www. primaryreview. org. uk/

Archibald, L.M.D. & Gathercole, S.E. (2006). Short-term and working memory in specific language impairment. *International Journal of Language and Communication Disorders, 41*, 675–693.

Baumann, J.F., Kame'enui, E.J., & Ash, G.E. (2003). Research on vocabulary instruction: Voltaire redux. *Handbook of Research on Teaching the English Language Arts, 2*, 752–785.

Beck, I.L., McKeown, M.G., & Kucan L. (2013). *Bringing Words to Life: Robust Vocabulary Instruction, 2nd ed.* New York, NY: The Guilford Press.

Biemiller, A. (2006). Vocabulary development and instruction: A prerequisite for school learning. *Handbook of Early Literacy Research, 2*, 41–51.

Bradley, R., Danielson, L., & Doolittle, J. (2005). Response to intervention. *Journal of Learning Disabilities, 38*, 485–486.

Cazden, C.B. & Beck, S.W. (2008). Classroom discourse. In: A.C. Graesser, M.A. Gernsbacher, & S.R. Goldman, S.R. (Eds), *Handbook of Discourse Processes*. New Jersey: Lawrence Erlbaum Associates.

Cohen, N.J., Vallance, D.D., Barwick, M., Im, N., Menna, R., Horodezky, N.B., & Isaacson, L. (2000). The interface between ADHD and language impairment: An examination of language, achievement, and cognitive processing. *Journal of Child Psychology and Psychiatry and Allied Disciplines, 41*, 353–362.

Dockrell, J.E. & Lindsay, G. (2001). Children with specific speech and language difficulties: The teachers' perspective. *Oxford Review of Education, 27*, 369–394.

Dockrell, J.E., Lindsay, G., & Connelly, V. (2009). The impact of specific language impairment on adolescents' written text. *Exceptional Children, 75*, 427–446.

Ehren, B.J. (2002). Speech-Language Pathologists contributing significantly to the academic success of high school students: A vision for professional growth. *Topics in Language Disorders, 22*, 60–80.

Ford-Connors, E. & Paratore, J.P. (2015). Vocabulary instruction in fifth grade and beyond: Sources of word learning and productive contexts for development. *Review of Educational Research, 85*, 50–91.

Graves, M.F. (2006). *The Vocabulary Book: Learning & Instruction*. New York, NY: Teachers College Press.

Guskey, T.R. & Yoon, K.S. (2009). What works in professional development? *Phi Delta Kappa, 90*, 495–500.

Hart, B. & Risley, T.R. (2003). The early catastrophe: The 30 million word gap by age 3. *American Educator, 27*, 4–9.

Hoffman, L.M. & Gillam, R.B. (2004). Verbal and spatial information processing constraints in children with specific language impairment. *Journal of Speech, Language, and Hearing Research*, 47, 114-125.

Hughes, D.M., Turkstra, L.S., & Wulfeck, B.B. (2009). Parent and self-ratings of executive function in adolescents with specific language impairment. *International Journal of Language and Communication Disorders*, 44, 901-916.

Joffe, V.L. (2006). Enhancing language and communication in language-impaired secondary school-aged children. In: J. Ginsborg & J. Clegg (Eds), *Language and Social Disadvantage*. Chichester: John Wiley & Sons.

Kan, P.F. & Windsor, J. (2010). Word learning in children with primary language impairment: A meta-analysis. *Journal of Speech, Language, and Hearing Research*, 53(3), 739-756.

Larson, V.L. & McKinley, N.L. (2003). Service delivery options for secondary students with language disorders. *Seminars in Speech and Language*, 24(3), 181-197.

Law, J., Rush, R., Schoon, I., & Parsons, S. (2009). Modeling developmental language difficulties from school entry into adulthood: Literacy, mental health and employment outcomes. *Journal of Speech, Language and Hearing Research*, 52, 1401-1416.

Lindsay, G. & Dockrell, J. (2008). Language intervention in the school years: A systemic approach. *Revista de Logopedia, Foniatria y Audiologia*, 28, 207-217

Marzano, R.J. (2009). The art and science of teaching: Six steps to better vocabulary instruction. *Educational Leadership*, 67, 84-85.

Moore, B. (2003). *The Australian Pocket Oxford Dictionary, 5th ed.* Melbourne: Oxford University Press.

Murphy, A., Franklin, S., Breen, A., Hanlon, M., McNamara, A., Bogue, A., & James, E. (2017). A whole class teaching approach to improve the vocabulary skills of adolescents attending mainstream secondary school, in areas of socioeconomic disadvantage. *Child Language Teaching and Therapy*, 33(2), 129–144.

Nash, M. & Donaldson, M.L. (2005). Word learning in children with vocabulary deficits. *Journal of Speech Language and Hearing Research*, 48, 439-458.

Nippold, M. (2007). *Later Language Development: School-Age Children, Adolescents, and Young Adults, 3rd ed.* Austin, TX: Pro-Ed.

Nippold, M. (2010). It's not too late to help adolescents succeed in school. *Language, Speech and Hearing Services in Schools*, 41, 137-138.

Nippold, M.A., Mansfield, T.C., Billow, J.L., & Tomblin, J.B. (2009). Syntactic development in adolescents with a history of language impairments: A follow-up investigation. *American Journal of Speech-Language Pathology*, 18, 241-251.

Paul, R. (2007). *Language Disorders from Infancy to Adolescence*. Missouri, MI: Mosby Elsevier.

Perfetti, C. & Strafura, J. (2014). Word knowledge in a theory of reading comprehension. *Scientific Studies of Reading*, 18, 22–37.

Prelock, P.A. (2000). Multiple perspectives for determining the roles of speech-language pathologists in inclusionary classrooms. *Language, Speech & Hearing Services in Schools, 31*, 213.

Rowe, M.B. (1986). Wait time: Slowing down may be a way of speeding up! *Journal of Teacher Education, 37*, 43-50.

Snowling, M.J., Adams, J.W., Bishop, D.V.M., & Stothard, S.E. (2001). Educational attainments of school leavers with a preschool history of speech-language impairments. *International Journal of Language and Communication Disorders, 36*, 173-183.

Starling, J. (2014). Linking language with secondary school learning. Retrieved June 2018 from: www.linksresources.com.au

Starling, J., Munro, N., Togher, L., & Arciuli, J. (2011). Recognising language impairment in secondary school student populations. *Australian Journal of Learning Difficulties, 16*, 145-158.

Starling, J., Munro, N., Togher, L., & Arciuli, J. (2012). Training secondary school teachers in instructional language modification techniques to support adolescents with language impairment: A randomized controlled trial. *Language, Speech, & Hearing Services in Schools, 43*, 474-495.

Steele, S.C. & Mills, M.T. (2011). Vocabulary intervention for school-age children with language impairment: A review of evidence and good practice. *Child Language Teaching and Therapy, 27*(3), 354-370.

Whitmire, K. (2000). Adolescence as a developmental phase: A tutorial. *Topics in Language Disorders, 20*, 1-14.

Wilson, G., Nash, M., & Earl, G. (2010). Supporting students with language learning difficulties in secondary schools through collaboration: The use of concept maps to investigate the impact on teachers' knowledge of vocabulary teaching. *Child Language Teaching and Therapy, 26*, 163-179.

12 Evaluating whole-school language programmes in secondary schools

Opportunities, challenges and learning

Mary Hartshorne

Learning outcomes

The chapter will enable readers to:

- Describe a three-tier approach to supporting adolescents with language difficulties

- Provide a clear rationale for supporting adolescents' language difficulties through adopting a whole-school programme

- Describe the current evidence base for whole-school programmes to support oracy skills across the curriculum

- Identify relevant factors when designing and implementing an evaluation of a whole-school language programme in secondary schools

- Discuss the challenges to evaluating whole-school approaches to supporting oracy skills, and present potential ways to address these challenges.

Introduction

Young people who develop good language and communication skills find learning easier in secondary school, where language demands of both the educational and social curriculum become increasingly complex (summarized in Hartshorne, 2012). However, around 10% of children have language difficulties which are long term or persistent (Law, McBean, & Rush, 2011), and in some areas of deprivation in the UK up to 83% of adolescents have problems with language which are likely to make learning hard (Spencer, Clegg, & Stackhouse, 2012: Stringer 2006). Despite this, specialist services in secondary schools are rare (Dockrell, Ricketts, & Lindsay, 2012), and often focused in early years and primary schools. A number of factors compound the limited support received by pupils at this age.

Education staff in secondary schools report they are under-confident in working with pupils' language and communication (Mercer, Warwick, & Ahmed, 2014), and in supporting those with needs (Department of Children, Schools and Families, 2008). Lack of services for secondary schools is often based on the assumption that early intervention lowers the priority for services in adolescence (Ehren, 2002; Lindsay, Desforges, Dockrell et al., 2008). There is also an acknowledged paucity of evidence in the field of older children and young people's language and language difficulties on which to draw. In their systematic review of intervention studies on school-age children with spoken language disorder only two out of 21 studies involved secondary-age pupils (Cirrin & Gillam, 2008). What evidence there is often focuses on specific disorder-based interventions (e.g., Ebbels, Maric, Murphy, & Turner, 2014) which is not representative of the curriculum-based support most likely to be offered to this age group (RCSLT, 2005).

More relevant curriculum or school-based approaches, however, present challenge in terms of their evaluation. Drawing on a range of examples of studies which have met this challenge, this chapter sets a case for whole-school approaches to support adolescents' language and language difficulties. It explores a range of factors found to be important in planning and implementing evaluations of these approaches, identifying the challenges, solutions and benefits.

A rationale for whole-school language programmes to support adolescents' language difficulties in secondary schools

Language, learning and the classroom

There is a close relationship between language and cognition, with language having a particular role in shaping thought, building ideas and accelerating thinking (Bruner, 1996; Vygotsky, 1962). This crucial role of language in developing thinking starts early, becomes more complex and is no less important as children get older. Adolescents need more complex language to manage the complex tasks and problem solving expected of them at this age (Nippold, 2009, 2014), when they are "required to integrate their linguistic, cognitive and social skills into coherent meaningful discourse" (Joffe, 2006).

In the classroom, language has been described as having a dual role educationally – as a tool for developing thinking, but also for accessing and taking part in learning. Barnes and Todd (1976) articulated the distinction between the two by describing what they called 'exploratory talk' (known as 'accountable talk' in the US). Marked by hesitations, revisions and rephrasings, this is talk for reasoning where there is suggestion and hypothesis, but also challenge and justification. Research over many years has demonstrated the central role of this type of talk in learning across the curriculum (Alexander, 2001; Barnes & Todd, 1976; Mercer, 2008). The term 'oracy' was coined by Wilkinson (1965), parallel to 'literacy', in an attempt to ensure that teachers treat spoken language as seriously as they do written language.

In addition to this, a critical role for language- or oracy-based classrooms is to provide a forum for supporting the development of skills in young people who present with language difficulties.

Supporting pupils with language difficulties – a three-tier model

Professional guidelines in both the UK and US stress that support for school-aged pupils with language difficulties should recognize the unique contribution of language to learning, and the opportunities the school environment provide (ASHA, 2010; RCSLT, 2005). Over the last decade, school-based services in the UK have worked within a model organized over three tiers (Gascoigne, 2006). At tier one, a strong oral environment can facilitate the identification of pupils needing more support. These identified pupils with language difficulties may need focused, short-term targeted support at tier two, or more specialist interventions for more persistent, complex difficulties at tier three (Dockrell & Lindsay, 2008).

In the US, 'Response to Intervention' is a similar multi-tiered approach whereby pupils who are not responding to classroom-based approaches can be identified as needing additional intervention (Ehren, Montgomery, Rudebusch, & Whitmore, 2006). The foundation is high-quality instruction and, on top of this, tailored support is offered to learners in response to their identified need, at increasing levels of intensity.

Both systems rely on a foundation of high-quality language learning environments where there are multiple opportunities to practise, recall and receive feedback in a real context (Kamhi, 2014). The recently-introduced Code of Practice for children with special educational needs in the UK (Department for Education, 2015) also highlights this high-quality teaching as crucial to identifying and supporting more significant needs. Ehren and Whitmire (2009) see this approach in schools as particularly important for secondary-aged pupils who may have previously had intervention, who may not now meet requirements for services and yet have language difficulties which impact on learning. With adolescents often reluctant to participate in out-of-class speech and language therapy (Ehren, 2002), this lesson-based, contextualized approach is one preferred by young people themselves (Dockrell & Lindsay, 2008).

The similarities between the language environments needed for learning, and universal approaches for supporting language difficulties in adolescents make a case for language focused classrooms. The fact that a focus on communication is judged to be an element of high-quality teaching (Ofsted, 2015) also adds strength to this case.

Language-focused classrooms

Despite this strong professional steer and the evidence for language as a tool for learning, high-quality language learning environments are rare, particularly in secondary schools. Likewise, the relative importance of language in learning is not always realized in practice. Applebee, Langer, Nystrand, and Gamoran (2003) carried out observations in 64 classrooms in secondary schools over a whole school year and found that open discussion averaged just 1.7 minutes per 60-minute lesson. A further study found that teachers in secondary science lessons asked on average two questions a minute, 91% of which were closed questions, and were unaware of how few questions their pupils asked – on average six times fewer questions than teachers (Albergaria-Almeida, 2010).

In their review of 225 studies of classroom dialogue published between 1972 and 2011, Howe and Abedin (2013) reported little change over the last 20 years. Likewise, reviewing support for language difficulties in classrooms across England, Lindsay et al. (2008) felt that, unlike primary schools, secondary schools did not prioritize whole-school language approaches.

There have been many reasons suggested for this. In England, oracy has received far less attention than reading and writing in schools (Mercer & Dawes, 2014), with Coultas (2015) suggesting that talk is undervalued because of a focus on Standard English as the language of knowledge rather than learning. Howe and Abedin (2003) describe a tension between encouraging flexibility through talk and having control and time to cover curriculum content. They also felt that the difficulty in actually describing talk-based approaches, and the limited evidence of effectiveness, were barriers.

Ehren (2002) suggests that secondary-school teachers do not typically think of academic difficulties as language related, so do not identify a need for these approaches in lessons. McLeod and McKinnon (2010) reviewed primary and secondary schools in New South Wales and found that, even when a need was identified, teachers were unlikely to adapt their teaching because of a lack of knowledge and skill in supporting adolescent language. Likewise, many speech and language therapists do not feel confident working in secondary schools, being unfamiliar with the curriculum, and with their knowledge of appropriate approaches (Ehren, 2002). In fact, a survey of 536 speech and language therapists found that only 8.4% worked with children older than 11 years of age (Roulstone,Wren, Bakopoulou et al., 2012).

An overarching concern, however, is the lack of an evidence base for working in secondary schools with pupils' language. In a UK survey, of 57 interventions identified as either currently in use by speech and language therapists or published in the research literature, none were aimed specifically at secondary-aged pupils (Law, Lee, Roulstone, et al., 2012). In their review of studies looking at talk in classrooms, Howe and Abedin (2013) found few across whole classes, most were small group studies. They proposed that teachers will only change if they can see a substantial case for change, demonstrated through a significant effect.

Whole-school approaches: The evidence

What is promising is that the number of studies in secondary schools is growing, with evidence of positive impacts both on pupils' language and their wider academic performance. Studies are organized at either whole-school or individual class level – and target either whole-school populations or are focused more specifically on those pupils identified with language difficulties.

Whole-school oracy programmes

Three notable programmes focus on the power of using talk as a tool for learning. Unlike many smaller-scale studies, these aim to embed a culture of oracy across whole-school populations.

Mannion and Mercer (2016) describe a study in a secondary school over three years embedding a whole-school *Learning to Learn (L2L)* approach. The approach makes learning visible to students by teaching metacognitive and self-regulation strategies shown to improve outcomes for students from disadvantaged backgrounds (Higgins, Kokotsaki, & Coe, 2011), and includes a strong oral language component. They adopted an approach where learning to learn strategies were both taught explicitly and embedded in subject areas throughout the curriculum.

School 21 in partnership with a team at the University of Cambridge (Mercer et al., 2014) built on this approach to develop the *Oracy Curriculum, Culture and Assessment Toolkit*. Oracy is planned into every lesson through a number of teaching and learning strategies, supported by a whole-school oracy culture and by a professional development package.

The *Talking Schools* programme (Howe, 2013) is less structured. Pupils are taught how to develop their skills in discussion and debate in a range of subjects with the aim of deepening their subject knowledge, sharpening their critical thinking skills, and supporting progress in writing. A group of subject specialists use a 'lesson study' approach, jointly planning lessons using a common set of teaching strategies and classroom activities, reviewing the impact and agreeing next steps.

L2L and the *Oracy Toolkit* were evaluated in controlled studies, while *Talking Schools* was a piece of action research. In all three of the programmes school attainment data were used to show increased pupil progress; Mannion and Mercer (2016) found this to be statistically significant after *L2L* was compared with the control group. Maxwell, Burnett, Reidy et al. (2015) also used a measure designed for and based on the *Oracy Toolkit* which suggested that pupils made significant progress. Mannion and Mercer (2016) reported striking differences across subject areas and between groups of pupils, with disadvantaged pupils outperforming their more affluent peers in some areas.

Whole-school vocabulary programmes

Supporting word learning in pupils has one of the strongest evidence bases in the field of language and communication (Justice, Schmitt, Murphy, et al., 2014). This, together with evidence-based links between both poor vocabulary and disadvantage (Snow, Prosche, Tabors, & Harris, 2007; Spencer et al., 2012) and between vocabulary performance and later academic proficiency (Feinstein & Duckworth 2006), provides a strong rationale for introducing whole-school approaches. Two key projects implemented in secondary schools have been evaluated as having a significant impact on word learning and wider school performance.

Word Generation (Snow, Lawrence, & White, 2009) operates across whole schools. Each week, over 24 weeks, five academic words are introduced and then reinforced in different subject areas through weekly units, each with a brief lesson plan. This provides a cross-curricula focus on a small number of words involving multiple exposure, debate and discussion, finishing at the end of the week in a written task.

Also targeting academic vocabulary, *Academic Language Instruction for All Students* (ALIAS) (Lesaux, Keiffer, Faller, & Kelley, 2010) is a class-based programme of daily lessons; a developmental sequence of activities builds up word knowledge incrementally over 18 weeks. It introduces academic words through written narrative, and includes a variety of whole-group, small-group, and independent activities designed to promote deep processing through opportunities for listening, speaking, reading, and writing with the words.

Both programmes were run in areas of social disadvantage. They were evaluated using a controlled trial design and provide evidence for the wider impact of a whole-school focus on vocabulary. Both found significant effects of the programme using researcher-developed measures based on taught vocabulary. In *ALIAS*, significant impacts were also found on a standardized reading comprehension measure (Lesaux et al., 2010). A randomized control trial of *Word Generation* in 28 secondary schools (Lawrence, Crosson, Paré-Blagoey, & Snow, 2015) showed the effects on word learning were sustained at least a year after the programme finished. The study also found large effects on classroom discussion quality, particularly in maths and science.

Whole programmes for pupils with language difficulties

Whole-school programmes addressing the needs of young people with language difficulties at a population level are rare; all three of the programmes described here include a training element, aiming for impacts beyond the programme itself.

Starling, Munro, Togher, & Airculi (2012) designed, delivered and evaluated a collaborative training programme, *Linking Language with Secondary School Learning* (LINK-S), where speech and language therapists train secondary-school teachers in ways to modify their approach to teaching so that it supports pupils with language impairment. Components include modifications to teachers' own spoken and written instruction, to how they support processing of complex language and to their teaching of vocabulary. Joffe (2011) trained teaching assistants to deliver *Enhancing Language and Communication in Secondary Schools (ELCISS)*, which comprised storytelling and vocabulary group sessions delivered either separately or in combination.

In both these studies, a randomized control trial found significant improvements to pupils' performance compared to a control group. In *ELCISS*, this was using non-standardized assessments; for Starling et al. (2012) there was a significant improvement in students' written expression and listening comprehension using standardized measures. Both studies found changes in the confidence of school staff as a result of the programme, but Starling et al. (2012) also used a tool designed to capture change in teaching attitudes and in their practice. After LINK-S, teachers' use of the targeted techniques significantly increased when compared to the non-intervention group.

Finally, I CAN's *Secondary Talk*, a whole-school development programme, uses an action research model to develop practice and teacher confidence in supporting all pupils including those with language difficulties. Practical materials are organized around three core principles: changing the amount and type of teacher talk; increasing pupil interaction; and supporting the teaching of academic vocabulary. The programme was evaluated using a within-school comparison design which found that it had an impact on aspects of teaching practice (Clegg, Leyden, & Stackhouse, 2011). A further evaluation (Hartshorne & Black, 2015) used interviews and observations to show that these changes were sustained over a 3-year period. This second evaluation included a small-scale comparison study to demonstrate significant changes to pupils' language and communication, with those with delayed language making most progress.

These whole-school programme evaluations demonstrate their effectiveness, and show the impact of a whole-school focus on outcomes for pupils, measured in different ways, using a range of measures, often with complex and multifaceted designs. Those programmes with a tighter, more defined set of activities can, on the whole, be evaluated using a more rigorous, controlled method. What all the studies share is the opportunity to reflect on the complexities of evaluating programmes implemented across secondary schools. From this reflection, key factors can be considered.

Factors in evaluating whole-school programmes in secondary schools

Crossing the divide between research and practice

Evaluating whole-school programme impact is not, in itself, enough. Olswang and Prelock (2015) recognize a gap between what we *know* and what we *do* in the field of speech and language, and a need to ensure that research is translated into practice. They describe this as an active process and suggest that 'implementation research', based on the concept of 'implementation science' is what is needed. Without also identifying the factors supporting effective implementation, there is a risk that the positive outcomes found through tightly-controlled studies cannot be replicated in real life (Lindsay et al., 2008). If a key aim of evaluations is to ensure the take-up of the programme in schools, real-world utility is crucial and has been addressed in a range of ways.

In *Secondary Talk*, thematic analysis of data from yearly interviews with a group of senior school leaders yielded key factors for implementation; these included barriers as well as facilitators. Maxwell et al. (2015) were able to collect similar evidence for the *Oracy Curriculum* through focus groups, interviews and observation. Teachers in the ALIAS project completed lesson implementation logs which recorded time taken and material covered but also strengths and weaknesses of the programme (Lesaux et al., 2010). Starling et al. (2012) used a framework which looks at the process of change when a new approach is introduced: the Concerns-Based Adoption Model (CBAM; Hord, Rutherford, Huling-Austin, & Hall, 2006) to monitor and document the process of change in a more structured way.

Where researchers are an integral part of the evaluation and programme implementation, this helps cross the research/practice divide. In *Learning to Learn*, Mannion and Mercer (2016) felt that having the researcher as part of the delivery team was essential in supporting this. In the *Talking Schools* project, the lesson study approach helped shape scaling up the approach across the whole school (Howe, 2013), while Mercer et al. (2014) used a three-way partnership between the developer, evaluators and school to develop the oracy curriculum. They worked closely together with piloting aspects of the programme, regularly reviewing and further developing the intervention. Although this then did compromise robust independent evaluation of impact (Maxwell et al., 2015), it fulfilled a main purpose of the evaluation: to inform future development.

Attributing impact – using a theory of change model

Many whole-school programmes contain an element of staff development, making attribution of impact particularly challenging given the distance between the input (training) and expected outcomes (changes to practice or to pupils' skills and outcomes). The theory of change model for *Secondary Talk* illustrates this (Figure12.1). Theory of change emerged as a concept in the 1990s in the field of community evaluations. Weiss (1995) felt that a key reason that complex programmes were so difficult to evaluate was that often there was a lack of clarity about how the change process would unfold. The model is a way of describing the assumptions between each step of a process, with clarity about the evidence (or theory of change) between each step, so strengthening the ability to claim credit for outcomes, or attribute outcomes to initial input.

Of course, movement from one step to the next is not automatic; merely increasing knowledge may not result in behaviour change (Wren, 2003). In fact, there is very little evidence of impact of staff development on outcomes for pupils, particularly in secondary schools (Yoon, Duncan, Lee et al., 2007).

Stoll, Harris and Handscombe (2012) identified the importance of 'starting out with the end in mind' when planning professional development. Maxwell et

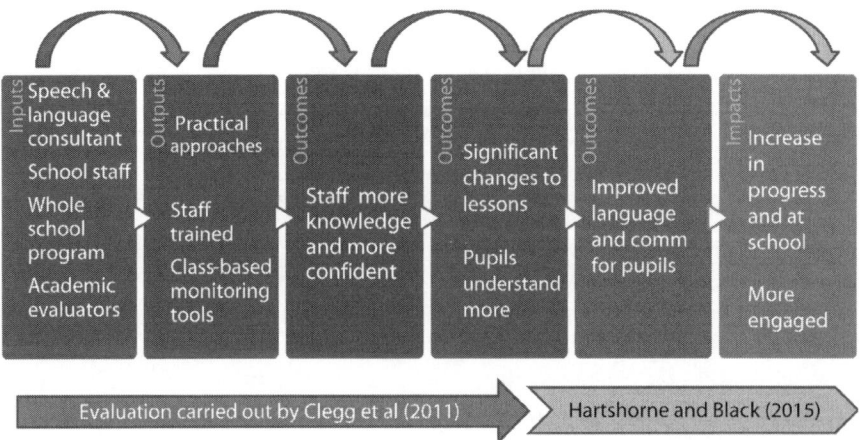

Figure 12.1 Theory of change model showing the evaluation phases of *Secondary Talk*.

al. (2015) considered that the training planned to develop an *Oracy Curriculum* did just this, being focused from the outset on intended student outcomes. They also recognized that encouraging discussion amongst teachers about what they had learned encouraged changes to practice.

More systematic attempts to attribute outcomes to inputs include a study in the Czech Republic, where Sedova, Sedlacek and Svaricek (2016) introduced dialogic teaching into classrooms and recorded pupil responses. They used regression analysis to confirm that the nature of student talk was determined by the communication behaviour of teachers, which changed as a result of programme input. For example, every additional 100 seconds of open discussion resulted in one more pupil 'utterance with reasoning'. Lawrence et al. (2015) carried out mediation analysis to find that 14% of the effect of progress in academic vocabulary made after the *Word Generation* project was mediated by improved discussion skills, supporting a causal relationship between a change in classroom practice and language outcomes. However, these attempts to attribute change using statistical analysis are rare in whole-school evaluations.

Lesaux et al. (2010) analyzed observational data comparing teachers delivering the intervention with teachers in control lessons to validate assumptions about the specific impact of ALIAS programme. They found that the intervention teachers only differed in their instruction in ways related to the intervention, and not on other criteria. They used this information to confirm that changes in instruction were a result of the programme.

The eventual impact on pupils' learning as a result of improved language can be even harder to attribute to programme inputs, and yet this is the most meaningful evidence for schools. In the *Talking Schools* project Howe (2013) felt that explicit teaching would be needed to translate the increased classroom talk into wider impacts such as improved writing. Interestingly, despite being cautious in their expectations following LINK-S, Starling et al. (2012) found significant changes to pupils' written expression and listening comprehension relative to pupils in a control group. Seemingly, this 'skipped' a link in the theory of change, as the impact on pupils' language was not significant. In contrast, the ELCISS programme, delivered in small groups by trained teaching assistants, was found to significantly impact on language (Joffe, 2011) and also, in a further evaluation (Styles & Bradshaw, 2015) to significantly impact on reading comprehension.

It will always be a challenge to directly attribute change when programmes are flexible and responsive, particularly where there is no rigorous control, when there are issues with collecting treatment fidelity data, and where the evaluation stretches over a number of years. In the evaluation of *Secondary Talk*, collecting a range of quantitative and qualitative data at the end of each year showed patterns in change and helped to corroborate findings. Lesaux et al. (2010) used evidence from teacher logs to triangulate findings, with teachers clearly identifying links between the vocabulary programme and improvements in writing through *ALIAS*. Perhaps some of the strongest informal evidence to support attribution comes from participants themselves. In *Secondary Talk*, interview data showed that staff linked activity in classrooms to impacts on pupils, and young people made similar links in their focus groups. Maxwell et al. (2015) relied on feedback from staff, who felt strongly that the focus on oracy introduced through the *Oracy Curriculum* was the cause of improved learning outcomes across the curriculum.

Designing robust evaluation studies

Seven of the eight studies described above used a control or comparison design to evaluate the impact of programmes introduced. All of them identified challenges in doing so, but found solutions to ensure design was as rigorous as possible.

Comparison groups

With pupils situated in intact classes and taught by subject teachers, it can be difficult to assign individuals to different conditions. In many school evaluations, this is addressed by assigning whole schools rather than pupils to different conditions (for example, Obsuth, Sutherland, Eisner, et al., 2015; Styles & Bradshaw, 2015). This challenge with this is to find a 'matched' comparison school. Lawrence et al. (2015) ranked schools within district on comparable variables to calculate a composite score to matched schools before randomization. Starling et al. (2012) used area sampling, selecting demographically similar schools.

However, by the very nature of their organization secondary schools offer an alternative. In their evaluation of the pilot of *Secondary Talk*, Clegg et al. (2011) used a within-school comparison design where subject lessons or class groups not taking part in the programme acted as comparison groups. Although this has been identified as potentially increasing the likelihood of cross-contamination of the control group (Lawrence et al., 2012), it does control for school demographic features such as levels of deprivation.

A third option was adopted in the *Learning to Learn* evaluation. Mercer and Mannion (2016) designed a controlled study where the comparison group was the previous school cohort, matched on their attainment schools at the end of primary schools, and on a standard cognitive abilities test.

The long-term evaluation of *Secondary Talk* (Hartshorne & Black, 2015) drew on both of the first two approaches, using an in-school comparison design to investigate continued changes to classroom practice, and a between-schools design to look at impact on pupils themselves. A small sample comparison study investigated groups of pupils in two schools, one that implemented *Secondary Talk* and one that did not.

Randomization was used in only two of the studies described above (ELCISS and LINK-S); increasing the level of rigour with randomization adds academic weight to findings (Lesaux et al., 2010).

Compounding factors

Secondary schools are dynamic, complex institutions, and they often introduce and run multiple initiatives regarding teaching practices. It is a significant challenge to control or account for the many variables that potentially impact on the impact of oracy programmes, especially at a whole-school level. For example, there may be staff changes, new curriculum guidelines or syllabuses, or other teacher training programmes running in parallel.

Organizational aspects of secondary schools can impact on evaluations' design. For example, in the evaluation of the *Oracy Framework and Curriculum*, difficulties with timetabling resulted in some pupils having already started the intervention by the time baseline measures were taken. In *Secondary Talk* regular and often rapid staff changes meant that key contact people often moved schools, resulting in difficulties collecting consistent, replicable observations and interview data. Even without these organizational factors, pressures to cover critical academic and exam curricula can make it difficult to engage school staff. Ensuring the evaluation is meaningful to the school can help to minimize some of these compounding factors, and researchers have used a range of ways to engage schools. Through teacher learning logs, Lesaux et al. (2010) observed that concerns diminished once they saw the impact of *ALIAS*; this feedback of impact was also important in the evaluation of *Secondary Talk*. Making clear links to wider school or regional initiatives ensures relevance and can also motivate and engage (Lesaux et al., 2010; Starling et al., 2012).

Whole-school programmes themselves are also dynamic and complex, bringing additional confounds. It can be difficult to separate out and examine specific aspects of multilayered programmes, particularly when a key aim is to embed oral language in every aspect of school. In the *Oracy Framework and Curriculum*, for example, Maxwell et al. (2015) found challenges in evaluating training which was integrated in the school's approach to oracy rather than a discrete identifiable activity. They carried out additional interviews and focus groups to explore what had supported teachers' professional learning. Likewise, given the developmental nature of *Secondary Talk*, interviews were used to identify perceptions about the most used and most impactful activities. The fact that *Secondary Talk* gradually spread in schools also impacted on research design and the within-school comparison design was only effective for the first year; in following years it was difficult to find a class where the programme had not been implemented in some way.

Time frame

School-based programmes are constrained by the school year and three-term system. In addition, timely evaluations can be challenged by the fact that programmes are working through a third party: school staff. To make an impact on pupils, teaching practice has to change and this takes time (Lubliner & Smetana, 2005). Similar evaluations in primary schools report considerable time to show an effect on pupil outcomes (Wren, 2003), but this can be even more so in secondary schools given their size and complexity (Humphrey, Lendrum, & Wigelsworth, 2011). Less than a year can impact negatively on results (Breen, 2014), with some programmes needing more than two years to embed change (*Words for Work*, National Literacy Trust, 2013). But this does vary. In the *Talking Schools* project, where there were multiple opportunities for students to use and practise discussion techniques introduced, Howe (2013) found change after two terms. To look at change over time, and also at how that change was sustained, *Secondary Talk* was evaluated over a 3-year period (Hartshorne & Black, 2015).

Ensuring fidelity to the programme

Implementation across whole schools can make it difficult to ensure that programmes are the same in each school, in each lesson, or with each teacher. Styles and Bradshaw (2015), for example, reported that teaching assistants involved in delivering narrative and vocabulary intervention programmes in secondary schools adapted the content to fit into timetabling. In many whole-school programmes, flexibility is viewed as a strength, and attempts have been made to address fidelity issues.

Lawrence et al. (2015) provided a comprehensive training programme for teachers delivering the programme, together with ongoing support and structured lesson-by-lesson materials. Lesaux (2010) also developed specific lesson formats and carried out specific fidelity checks. The team carried out lesson observations and found fidelity to be high, correlating with teacher reports collected through weekly teacher logs.

Starling et al. (2012) produced a clear manual, with rationales and protocols for activities, and clear examples of applications of the programme. They also used a standard format for lesson observations, and developed a moderating system for ensuring that any modifications of resources were used consistently across the teacher group. The generation of new ideas, independently, by teachers was an important feature of the programme. This is also typical in *Secondary Talk*, which encourages school staff to adapt the programme to identified need, inevitably resulting in variation in how it is presented in schools. *Secondary Talk* attempts to address this by adopting a pedagogy of evidence and principle rather than prescription (Alexander, Doddingon, Gray, et al., 2010), emphasizing fidelity to the core principles on which it is based rather than on prescribed activities.

Selecting meaningful outcome measures to capture change

Carrying out assessment of adolescent language in a way that reflects functional communication and learning can be challenging. While standardized assessments may provide more reliable data, they can be susceptible to bias (Spencer et al., 2012), provide limited information about the strategies pupils use (Breen, 2014), and finding an assessment that accurately measures oracy skills in secondary classrooms is unlikely (Maxwell et al., 2015). Most critically, those tests available are often not designed to measure progress over a short timeframe (Breen, 2014) and are not sensitive enough to pick up changes following intervention in adolescents' language and communication (Lesaux et al., 2010; Spencer et al., 2012; Stothard, Snowling, Bishop, et al., 1998).

Researcher-created tests have the potential to pick up these more subtle changes, and to inform classroom practice. In evaluating small group interventions for narrative and vocabulary, Joffe (2011) found significant differential impacts on students' language skills using six non-standardized tests; impacts not seen using standardized language assessments (Styles & Bradshaw, 2015). Likewise, Leasaux et al. (2010) found significant effects using researcher-developed vocabulary measures, but not on a standardized measure of reading vocabulary. Mercer et al.'s (2014) specifically designed oracy assessment toolkit, closely aligned to the programme being evaluated, was felt to have strong validity as an impact measure. However, at the same time it was criticized for not being standardized (Maxwell et al., 2015).

There are risks in designing tools *so* close to the intervention that the intervention itself can be criticized as 'teaching to the test' and their objectivity is lost. But equally, without these more bespoke tools, we risk measuring what is easiest to measure rather than what is useful (Ahmed, 2015) or selecting the wrong measure. Maxwell et al. (2015) used a nonverbal standardized assessment in their evaluation of the *Oracy Curriculum*, and reflected afterwards that it limited the confidence placed on results as it was not aligned to the programme. Interestingly, students themselves reacted critically to undergoing the assessment, questioning its relevance to oracy.

There is an alternative used by a number of the studies described in this chapter. Schools collect whole-school attainment data regularly, and also predict performance in curriculum subjects. Although based on teacher judgement rather than objective assessment, used in conjunction with other data school data can add strength, and has the added bonus of being meaningful to schools. Mannion and Mercer (2016) collected summative data each term pupils were involved in the *Learning 2 Learn* programme. Using this they found that, over three years, pupils in the intervention group made a statistically significant increase in the proportion either meeting or exceeding their target grades compared with the control group.

Howe (2013) in the *Talking School* project also looked at progress and attainment data in English, humanities and science. However, he supported this with data from observations, which he felt were essential to measure progress in spoken language. To make this meaningful to schools, he correlated students' spoken language levels with curriculum levels. Lawrence et al. (2015) also used lesson observation to look specifically at the impact of the *Word Generation* programme on the quality of classroom discussion, randomly sampling 168 observations across lessons. They used a rubric to look at dimensions of quality whose indicators were observable and low incidence to ensure consistency.

In the evaluation of *Secondary Talk*, Hartshorne and Black (2015) used a combination of standardized assessments and non-standardized tools designed by the research team, such as a word-learning task looking at strategies pupils used to deduce word meanings. Following each assessment activity, pupils were encouraged to reflect on their communication and learning, providing a rich source of data. Spencer, Clegg and Stackhouse (2010) used a similar consultative approach, carrying out interviews with pupils giving them the opportunity to discuss issues related to their communication skills. This corroborated information found through standardized assessments but also yielded additional, more subtle findings.

Involving pupils in the evaluation

In England, all schools are expected to take account of pupils' views (Ofsted, 2015), and they have been a central driver in the recent overhaul of the special educational needs system (Department for Education and Department of Health, 2015). Using rating or interviews to get pupils' views of teaching practice is also becoming more common. These are sometimes not considered a valid source of information because of potential biases and lack of knowledge about the full context of teaching (Goe et al., 2014). However, pupils provide rich information about their experiences, and can offer valuable insight into their language skills and areas of language difficulty (Spencer et al., 2010).

Maxwell et al. (2015), in their evaluation of an oracy curriculum, carried out regular pupil focus groups and found them to have a good grasp of oracy. Drawing on pupils' experience helped the evaluation team to, for example, tease out the fact that there was more focus on language for presentation rather than for learning.

Like many others (Burrows & Yiga, 2012; Joffe & Black, 2012; Melvin, 2010), the evaluation of *Secondary Talk* showed that students with poor language found it hard to accurately reflect on their performance. In fact, there was a strong negative correlation between pupils' language skills and their confidence in communicating: the weaker pupils' language skills, the more confident they were about their communication performance (Hartshorne & Black. 2015). Snowling, Bishop, Stothard, et al. (2006) suggest that this may be because their weak language skills make responses in questionnaires unreliable. Humphrey et al. (2010) felt that intervention may make pupils more aware of their difficulties, so lowering scores.

There may be different ways of gathering information from students, some more effective than others. Within the evaluation of *Secondary Talk*, self-rating using a 5-point scale was used, along with a sorting activity. This latter activity yielded more interaction and a more considered approach than merely asking students to rate their abilities. Roulstone, Harding and Morgan (2016) recommended this dynamic approach instead of something purely verbal in their review of ways to consult with young people. Melvin (2010) found that providing the scaffolding to develop self-rating skills in young people can enable them to more accurately be involved in self-rating – helping them to give feedback and contribute to decisions made about them.

Where students have language difficulty, what seems to be crucial is that this is done by an assessor skilled in working with adolescents' language and communication (as recommended by Joffe & Black, 2012; Palikara et al., 2009; Spencer et al., 2010), ensuring that instructions are in pupil-friendly language, and appropriate materials used.

Concluding comments

Supporting young people's language and communication in schools depends on a good language-focused environment on which to base more targeted approaches. This can be provided via whole-school approaches, but for these to be taken up they must be shown to be both effective and efficient. Evaluating flexible, multilevel whole-school models of intervention can be challenging, but it is not impossible. If we do not take up the challenge, we risk gathering limited evidence of the impact of valuable whole-school programmes for teaching practice, pupil skills, and attainment over time.

Reflective questions

- What is the rational for delivering whole-school programmes for oracy?

- What are the key elements of designing an evaluation of whole-school intervention programmes?

- How might the evidence generated by evaluation of whole-school approaches be used to influence service delivery?

References

Albergaria-Almeida. P. (2010). Classroom questioning: Teachers' perceptions and practices. *Procedia: Social and Behavioural Sciences, 2,* 305-309.

Alexander, R.J. (2001). *Culture and Pedagogy: International Comparisons in Primary Education.* Oxford: Blackwell.

Alexander, R., Doddington, C., Gray, J., Hargreaves, L., & Kershner, R. (2010). *The Cambridge Primary Review Research Surveys.* London: Routledge.

American Speech, Language and Hearing Association (ASHA) (2010). Roles and responsibilities of speech-language pathologists in schools. Accessed online at http://www.asha.org/policy/PI2010-00317/

Applebee, A.N., Langer, J.A., Nystrand, M., & Gamoran, A. (2003). Discussion based approaches to developing understanding: Classroom based instruction and student performance in middle and high school English. *American Journal of Educational Research, 40*(3), 685-730.

Barnes, D. & Todd, F. (1976). *Communication and Learning in Small Groups.* London: Routledge & Kegan Paul.

Breen, A.M. (2014). Whole class intervention to improve vocabulary learning skills in post primary school students. University of Limerick. Accessed online at https://ulir.ul.ie/bitstream/handle/10344/4080/Breen_2014_speech.pdf?sequence=5

Bruner, J.S. (1996). *The Culture of Education.* Cambridge, MA: Harvard University Press.

Burrows, S. & Yiga, I. (2012). *Youth Offending and Speech and Language Therapy (A Controlled Study).* London: The London Borough of Ealing.

Cirrin F.M. & Gillam R.B. (2008). Language intervention practices for school-age children with spoken language disorders: A systematic review *Language, Speech & Hearing Services in Schools, 41,* 233-264.

Clegg, J., Leyden, J., & Stackhouse, J. (2011). An evaluation of the I CAN Secondary Talk Programme. Sheffield University. https://www.ican.org.uk/secondarytalk

Coultas, V. (2105). Revisiting debates on oracy: Classroom Talk – Moving towards a democratic pedagogy? Changing English. *Studies in Culture and Education, 22*(1), 72-86.

Department for Children, Schools and Families (2008). *The Bercow Report: A Review of Services for Children and Young People (0-19) with Speech, Language and Communication Needs.* London: The Stationery Office.

Department for Education (2010). *The Importance of Teaching*: The Schools White Paper. London: The Stationery Office.

Department for Education and Department of Health (2015). *Special Educational Needs and Disability Code of Practice: 0 to 25 Years.* London: The Stationery Office.

Dockrell, J.E. & Lindsay, G. (2008). Inclusion versus specialist provision: Ideology versus evidence based practice for children with developmental language disorders. In: C.F. Norbury, J.B. Tomblin, & D.V.M. Bishop (Eds), *Understanding Developmental Language Disorders: From Theory to Practice.* Hove: Psychology Press.

Dockrell, J.E., Ricketts, J., & Lindsay, G. (2012). *Understanding SLCN: Profiles of Need and Provision*. Research Report RR247 BCRP4. London: Department for Education.

Ebbels, S.H., Marić, N., Murphy, A., & Turner, G. (2014). Improving comprehension in adolescents with severe receptive language impairments: A randomized control trial of intervention for coordinating conjunctions. *International Journal of Language and Communication Disorders, 31*(1), 30‑48.

Ehren, B. (2002). Speech-language pathologists contributing significantly to the academic success of high school students: A vision for professional growth. *Topics in Language Disorders, 22*(2), 60–80.

Ehren, B.J. & Whitmire, K. (2009). Speech-Language Pathologists as primary contributors to response to intervention at the secondary level. *Seminars in Speech and Language, 30*(2), 90–104.

Ehren, B.J., Montgomery, J., Rudebusch, J., & Whitmire, K. (2006). Responsiveness to intervention: New roles for Speech-Language Pathologists. In: *New Roles in Response to Intervention: Creating Success for Schools and Children*. International Reading Association.

Gascoigne, M. (2006). Supporting children with speech, language and communication needs within integrated children's services: Position paper. London: RCSLT.

Goe, L, Bell, C., & Little, O. (2008) Approaches to evaluating teacher effectiveness: A research synthesis. National Comprehensive Center for Teacher Quality. Accessed 27th July 2015 at http://files.eric.ed.gov/fulltext/ED521228.pdf

Hartshorne, M. (2012). Speech, language and communication in secondary aged pupils. *I CAN Talk Series*, issue 10.

Hartshorne, M. & Black, R. (2015). I CAN Secondary Talk: An evaluation over three years, *I CAN*. Accessed online at http://www.ican.org.uk/~/media/Ican2/Training/Downloads/Secondary%20Talk%20full%20final%20evaluation%20report.ashx. Downloaded 26.06.16

Higgins, S., Kokotsaki, D., & Coe, R. (2011). *Toolkit of Strategies to Improve Learning: Summary for Schools Spending the Pupil Premium*. London: Sutton Trust/Education Endowment Foundation.

Hord, S.M., Rutherford,W.L., Huling-Austin, L., & Hall, G.E. (2006). *Taking Charge of Change*. Austin, TX: Southwest Educational Development Laboratory.

Howe, A. (2013). *Developing the Talking School: Action Research at Oxford Spires and St Mark's Church of England Academies: Research Report*. CfBT Education Trust. Accessed online at https://www.educationdevelopmenttrust.com/~/media/EDT/Reports/Research/2013/r-talking-schools-report-2013.pdf downloaded 1.05.16

Howe, C. & Abedin, M. (2013). Classroom dialogue: A systematic review across four decades of research. *Cambridge Journal of Education, 43*(3), 325–356.

Humphrey, N., Lendrum, A., & Wigelsworth, M. (2010). *Social and Emotional Aspects of Learning (SEAL) Programme in Secondary Schools: National Evaluation*. London: Department for Education.

Joffe, V. (2006). Enhancing language and communication in language-impaired secondary school-aged children. In: J. Clegg & J. Ginsborg, J. (Eds), *Language and Social Disadvantage: Theory Into Practice*. Chichester: John Wiley & Sons.

Joffe, V. (2011). Secondary school is not too late to support and enhance language and communication. *Afasic Abstract Winter Edition 2011*. Accessed online at http://www.nuffieldfoundation.org/sites/default/files/files/NEW%20Victoria%20Joffe%20Afasic%20NL%20Winter%202011[1].pdf downloaded on 1.05.16

Joffe, V. & Black, E. (2012). Social, emotional and behavioural functioning in secondary school students with low academic and language performance: Perspectives from students, teachers and parents. *Language, Speech, & Hearing Services in Schools, 43*(4), 461–473.

Justice, L.M., Schmitt, M.B., Murphy, K.A., Pratt, A., & Biancone, T. (2014). The 'robustness' of vocabulary intervention in the public schools: Targets and techniques employed in speech-language therapy. *International Journal of Language and Communication Disorders, 49*(3), 208–303.

Kamhi, A. (2014) Improving clinical practices for children with language and learning disorders. *Language, Speech & Hearing Services in Schools, 45*, 92–103.

Law, J., Lee, W., Roulstone, S , Wren, Y., Zeng, B., & Lindsay, G. (2012). 'What Works': *Interventions for Children and Young People with Speech, Language and Communication Needs*. Research Report DFE-RR247-BCRP10. London: Department for Education.

Law, J., McBean, K., & Rush, R. (2011). Communication skills in a population of primary school-aged children raised in an area of pronounced social disadvantage. *International Journal of Language and Communication Disorders, 46*(6), 657–664.

Lawrence, J.F., Crosson, A.C., Paré-Blagoev, E.J., & Snow, C.E. (2015) Word generation randomized trial: Discussion mediates the impact of program treatment on academic word Learning. *American Educational Research Journal, 52*(4), 750–786.

Lesaux, N.K., Kieffer, M.J., Faller, S.E., & Kelley, J.G. (2010) The effectiveness and ease of implementation of an academic vocabulary intervention for linguistically diverse students in urban middle schools. *Reading Research Quarterly, 45*(2), 196–228.

Lindsay, G., Desforges, M., Dockrell, J., Law, J., Peacey, N., & Beecham, J. (2008). *Effective and Efficient Use of Resources in Services for Children and Young People with Speech, Language and Communication Needs*. Research Report DCSF-RW053. London: Department for Children, Schools and Families.

Lubliner, S. & Smetana, L (2005). The effects of comprehensive vocabulary instruction on title I students' metacognitive word-learning skills and reading comprehension. *Journal of Literacy Research, 37*, 163–200.

Mannion, J. & Mercer, N. (2016). Learning to learn: Improving attainment, closing the gap at Key Stage 3. *The Curriculum Journal, 27*(2), 246–271.

Maxwell, B., Burnett, C., Reidy, J., Willis, B., & Demack, S. (2015). *Oracy Curriculum, Culture and Assessment Toolkit Evaluation Report and Executive Summary*. Sheffield: Education Endowment Foundation and Sheffield Hallam University.

McLeod, S. & McKinnon, H. (2010). Support required for primary and secondary students with communication disorders and/or other learning needs *Child Language Teaching and Therapy, 26*(2), 123–143.

Melvin, S. (2010). *Words for Work Evaluation Report*. London: National Literacy Trust.

Mercer, N. (2008). Talk and the development of reasoning and understanding. *Human Development, 51*, 90-100.

Mercer, N. & Dawes, L. (2014). The study of talk between teachers and students, from the 1970s until the 2010s. *Oxford Review of Education, 40*(4), 430-445.

Mercer, N., Warwick, P., & Ahmed, A. (2014) *Developing a Toolkit to Assess Spoken Language Skills in the Classroom*. Final report of a project carried out in partnership with School 21 and funded by the Educational Endowment Foundation. Cambridge: University of Cambridge.

Nippold, M. (2009). School age children talk about chess: Does knowledge drive syntactic complexity? *Journal of Speech, Language and Hearing Research, 52*(4), 856-871.

Nippold, M. (2014). Language intervention at the middle school: Complex talk reflects complex thought. *Language, Speech, & Hearing Services in Schools, 45*, 153-156.

Obsuth, I., Sutherland, A., Eisner, M., Cope, A., & Pilbeam, L. (2015). *London Education Inclusion Programme: Evaluation Report and Executive Summary*. Cambridge: University of Cambridge and Education Endowment Foundation.

Ofsted (2015). *School Inspection Handbook*. London: Ofsted.

Olswang, L.B. & Prelock, P.A. (2015). Bridging the gap between research and practice: Implementation science. *Journal of Speech, Language and Hearing Science*, 58, S1818-S1826.

Payne, J. (2002). *Attitudes to Education and Choices at Age 16: A Brief Research Review*. London: Policies Studies Institute.

Qualifications and Curriculum Authority (undated). Personal learning and thinking skills. Accessed online at http://webarchive.nationalarchives.gov.uk/20110223175304/http://curriculum.qcda.gov.uk/uploads/PLTS_framework_tcm8-1811.pdf

Roulstone, S., Harding, S., & Morgan, L. (2016). *Exploring the Involvement of Children and Young People with Speech, Language and Communication Needs and Their Families in Decision Making. A Research Project*. London: The Communication Trust.

Roulstone, S., Wren, Y., Bakopoulou, I., Goodlad, S., & Lindsay, G. (2012). *Exploring Interventions for Children and Young People with Speech, Language and Communication Needs: A Study of Practice*. Research Report RR247 BCRP13. London: Department for Education.

Royal College of Speech and Language Therapists (2005). *Clinical Guidelines*. Milton Keynes: Speechmark.

Sedova, K., Sedlacek, M., & Svaricek, R. (2016). Teacher professional development as a means of transforming student classroom talk. *Teacher and Teacher Education, 57*, 14-25.

Snow, C.E., Prosche, M., Tabors, P O., & Harris, S.R. (2007). *Is Literacy Enough?: Pathways to Academic Success for Adolescents*. Baltimore, MD: Brookes Publishing.

Snow, C.E., Lawrence, J.F., & White, C. (2009). Generating knowledge of academic language among urban middle school students. *Journal of Research on Educational Effectiveness, 2*(4), 325-344.

Snowling, M.J., Bishop, D.V.M., Stothard, E., Chipchase, B., & Kaplan, C. (2006). Psychosocial outcomes at 15 years of children with a preschool history of speech-language impairment. *Journal of Child Psychology and Psychiatry*, *47*(8), 759-765.

Spencer, S., Clegg, J., & Stackhouse, J. (2010). 'I don't come out with big words like other people': Interviewing adolescents as part of communication profiling. *Child Language Teaching and Therapy*, *26*(2), 144-162.

Spencer, S., Clegg, J., & Stackhouse, J. (2012). Language and disadvantage: A comparison of the language abilities of adolescents from two different socioeconomic areas. *International Journal of Language and Communication Disorders*, *47*(3), 274-284.

Starling, J., Munro, N., Togher, L., & Arciuli, J. (2012) Training secondary school teachers in instructional language modification techniques to support adolescents with language impairment: A randomised control trial. *Language, Speech, & Hearing Services in Schools*, *43*, 474-495.

Stothard, S.E., Snowling, M.J., Bishop, D.V.M., Chipchase, B.C., & Kaplan, C.A. (1998). Language-impaired preschoolers: A follow-up into adolescence. *Journal of Speech, Language and Hearing Research*, *41*(2), 407-418.

Stringer, H. (2006) Facilitating narrative and social skills in secondary school students with language and behaviour difficulties. In: J. Clegg & J. Ginsborg (Eds), *Language and Social Disadvantage: Theory into Practice*. Chichester: John Wiley & Sons.

Stoll, L., Harris, A., & Handscombe, G. (2012) Great professional development which leads to great pedagogy: Nine claims from research. London: National College for School Leadership. Downloaded 22nd June 2015 from: https://www.gov.uk/government/uploads/system/uploads/attachment_data/file/335707/Great-professional-development-which-leads-to-great-pedagogy-nine-claims-from-research.pdf

Styles, B. & Bradshaw, S. (2015). Talk for Literacy: Evaluation Report and Executive Summary. London: EEF and NfER. Downloaded 28th July 2015 from https://educationendowmentfoundation.org.uk/uploads/pdf/Talk_For_Literacy_(Final).pdf. Vygotsky, L. S. (1962) Thought and Language. *Cambridge, MA: MIT*

Weiss, C. (1995). Nothing as practical as good theory: Exploring theory-based evaluation for comprehensive community initiatives for children and families. In: J. Connell, A. Kubisch, L. Schorr, & C. Weiss (Eds), *New Approaches to Evaluating Community Initiatives*. Washington, DC: Aspen Institute.

Wilkinson, A. (1965). *Spoken English*. Birmingham: University of Birmingham Press.

Wren Y. (2003). Using scenarios to evaluate a professional development programme for teaching staff. *Child Language Teaching and Therapy*, *19*(2), 115-134.

Yoon, K.S., Duncan, T., Lee, S.W., Scarloss, B., & Shapley, K.L. (2007). *Reviewing the Evidence on how Teacher Professional Development Affects Student Achievement*. REL 2007-003. Washington, DC: US Department of Education. Downloaded 22nd June 2015 from http://files.eric.ed.gov/fulltext/ED498548.pdf ()

13 The Strategic Adolescent Reading Intervention

Using oral language to boost reading comprehension

Jenny Thomson, Lowry Hemphill and Catherine Snow

Learning outcomes

This chapter will enable readers to:

- Describe potential challenges that adolescents may have with written language

- Discuss the current evidence for supporting adolescents' written language difficulties

- Give an overview of the Strategic Adolescent Reading Intervention (STARI) programme

- Outline the core components of STARI and present their theoretical rationale.

Introduction

Reading, a process central to academic success, has sometimes been described as speech written down, and this characterization makes salient a core connection between oral and written language. A consequence of this connection is that oral language difficulties have the potential to negatively impact reading development. By the teenage years, an individual with language difficulties will have experienced several years of explicit reading instruction as well as three to four subsequent years of using written text to learn across the curriculum. Difficulties in either word decoding and/or reading comprehension may have been encountered during this process, exacerbating the negative impact of any underlying language issues. To support these young adults, multitarget intervention is needed. This chapter describes one such approach, the Strategic Adolescent Reading Intervention (STARI). STARI aims not only to support the ongoing development of oral language skills, address gaps in reading skills, but also break down the negative associations these teenagers have built up towards text and the act of reading.

Written language challenges in adolescence

Learning to read is a process relying upon multiple factors, including adequate vision, vocabulary and background knowledge, letter knowledge, inferential comprehension and working memory (Cain & Oakhill, 2012). Studies examining the impact of these factors on children's reading success suggest that two skills are particularly critical: single word recognition and listening comprehension (Gough & Tumner, 1986; Melby-Lervåg & Lervåg, 2014). The role of these two factors, whose importance is put forward in the Simple View of Reading (Gough & Tumner, 1986), has a developmental progression. Early literacy instruction focuses heavily on equipping children with word recognition skills, which then opens the gateway to text comprehension, itself highly dependent upon oral language comprehension skills. This developmental progression has been described as the transition from "learning to read" to "reading to learn" (Chall, 1983).

As students move from the early primary years, into Key Stages 2 and 3 (UK)/the middle school grades 6–8 (US), explicit reading instruction typically stops and there is more onus on the individual student to acquire new word knowledge. Students increasingly use their knowledge of how language maps to print (orthographic knowledge) to identify unfamiliar words, while inferencing at the sentence and discourse level facilitates access to meaning.

Texts read at this stage more often address worlds beyond the readers' direct experience. Reading more complex text builds, but also relies upon the individual reader's background knowledge (Cromley & Azevedo, 2007). In parallel, 'academic language' structures, such as complex noun phrases and subordinate clauses, increasingly predominate in written text (Fang, 2012), structures which are not acquired in everyday oral communication (Miller & Weinert, 1998).

For a teenager with language difficulties, the critical role of language in many of the above processes is clear. Students with language difficulties in their native language have a higher risk than their typically developing peers of poor phonological awareness skills at the time of school entry (Claessen, Leitão, Kane, & Williams, 2013; Vandewalle, Boets, Ghesquière, & Zink, 2012). Phonological awareness, the ability to reflect on the sound structure of a language, is an important precursor of acquiring the letter-sound correspondences needed in early word decoding (Bradley & Bryant, 1983). Some teenagers with language difficulties may have residual decoding problems, or a lack of automaticity in their word recognition skills (Lewis, Freebairn, Tag, Ciesla, et al., 2015). Another key group of teenagers whose academic skills may be delayed in the language of instruction are students for whom English is an additional language (EAL). Several studies have now shown that this group, as a whole, can learn to decode in English as well as their typically developing monolingual peers (Kieffer & Vukovic, 2013; Mancilla-Martinez & Lesaux, 2011); however, for students where the phonology or orthography of their home language is very contrastive with the language of instruction, there may be key gaps in knowledge or specific decoding difficulties (Marx, Stanat, Roick, Segerer, Marx, & Schneider, 2015; Pasquarella, Chen, Gottardo, & Geva, 2015). For example, for students exposed to first languages that do not contain consonant clusters (e.g., [str][pl]), both perceiving the sounds in these clusters as well as linking the sounds to multiple letter patterns can be a specific challenge (Altenberg, 2005).

Arguably a more pervasive issue for teenagers with written language difficulties is the high level of oral language competence needed to process text at the secondary education level (Cain & Oakhill, 2012; Karasinski & Ellis-Weismer, 2010). This group may struggle with the processes of inference generation, abstract language, higher level vocabulary and complex grammar in their spoken language – all facets of Gough and Tumner's "listening comprehension" in the Simple View of Reading, which in turn will create significant barriers to reading comprehension. If such issues are added to a potential lack of decoding automaticity, which makes the mechanical act of reading slower and more effortful, the level of reading challenge for these teenagers is huge, and potentially demoralizing.

As has been discussed in other chapters of this volume, language difficulties in the teenage years cannot be fully understood without acknowledging the potential interaction with motivational and engagement processes. For students *without* overt literacy difficulties it has been documented that reading motivation and engagement show decline on average as students move through early years of schooling and into adolescence (McKenna, Kear, & Ellsworth, 1995; Unrau & Schlackman, 2006). A history of struggle with reading acquisition can result in additional vicious cycles related to motivation and engagement (Hidi & Harackiewicz, 2000); for example, students who are less engaged by texts they encounter may show less flexibility and persistence in sense-making (Mol & Bus, 2011).

Literacy interventions in adolescence and STARI

The above section makes clear that any attempt to support a struggling adolescent reader, especially one with underlying language difficulties, will need to include multiple components to address the potential barriers at the levels of decoding, background knowledge, comprehension and, in addition, motivation.

Multicomponent interventions have been developed for struggling older readers; however, their impact overall has often been small, especially when tested at scale in low-performing schools and with a teacher, as opposed to researcher implementation (Solis et al., 2014; Somers et al., 2010; Wanzek et al., 2013). For example, a US evaluation of the multicomponent Content Literacy Continuum (Corrin et al., 2012) showed no significant differences between participants' and nonparticipants' reading comprehension gains and only modest advantages for participants' vocabulary growth. Adolescents enrolled in a large-scale trial of two multicomponent interventions, Reading Apprenticeship Academic Literacy (RAAL) and XTreme Reading, showed only a small advantage over nonparticipants in reading comprehension and none in reading vocabulary (Somers et al., 2010). Approaches to reading intervention have been critiqued as not engaging enough (Kamil et al., 2008; O'Brien, Beach, & Scharber, 2007) and as insufficiently focused on competencies needed for deep comprehension of text (Compton, Miller, Elleman, & Steacy, 2014).

The Strategic Adolescent Reading Intervention (STARI) was created to meet this challenge. STARI is a multicomponent, supplemental reading programme, designed to be delivered five days a week for one class period over an entire school year. As well as addressing essential skills of decoding, fluency and literal comprehension, STARI endeavours to integrate remedial instruction with content that: engages and cognitively stretches students;

provides extensive opportunities for peer collaboration in meaning-making; and develops the background knowledge needed to comprehend full-length, complex texts. STARI is targeted towards students who have below-average reading skills, which may be for a variety of reasons including poor oral language skills, English as an additional language, and/or inconsistent access to instruction. Given the text- and language-rich materials, however, it is not intended as a primary intervention for students with very limited English, or students who require an intensive phonics-based reading intervention.

STARI is delivered as a set of four thematic units organized around a central question, such as, "how can we find a place where we really belong?" Unit topics, such as sports in society, the war in Iraq, or the immigration debate, are designed to be of high interest, personally relevant to adolescents and complex enough to encourage discussion and debate. Each unit includes a central novel and one or more full-length works of nonfiction. Accompanying this is a student workbook for each unit which includes activities for fluency, decoding and comprehension practice, along with detailed daily lesson plans for teachers.

In the section that follows, we outline the core components of STARI and their theoretical rationale.

The Strategic Adolescent Reading Intervention (STARI)

Word study and fluency

Difficulties in word decoding and/or fluency have been observed in up to 50% of adolescent struggling readers (Brasseur-Hock, Hock, Kieffer, Biancarosa, & Deshler, 2011; Cirino et al., 2013). Students who read text very slowly or inaccurately often have trouble building up a coherent representation of text content. In addition, slow and inaccurate word reading affects students' ability to sustain attention while reading longer and more challenging texts. In order to limit the impact these difficulties might have on reading comprehension, as well as develop students' vocabulary and background knowledge, word study and fluency activities are a daily component of the STARI intervention.

To promote teenagers' interest and motivation, STARI embeds word study and fluency work in high-interest readings related to the unit themes. For example, in a unit focused on sports and society, students practise fluency and decoding strategies in passages about the trend towards an early focus

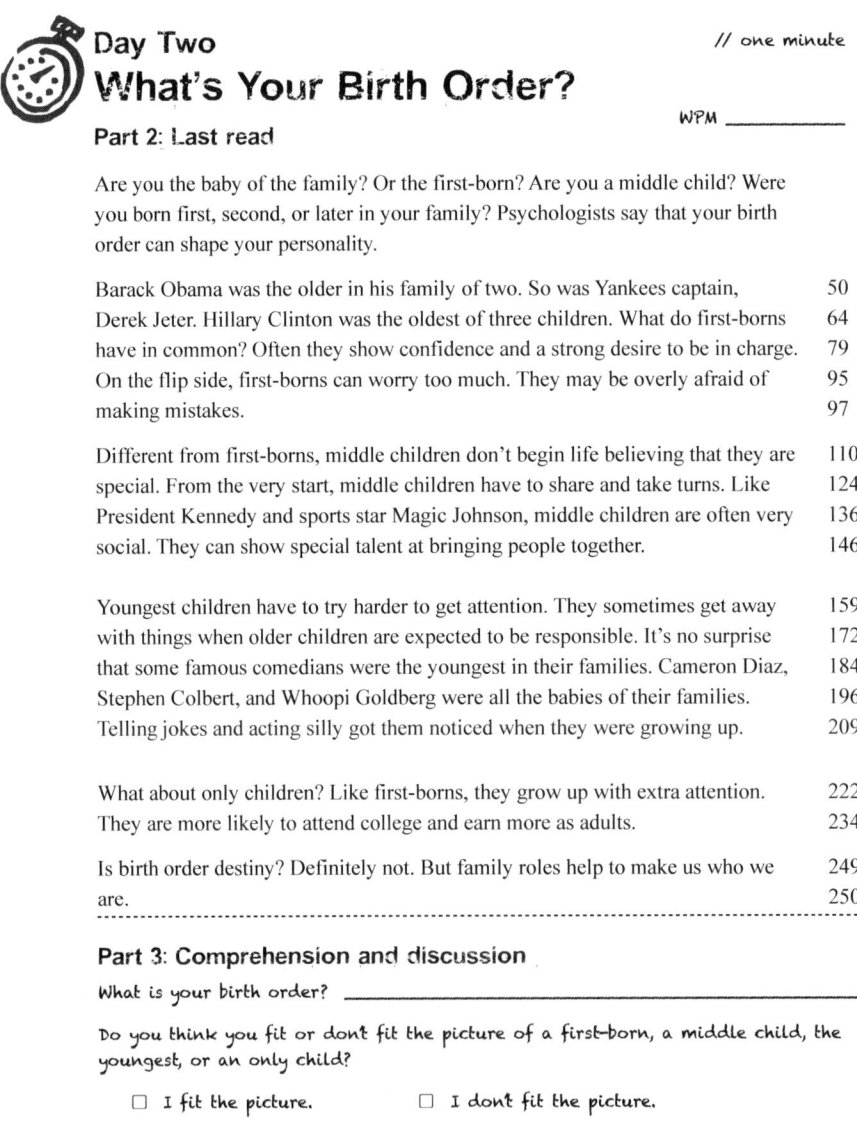

Day Two
What's Your Birth Order?

// one minute

WPM _____

Part 2: Last read

Are you the baby of the family? Or the first-born? Are you a middle child? Were you born first, second, or later in your family? Psychologists say that your birth order can shape your personality.

Barack Obama was the older in his family of two. So was Yankees captain,	50
Derek Jeter. Hillary Clinton was the oldest of three children. What do first-borns	64
have in common? Often they show confidence and a strong desire to be in charge.	79
On the flip side, first-borns can worry too much. They may be overly afraid of	95
making mistakes.	97

Different from first-borns, middle children don't begin life believing that they are	110
special. From the very start, middle children have to share and take turns. Like	124
President Kennedy and sports star Magic Johnson, middle children are often very	136
social. They can show special talent at bringing people together.	146

Youngest children have to try harder to get attention. They sometimes get away	159
with things when older children are expected to be responsible. It's no surprise	172
that some famous comedians were the youngest in their families. Cameron Diaz,	184
Stephen Colbert, and Whoopi Goldberg were all the babies of their families.	196
Telling jokes and acting silly got them noticed when they were growing up.	209

What about only children? Like first-borns, they grow up with extra attention.	222
They are more likely to attend college and earn more as adults.	234

Is birth order destiny? Definitely not. But family roles help to make us who we	249
are.	250

Part 3: Comprehension and discussion

What is your birth order? _____

Do you think you fit or don't fit the picture of a first-born, a middle child, the youngest, or an only child?

☐ I fit the picture.   ☐ I don't fit the picture.

Share answers with your partner!

☐ I read my answer to my partner.

Figure 7.1 Unit 1.1. Workbook p.23. Example of STARI fluency passage.

on a single sport, siblings who achieved Olympic success, and problems with betting on football. The content of the fluency passages is carefully designed to build background knowledge and vocabulary needed for understanding the longer texts (novels, short stories, nonfiction books) read in each unit.

In most STARI lessons, students practise fluent reading with topical 250-word nonfiction passages (10 passages per unit; see Figure 13.1 for an example). In line with evidence supporting the value of repeated reading (O'Connor, Swanson, & Geraghty, 2010; Rasinski, Homan, & Biggs, 2009), passages are read out loud with a partner, re-read the same lesson, and then re-read the following day to encourage improvement in reading rate (which is timed by the partner) and accuracy. Recording and tracking incremental progress in reading rate is intended to support confidence in attempting more challenging text reading. Each fluency passage ends with partner comprehension activities to promote more active and critical reading.

STARI draws from research that suggests important contributions of prosody to overall oral reading fluency, and which documents an independent contribution of good phrasing and intonation to comprehension (Kuhn, Schwanenflugel, & Meissinger, 2012; Valencia et al., 2010). The STARI repeated reading routine also includes oral reading of phrase-cued versions of the passages. Phrase breaks signal meaning units and help students practise reading and processing text in larger units, rather than reading word-by-word (see Figure 13.2). Attention to phrase and clause units will also help bolster syntactic awareness, another skill domain that is often vulnerable for struggling adolescent readers (Gaux & Gombert, 1999).

Struggling readers make greater progress in fluency when text difficulty is matched to readers' current instructional levels (O'Connor et al., 2002). Therefore, to accommodate differences in decoding ability, fluency passages are provided at four different levels, ranging from 3rd grade (Level A, 500–590 lexile) to 6th grade reading level (Level D, 800–890 lexile). Passages have similar content, length, and design across levels but vary in average sentence length and density of less familiar words. Passages within each level are designed to gradually increase in difficulty across the unit. Students can be placed at any of the four levels, depending on the teacher's assessment.

To support word decoding, isolated practice in identifying and reading aloud challenging words in the fluency passages is provided (see Figure 13.3). In addition, fluency passages are deliberately loaded with word patterns that are featured in each STARI unit as part of the word study strand.

Day One
What's Your Birth Order?
Part 3: Phrase-cued reading

→ Read the passage **out loud** in phrases to your partner.

→ Pause at each / mark for a phrase.

→ Also pause at each // mark that shows the end of a sentence.

Are you the baby of the family? // Or the first-born? // Are you a middle child? // Were you born first, / second, / or later in your family? // Psychologists say that your birth order / can shape your personality. //

Barack Obama was the older / in his family of two. // So was Yankees captain, / Derek Jeter. // Hillary Clinton was the oldest of three children. // What do first-borns have in common? // Often they show confidence / and a strong desire to be in charge. // On the flip side, / first-borns can worry too much. // They may be overly afraid of making mistakes. //

Different from first-borns, / middle children don't begin life / believing that they are special. // From the very start, / middle children have to share / and take turns. // Like President Kennedy / and sports star Magic Johnson, / middle children are often very social. // They can show special talent / at bringing people together. //

Youngest children have to try harder / to get attention. // They sometimes get away with things / when older children are expected to be responsible. // It's no surprise that some famous comedians / were the youngest in their families. // Cameron Diaz, / Stephen Colbert, / and Whoopi Goldberg / were all the babies of their families. // Telling jokes and acting silly / got them noticed when they were growing up. //

What about only children? // Like first-borns, / they grow up with extra attention. // They are more likely to attend college / and earn more as adults. //

Is birth order destiny? // Definitely not. // But family roles help to make us / who we are. //

☐ I read the passage in phrases out loud to my partner.

Figure 13.2 Unit 1.1 Workbook p.19. Example of STARI fluency passage with phrase-cues.

Day Two
What's Your Birth Order?
Part 1: Tricky phrases and words

→ Read these phrases and words **out loud** to your partner.

→ Put a check ✓ in each box as you read the word or phrase.

☐   Psychologists say that your birth order

☐   What do first-borns have in common?

☐   They may be overly afraid of making mistakes

☐   when older children are expected to be responsible

☐   It's no surprise that some famous comedians

☐   psychologists   sye | **KOL** | uh | jists

☐   personality   per | sun | **AL** | ih | tee

☐   confidence   **KON** | fuh | denss

☐   comedians   kuh | **MEE** | dee | enz

☐   definitely   **DEF** | ih | nit | lee

Word study:

Each word below has a base word. A base word is a word part that shows the core meaning. Circle the base word. The first one is done for you:

(over)ly   oldest

     personality   harder

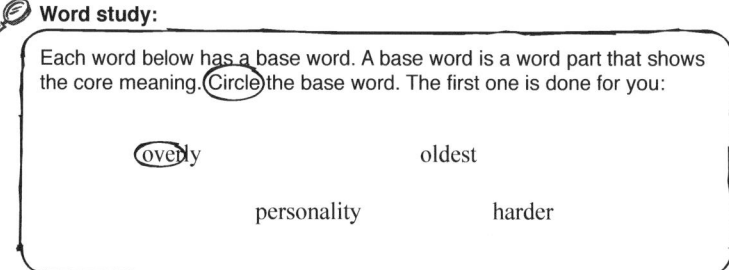

Figure 13.3 Unit 1.1 Workbook p.22. Example of STARI decoding support for more challenging words within fluency passages.

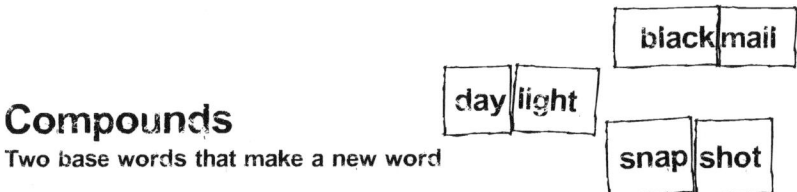

Compounds

Two base words that make a new word

Many words are compounds. Compounds are words like "homework" that are made up of two shorter words called base words. In the word "homework," the base words are home + work.

In the words below, circle the two base words.

everyone	network	runaway	skateboard
broadcast	toolkit	shortcut	teammate
weekend	schoolwork	sunflower	hotline
eyebrows	boyfriend	daydream	whatever

Figure 13.4 Unit 1.1 Workbook p22. Example of STARI word study activity.

Word study component

The word study component of the curriculum includes instruction in decoding patterns, for example, long vowel spellings, consonant clusters, and syllable chunking rules (mag-net). Students also receive direct instruction in morphological analysis, for example recognizing base words within compound words (basket-ball, earth-quake) and morphologically complex words, chunking common prefixes and suffixes (il-legal, amaze-ment), and learning how affixes change the meaning or grammatical role of the base word.

Decoding strategies are taught directly in teacher-scaffolded lessons, practised with workbook activities (see Figure 13.4), practised again in fluency work, and reinforced through teacher modelling and questioning in guided reading with the unit novels. The specific decoding and morphological features selected for inclusion in the units were chosen from a process of triangulation between research on persisting areas of difficulty for older readers (Carlisle & Stone, 2005; Diliberto, Beattie, Flowers, & Algozzine, 2009; Mahony, 1994), initial teacher reports of common error patterns, and further teacher feedback after using pilot versions of the curriculum.

Comprehension

Comprehension difficulties are characteristic of most adolescent struggling readers (Brasseur-Hock et al., 2011; Catts, Hogan, & Adlof, 2005). Problems with accurate word reading, along with gaps in vocabulary and understanding of sentence structure, can affect students' ability to create coherent mental representations of literal text content, the central process in basic reading for meaning. Struggling readers also show marked challenges in integrating background knowledge to make inferences and interpretations, processes that become increasingly important for understanding the more sophisticated texts encountered in adolescence (Barth, Barnes, Francis, Vaughn, & York, 2015). Challenges with inferencing may reflect underdeveloped background knowledge (Cain, Oakhill, Barnes, & Bryant, 2001), a consequence of many struggling readers' limited reading histories and social disadvantage. However, weaker adolescent readers may also lack experience and confidence using the cognitive strategies involved in integrating and extending understandings of a text. In survey studies, adolescents with reading difficulties report less use of strategies such as questioning, predicting, and making connections (Denton et al., 2015; Mokhtari & Reichard, 2002) and more use of basic strategies such as skipping over challenging text or asking for help. Thus, STARI lessons focus on direct teaching and guided practice with comprehension strategies needed for developing basic and deeper understanding of text alongside work on strengthening foundational components: decoding skills, background knowledge, and vocabulary.

Similar to the approach for teaching decoding skills in STARI, comprehension strategy instruction is embedded in content-focused units of study. A significant body of research suggests that adolescents are motivated to engage more deeply when they read varied texts on a single theme, for example

Summarizing with the 5 Ws

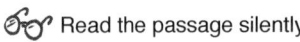 Read the passage silently.

Yadier Molina

On April 28, 2012, Yadier (yad-ee-AIR) Molina won a coveted award. He was honored with baseball's Platinum Glove. Molina was voted the best defensive player of the year. He received the award at Busch Stadium in St. Louis, Missouri.

Yadier is the youngest of three brothers. All are major league catchers. Big brother Bengie was a Giant, and middle brother José plays for Tampa Bay. Like Yadi, his two brothers have World Series rings.

Were Yadi's brothers jealous of his Platinum Glove award? They were the first to congratulate him on his honor.

WHO is this about? _____

WHAT did he/she do? _____

_____

WHEN did this happen? _____

WHERE did this happen? _____

WHY did this happen? _____

_____

Figure 13.5 Unit 1.1 Workbook p.28. Yadier Molina. Example of STARI reading comprehension strategy.

poetry, nonfiction, and novels, and when the texts selected are intrinsically interesting (Guthrie & Cox, 2001; Wade, Buxton, & Kelly, 2009).

STARI teachers directly model the set of four comprehension strategies (summarizing, clarifying, predicting, and questioning) whose value has been demonstrated in research on Reciprocal Teaching (Greenway, 2002; Klingner & Vaughn, 1996; Palincsar & Brown, 1984; Rosenshine & Meister, 1994; Spörer, Brunstein, & Kieschke, 2009). Students are exposed to all four strategies from the beginning of the first unit through teacher modelling and think-alouds. However, students practise one or two Reciprocal Teaching strategies at a time, gradually building up a repertoire of strategies that can be used flexibly at different points when reading a text.

Students first practise comprehension strategies such as summarizing through teacher-led workbook activities with simpler text, linked to unit themes (see Figure 13.5). They are then prompted to apply particular comprehension strategies during teacher-led guided reading of unit novels, as in this example from the teacher lesson plans for unit 1.1:

> What happened to Maleeka on her way home from Charlese's house? Let's **summarize**. What is important? What is new? What should we remember?

The teacher plans for guided reading include commentary (e.g., "What is important, what is new, what should we remember?") that highlights for students why a given comprehension strategy is relevant at that place in the text.

While guided reading provides scaffolded experience with more complex text, STARI students also practise using comprehension strategies with peers, an approach validated in the research on Reciprocal Teaching (Rosenshine & Meister, 1994; Spörer et al., 2009). To provide more opportunities for independent use of strategies, teacher-led guided reading in STARI alternates with partner reading of novels, short stories, and nonfiction books. Partners prompt each other to summarize, clarify, predict, and question, guided by collaborative workbook tasks.

Because struggling readers often engage with texts at a literal and limited level (Laing & Kamhi, 2002; McMaster et al., 2012), STARI lessons expand on the Reciprocal Teaching strategy of questioning, guiding students, while reading, to ask and answer questions that require inferences and interpretation. Using an approach adapted from Raphael and Au's Question and Answer Relationship (Raphael & Au, 2005), students learn to ask and answer literal, text-based questions whose answer can be found in one place in a text, questions that require the integration of information found in several places in a text, and questions that require the integration of textual information with reader background knowledge.

Discussion and debate

A growing body of research suggests that classroom discussions of literature can support adolescents' ability to respond more deeply to what they read (Applebee, Langer, Nystrand, & Gamoran, 2003; Murphy, Wilkinson, Soter, Hennessey, & Alexander, 2009; Soter et al., 2008). Classroom discussion benefits teenagers' reading comprehension through several distinct but related mechanisms. At the most basic level, putting understandings about a text into one's own words, a key practice in classroom discussion, aids in the process of meaning construction. Articulating a stance on a text requires students to distill what's important in what has been read and present their understanding in full enough language to be comprehensible to others. In true classroom discussion, readers articulate their own understandings but are also exposed to divergent peer perspectives. Peers may extend or even challenge what a classmate has offered. Exposure to diverse peer perspectives in discussion can help move students away from limited and literal understandings of text content, a shift that has been demonstrated to be especially important for struggling readers (Wilkinson & Fung, 2001).

STARI promotes discussion of text across several contexts. Unit texts are selected for qualities of 'openness' (Eco, 1984), the degree to which a text supports diverse reader interpretations. In daily guided reading with unit novels, short stories, and nonfiction books, students read several pages silently and then participate in a teacher-led discussion about meaning, a process that is repeated several times in each lesson. Similar to the kinds of teacher prompts used in studies of Questioning the Author (QtA, Beck & McKeown, 2006; McKeown, Beck, & Blake, 2009), STARI lesson plans prompt teachers to pose challenging, open-ended questions. Although teachers check on basic understandings of text content, guided reading discussion is focused on questions that require integration of information in the text and personal stances.

> What do you think about Maleeka and Charlese's friendship?
>
> Why do you think Miss Saunders wants her students to "know what it feels like to live in somebody else's skin"?
>
> What would happen if people stopped doing what Charlese told them to do?

STARI teachers are coached to ask follow up questions that elicit 'cross-talk':

Summarizing with "Blackmail"

Read the last lines of "Blackmail" on page 12 starting with the words "Under the orange glare…" to the end of the story.

Draw what you'd see if you were there on the porch with Angel:

Turn and talk to your partner. Summarize what happened with Pleitos the cat at the end of the story. Use the 5 Ws to write a summary.

WHO _____

DID WHAT _____

WHEN _____

WHERE _____

WHY _____

Figure 13.6 Unit 1.1. Workbook p.139. Example of STARI partner discussion activity.

Who can add something?

Who has a different idea?

Through provision of repeated, structured opportunities to engage beyond the surface of content-linked texts, STARI students learn to build and revise more complex models of extended text.

Partner work

To allow all students a chance to participate in discussion of passage content, partner workbook activities for fluency passages and reading with the unit novels include open-ended questions, often followed by prompts to compare responses with the partner (see Figures 13.1 and 13.6). Partner activities are designed to support 'mini debates', where students actively trade views about their interpretations of what they have read.

Unit debates

Unit debates are a final context for text discussion in STARI. 'Purpose-driven' reading can promote students' interest, their ability to sustain attention while reading and, in turn, their understanding of what has been read (Guthrie, McRae, & Klauda, 2007; Schraw & Dennison, 1994). In STARI, purpose-driven reading occurs during debates about key issues, such as whether it's a good idea for young teens to work. Debates motivate students to read and re-read across a range of unit texts, 'mining' what they have read for evidence that will make their team's position convincing and effective (see Figure 13.7).

Debates create a social purpose for close reading of text, and support integrating content across a range of unit readings. The strength of each STARI debate team's evidence is evaluated by peers. Peer feedback helps students learn about the effectiveness and impact of their interpretation of text.

What do we know about the efficacy of STARI?

At the beginning of the previous section, we discussed how studies exploring the impact of adolescent reading interventions have often reported modest results, especially when an attempt has been made to deliver the intervention

Debate speech
Who is more powerful?

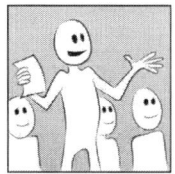

Introduction

Our team believes that _____
is more powerful. She is _____
_____
_____
_____.

Describe your character briefly and in general. *Example: strong, truthful, knows how to get what she wants.*

Evidence

The first reason we believe that _____
is more powerful is because _____
_____
_____
_____. This
example shows that _____ is more
powerful because _____
_____
_____
_____.

Find evidence and quotes from the text.

Describe WHY this evidence shows your character is powerful. *Example: The moment when Maleeka chose to defend John-John shows that she is willing to fight and she is brave, because she could be hurt by defending him.*

In addition, _____ is more powerful
because_____
_____
_____.
This shows that _____ is more powerful
because _____
_____
_____
_____.

Find evidence and quotes from the text.

Describe WHY this evidence shows your character is powerful.

Figure 13.7 Unit 1.2 Woekbook p.56. Example of STARI debate activity.

in a real-world setting, administered by teachers as opposed to researchers and delivered over a large number of individuals.

With STARI our aim has been to use a novel approach to try to achieve greater gains. As well as the integrated instructional approaches described above, it was important to consider the challenges a teacher might face in administering this programme. To this end, a comprehensive professional development and coaching package has been created to support implementation that includes summer institutes, workshops, and weekly access to STARI coaches, as well as graduate-level study courses.

A randomized controlled trial (RCT) of STARI has been carried out in the Northeast of the US with initial results reported (Kim et al., 2016). Early indicators suggest that across a sample of 402 struggling readers in Grades 6 to 8 (age 11-14), significant gains were observed for STARI participants in decoding, morphology and reading comprehension. Observations of teacher implementation also support the conclusion that generalist teachers can implement STARI with fidelity when robust professional development and coaching are provided.

Such promising results tell us that while the difficulties of adolescent struggling readers may be more complex and long-standing than for younger struggling readers, progress can be made. Key to this progress is the delivery of a multi-componential programme in an integrated manner, with attention paid to the support that *both* teachers and students need in such a process. Teacher training for subject-area teachers does not yet contain the preparation in reading instruction needed for confidence in this area and so coaching is an essential aspect of the programme.

Finally, although this programme aimed to build on previous interventions in *multiple* ways – through highly motivating materials, an increased focus on oral discussion, debate and meaning-making, development of background knowledge – the enhanced emphasis on oral language development as a driver of reading comprehension development is particularly pertinent to this volume. The language complexity within written text for post-primary students cannot be underestimated. Continued attention to oral language development in the classroom is thus important, not only to teenagers with identified language difficulties, but for a much wider group of underperforming students.

Reflective questions

1. Think of a teenager you know with a language disorder.

a. What is the nature of their difficulties with written language?

b. How could you apply principles of STARI to support this teenager?

c. Think about how (i) you could differentiate the application of principles to their levels of needs, and (ii) how you could tailor the content to their interests and motivations.

2. STARI was delivered for one lesson a day, five days per week, for one year. What are the advantages and challenges of delivering whole-class interventions in secondary schools with this level of input?

References

Altenberg, E.P. (2005). The judgment, perception, and production of consonant clusters in a second language. *IRAL - International Review of Applied Linguistics in Language Teaching, 43*(1). doi:10.1515/iral.2005.43.1.53

Andreassen, R. & Bråten, I. (2011). Implementation and effects of explicit reading comprehension instruction in fifth-grade classrooms. *Learning and Instruction, 21*(4), 520-537. doi:10.1016/j.learninstruc.2010.08.003

Applebee, A.N., Langer, J.A., Nystrand, M., & Gamoran, A. (2003). Discussion-based approaches to developing understanding: Classroom instruction and student performance in middle and high school English. *American Educational Research Journal, 40*(3), 685-730. doi:10.3102/0002831204000368

Barth, A.E., Barnes, M., Francis, D., Vaughn, S., & York, M. (2015). Inferential processes among adequate and struggling comprehenders and relations to reading comprehension. *Reading and Writing Quarterly, 28*, 587-609. doi: 10.1007/s11145-014-9540-1

Beck, I.L. & McKeown, M.G. (2006). Improving comprehension with questioning the author: A fresh and expanded view of a powerful approach. *Education Review/Reseñas Educativas.* doi.org/10.14507/er.v0.762

Bradley, L. & Bryant, P.E. (1983). Categorizing sounds and learning to read: A causal connection. *Nature, 301*(5899), 419-421. doi: 10.1038/301419a0

Brasseur-Hock, I.F., Hock, M., Kieffer, M., Biancarosa, G., & Deshler, D.D. (2011). Adolescent struggling readers in urban schools: Results of a latent class analysis. *Learning and Individual Differences, 21*(4), 438-452. doi:10.1016/j.lindif.2011.01.008

Cain, K. & Oakhill, J. (2012). Reading comprehension development from 7 to 14 years: Implications for assessment. In: J.P. Sabatini, E. Albro, & T. O'Reilly (Eds), *Measuring Up: Advances in How We Assess Reading Ability* (pp.59-76). Lanham, MD: Rowman & Littlefield.

Cain, K., Oakhill, J.V., Barnes, M.A., & Bryant, P.E. (2001). Comprehension skill, inference-making ability, and the relation to knowledge. *Memory & Cognition, 29*(6), 850-859. doi: 10.3758/BF03196414

Carlisle, J.F. & Stone, C.A. (2005). Exploring the role of morphemes in word reading. *Reading Research Quarterly, 40*(4), 428-449. doi:10.1598/rrq.40.4.3

Catts, H.W., Hogan, T.P., & Adlof, S.M. (2005). Developmental changes in reading and reading disabilities. In: H.W. Catts & A.G. Kamhi (Eds), *The Connections Between Language and Reading Disabilities* (pp.25-40). Mahwah, NJ: Lawrence Erlbaum Associates.

Chall, J.S. (1983). *Stages of Reading Development.* New York: McGraw-Hill.

Cirino, P.T., Romain, M.A., Barth, A.E., Tolar, T., Fletcher, J., & Vaughn, S. (2013). Reading skill components and impairments in middle school struggling readers. *Reading and Writing, 26*(7), 1059-1086. doi:10.1007/s11145-012-9406-3

Claessen, M., Leitão, S., Kane, R., & Williams, C. (2013). Phonological processing skills in specific language impairment. *International Journal of Speech-Language Pathology, 15*(5), 471-483. doi:10.3109/17549507.2012.75311

Compton, D.L., Miller, A.C., Elleman, A.M., & Steacy, L.M. (2014). Have we forsaken reading theory in the name of 'quick fix' interventions for children with reading disability? *Scientific Studies of Reading, 18*(1), 55-73. doi:10.1080/10888438.2013.836200

Corrin, W., Somers, M.-A., Myers, N., Meyers, C.V., Condon, C., & Smith, J.K. (2012). *Evaluation of the Content Literacy Continuum: Report on Program Impacts, Program Fidelity, and Contrast.* (NCEE2013-4001). Washington, DC: National Center for Education Evaluation and Regional Assistance, Institute of Education Sciences, U.S. Department of Education.

Cromley, J.G. & Azevedo, R. (2007). Testing and refining the direct and inferential mediation model of reading comprehension. *Journal of Educational Psychology, 99*, 311-325.

Denton, C.A., Wolters, C.A., York, M.J., Swanson, E., Kulesz, P.A., & Francis, D.J. (2015). Adolescents' use of reading comprehension strategies: Differences related to reading proficiency, grade level, and gender. *Learning and Individual Differences, 37*, 81-95. doi:10.1016/j.lindif.2014.11.01

Diliberto, J.A., Beattie, J.R., Flowers, C.P., & Algozzine, R.F. (2009). Effects of teaching syllable skills instruction on reading achievement in struggling middle school readers. *Literacy Research and Instruction, 48*(1), 14-27. doi:10.1080/19388070802226253

Eco, U. (1984). *The Role of the Reader: Explorations in the Semiotics of Texts.* Bloomington, IN: Indiana University Press.

Edmonds, M.S., Vaughn, S., Wexler, J., Reutebuch, C., Cable, A., Tackett, K.K., & Schnakenberg, J.W. (2009). A synthesis of reading interventions and effects on reading comprehension outcomes for older struggling readers. *Review of Educational Research, 79*(1), 262-300. doi:10.3102/0034654308325998

Fang, Z. (2012). Language correlates of disciplinary literacy. *Topics in Language Disorders, 32*(1), 19-34. doi:10.1097/TLD.0b013e31824501de

Gaux, C. & Gombert, J.E. (1999). Implicit and explicit syntactic knowledge and reading in pre-adolescents. *British Journal of Developmental Psychology*, *17*(2), 169–188. doi:10.1348/026151099165212

Gough, P.B. & Tunmer, W.E. (1986). Decoding, reading, and reading disability. *RASE: Remedial and Special Education*, *7*(1), 6–10.

Greenway, C. (2002). The process, pitfalls and benefits of implementing a reciprocal teaching intervention to improve the reading comprehension of a group of year 6 pupils. *Educational Psychology in Practice*, *18*(2), 113-137. doi:10.1080/02667360220144557

Guthrie, J.T. & Cox, K.E. (2001). Classroom conditions for motivation and engagement in reading. *Educational Psychology Review*, *13*(3), 283-302. doi:10.1023/a:1016627907001

Guthrie, J., McRae, A., & Klauda, S.L. (2007). Contributions of Concept-Oriented Reading Instruction to knowledge about interventions for motivations in reading. *Educational Psychologist*, *42*(4), 237-250. doi:10.1080/00461520701621087

Hidi, S. & Harackiewicz, J.M. (2000). Motivating the academically unmotivated: A critical issue for the 21st century. *Review of Educational Research*, *70*, 151-179.

Kamil, M.L., Borman, G.D., Dole, J., Kral, C.C., Salinger, T., & Torgesen, J. (2008). *Improving Adolescent Literacy: Effective Classroom and Intervention Practices: A Practice Guide* (NCEE #2008-4027). Washington DC: National Center for Education Evaluation and Regional Assistance, Institute of Education Sciences, U.S. Department of Education.

Karasinski, C. & Weismer, S.E. (2010). Comprehension of inferences in discourse processing by adolescents with and without language impairment. *Journal of Speech, Language, and Hearing Research*, *53*(5), 1268-1279. doi:10.1044/1092-4388

Kieffer, M.J. & Vukovic, R.K. (2013). Growth in reading-related skills of language minority learners and their classmates: More evidence for early identification and intervention. *Reading and Writing*, *26*(7), 1159-1194. doi:10.1007/s11145-012-9410-7

Kim, J., Hemphill, L., Troyer, M., Jones, S., LaRusso, M., Kim, H.-Y., Donovan, S., & Snow, C.E. (2016, March). Experimental effects of the Strategic Adolescent Reading Intervention on reading outcomes in high poverty middle schools. Paper presented at the Spring Conference of the Society for Research in Educational Effectiveness, Washington, DC.

Klingner, J.K. & Vaughn, S. (1996). Reciprocal teaching of reading comprehension strategies for students with learning disabilities who use English as a second language. *The Elementary School Journal*, *96*(3), 275-293. doi:10.1086/461828

Kuhn, M.R., Schwanenflugel, P.J., & Meisinger, E.B. (2010). Aligning theory and assessment of reading fluency: Automaticity, prosody, and definitions of fluency. *Reading Research Quarterly*, *45*(2), 230-251. doi:10.1598/rrq.45.2.4

Laing, S.P. & Kamhi, A.G. (2002). The use of think-aloud protocols to compare inferencing abilities in average and below-average readers. *Journal of Learning Disabilities*, *35*-(5), 436-447. doi:10.1177/00222194020350050401

Lewis, B.A., Freebairn, L., Tag, J., Ciesla, A.A., Iyengar, S.K., Stein, C.M., & Taylor, H.G. (2015). Adolescent outcomes of children with early speech sound disorders with and without language impairment. *American Journal of Speech-Language Pathology, 24*(2), 150-163. doi:10.1044/2014_ajslp-14-007

Mahony, D.L. (1994). Using sensitivity to word structure to explain variance in high school and college level reading ability. *Reading and Writing, 6*(1), 19-44. doi:10.1007/BF01027276

Mancilla-Martinez, J. & Lesaux, N.K. (2011). The gap between Spanish speakers' word reading and word knowledge: A longitudinal study. *Child Development, 82*(5), 1544-1560. doi:10.1111/j.1467-8624.2011.01633.x

Marx, A., Stanat, P., Roick, T., Segerer, R., Marx, P., & Schneider, W. (2015). Components of reading comprehension in adolescent first-language and second-language students from low-track schools. *Reading and Writing, 28*(6), 891-914. doi:10.1007/s11145-015-9554-3

McGeown, S.P., Duncan, L.G., Griffiths, Y.M., & Stothard, S.E. (2015). Exploring the relationship between adolescents' reading skills, reading motivation and reading habits. *Reading and Writing, 28*(4), 545-569. doi:10.1007/s11145-014-9537-9

McKenna, M.C., Kear, D.J., & Ellsworth, R.A. (1995). Children's attitudes toward reading: A national survey. *Reading Research Quarterly, 30*(4), 934-956. doi:10.2307/748205

McKeown, M.G., Beck, I.L., & Blake, R.K. (2009). Rethinking reading comprehension instruction: A comparison of instruction for strategies and content approaches. *Reading Research Quarterly, 44*(3), 218-253. doi:10.1598/rrq.44.3.1

McMaster, K.L., van den Broek, P., Espin, C.A., White, M.J., Rapp, D.N., Kendeou, P., & ... Carlson, S. (2012). Making the right connections: Differential effects of reading intervention for subgroups of comprehenders. *Learning and Individual Differences, 22*(1), 100-111. doi:10.1016/j.lindif.2011.11.017

Melby-Lervåg, M. & Lervåg, A. (2014). Effects of educational interventions targeting reading comprehension and underlying components. *Child Development Perspectives, 8*(2), 96-100. doi:10.1111/cdep.12068

Miller, J. & Weinert, R. (1998). *Spontaneous Spoken Language: Structure and Discourse.* New York: Oxford University Press.

Mokhtari, K. & Reichard, C.A. (2002). Assessing students' metacognitive awareness of reading strategies. *Journal of Educational Psychology, 94*(2), 249-259. doi:10.1037/0022-0663.94.2.249

Mol, S.E. & Bus, A.G. (2011). To read or not to read: A meta-analysis of print exposure from infancy to early adulthood. *Psychological Bulletin, 137*(2), 267-296. doi:10.1037/a0021890

Murphy, P.K., Wilkinson, I.A., Soter, A.O., Hennessey, M.N., & Alexander, J.F. (2009). Examining the effects of classroom discussion on students' comprehension of text: A meta-analysis. *Journal of Educational Psychology, 101*(3), 740-764. doi:10.1037/a0015576

O'Brien, D., Beach, R., & Scharber, C. (2007). "Struggling" middle schoolers: Engagement and literate competence in a reading writing intervention class. *Reading Psychology, 28*(1), 51-73. doi:10.1080/02702710601115463

O'Connor, R.E., Bell, K.M., Harty, K.R., Larkin, L.K., Sackor, S., & Zigmond, N. (2002). Teaching reading to poor readers in the intermediate grades: A comparison of text difficulty. *Journal of Educational Psychology, 94,* 474–485. doi:10.1037/0022-0663.94.3.474

O'Connor, R.E., Swanson, H.L., & Geraghty, C. (2010). Improvement in reading rate under independent and difficult text conditions: Influences on word and comprehension skills. *Journal of Educational Psychology, 102*(1), 1–19. doi:10.1037/a0017488

Palincsar, A.S. & Brown, A.L. (1984). Reciprocal teaching of comprehension-fostering and comprehension-monitoring activities. *Cognition and Instruction, 1*(2), 117–175. doi:10.1207/s1532690xci0102_1

Pasquarella, A., Chen, X., Gottardo, A., & Geva, E. (2015). Cross-language transfer of word reading accuracy and word reading fluency in Spanish-English and Chinese-English bilinguals: Script-universal and script-specific processes. *Journal of Educational Psychology, 107*(1), 96–110. doi:10.1037/a0036966

Raphael, T.E. & Au, K.H. (2005). QAR: Enhancing comprehension and test taking across grades and content areas. *The Reading Teacher, 59,* 206–221. doi:10.1598/rt.59.3.1

Rasinski, T., Homan, S., & Biggs, M. (2009). Teaching reading fluency to struggling readers: Method, materials, and evidence. *Reading & Writing Quarterly: Overcoming Learning Difficulties, 25*(2-3), 192–204. doi:10.1080/10573560802683622

Reed, D.K. & Vaughn, S. (2012). Retell as an indicator of reading comprehension. *Scientific Studies of Reading, 16*(3), 187–217. doi:10.1080/10888438.2010.538780

Rosenshine, B. & Meister, C. (1994). Reciprocal teaching: A review of the research. *Review of Educational Research, 64*(4), 479–530. doi:10.2307/1170585

Schraw, G. & Dennison, R.S. (1994). The effect of reader purpose on interest and recall. *Journal of Reading Behavior, 26*(1), 1–18. doi:10.1080/10862969409547834

Solis, M., Ciullo, S., Vaughn, S., Pyle, N., Hassaram, B., & Leroux, A. (2012). Reading comprehension interventions for middle school students with learning disabilities: A synthesis of 30 years of research. *Journal of Learning Disabilities, 45*(4), 327–340. doi: 10.1177/0022219411402691

Solis, M., Miciak, J., Vaughn, S., & Fletcher, J.M. (2014). Why intensive interventions matter: Longitudinal studies of adolescents with reading disabilities and poor reading comprehension. *Learning Disability Quarterly, 37*(4), 218–229. doi:10.1177/0731948714528806

Somers, M.-A., Corrin, W., Sepanik, S., Salinger, T., Levin, J., Zmach, C., & Wong, E. (2010). *The Enhanced Reading Opportunities (ERO) Study Final Report: The Impact of Supplemental Literacy Courses for Struggling Ninth Graders* (NCEE 2010-4021). Washington, DC: National Center for Education Evaluation and Regional Assistance, Institute of Education Sciences, U.S. Department of Education.

Soter, A.O., Wilkinson, I.A., Murphy, P.K., Rudge, L., Reninger, K., & Edwards, M. (2008). What the discourse tells us: Talk and indicators of high-level comprehension. *International Journal of Educational Research, 47*(6), 372–391. doi:10.1016/j.ijer.2009.01.001

Spörer, N., Brunstein, J.C., & Kieschke, U. (2009). Improving students' reading comprehension skills: Effects of strategy instruction and reciprocal teaching. *Learning and Instruction*, *19*(3), 272-286. doi:10.1016/j.learninstruc.2008.05.003

Uccelli, P., Phillips Galloway, E., Barr, C.D., Meneses, A., & Dobbs, C.L. (2015). Beyond vocabulary: Exploring cross-disciplinary academic-language proficiency and its association with reading comprehension. *Reading Research Quarterly*, *50*(3), 337-356. doi:10.1002/rrq.104

Unrau, N. & Schlackman, J. (2006). Motivation and its relationship with reading achievement in an urban middle school. *The Journal of Educational Research*, *100*(2), 81-101. doi:10.3200/joer.100.2.81-101

Valencia, S.W., Smith, A.T., Reece, A.M., Li, M., Wixson, K.K., & Newman, H. (2010). Oral reading assessment: Issues of construct, criterion, and consequential validity. *Reading Research Quarterly*, *45*(3), 270-291. doi:10.1598/rrq.45.3.1

Vandewalle, E., Boets, B., Ghesquière, P., & Zink, I. (2012). Development of phonological processing skills in children with specific language impairment with and without literacy delay: A 3-year longitudinal study. *Journal of Speech, Language, and Hearing Research*, *55*(4), 1053-1067. doi:10.1044/1092-4388(2011/10-0308)

Wade, S.E., Buxton, W.M., & Kelly, M. (1999). Using think-alouds to examine reader-text interest. *Reading Research Quarterly*, *34*(2), 194-216. doi:10.1598/rrq.34.2.4

Wanzek, J., Vaughn, S., Scammacca, N., Metz, K., Murray, C.S., Roberts, G., & Danielson, L. (2013). Extensive reading interventions for students with reading difficulties after grade 3. *Review of Educational Research*, *83*(2), 163-195. doi:10.3102/0034654313477212

Wilkinson, I.A. & Fung, I.Y. (2002). Small-group composition and peer effects. *International Journal of Educational Research*, *37*(5), 425-447. doi:10.1016/s0883-0355(03)00014-4

Index